THE PREVENTION AND TREATMENT OPTIONS YOUR DOCTOR MAY NOT TELL YOU ABOUT:

- Natural progesterone—the natural way to help prevent breast cancer
- How soy can help reduce the risk of breast cancer—and the healthiest forms and amounts for you
- Nutritional choices—the dos and don'ts—that can make the difference
- Creating a non-toxic environment that discourages cancer growth . . . and much more!

PRAISE FOR DR. JOHN LEE'S BESTSELLING
WHAT YOUR DOCTOR MAY NOT TELL YOU ABOUT MENOPAUSE

"A must-read for every woman over forty."
—Dr. Earl Mindell, author of *The Vitamin Bible*

"With a penetrating eye for truth and a courageous disregard for self-interest, John Lee makes clear sense out of the confusing area of women's hormone therapy."
—Philip Incao, M.D., family practice physician

"Natural progesterone has been an important, exciting, and innovative addition to my wellness practice in women's health care. . . . Now that we have begun to realize the dangers of environmental chemicals that mimic estrogen, I am even more grateful to discover that natural progesterone helps to safely restore healthy hormone balance."
—Jesse Hanley, M.D., director,
Malibu Health and Rehabilitation

WHAT YOUR DOCTOR MAY *NOT* TELL YOU ABOUT
BREAST CANCER

How Hormone Balance Can Help Save Your Life

JOHN R. LEE, M.D.
DAVID ZAVA, PH.D.
AND VIRGINIA HOPKINS

WARNER BOOKS

An AOL Time Warner Company

Publisher's Note: This book is not intended to replace a one-on-one relationship with a qualified health care professional and is not intended as medical advice, but as a sharing of knowledge and information from the research and experience of the authors. You are advised and encouraged to consult your health care professional with regard to matters relating to your health and, in particular, to symptoms that may require diagnosis or immediate attention.

Author's Note: Unless it is explicitly stated otherwise, the personal details of the experiences shared by women in this book have all been changed so as to protect their identities, but the essential experiences remain the same.

Some of the material in this book originally appeared in the *John R. Lee, M.D., Medical Letter,* and on www.johnleemd.com.

The Appendix originally appeared in *What Your Doctor May Not Tell You about Menopause.*

Copyright © 2002 John R. Lee, M.D., Virginia Hopkins, M.A., and David T. Zava, Ph.D. All rights reserved.

The title of the series What Your Doctor May *Not* Tell You About . . . and the related trade dress are trademarks owned by Warner Books, Inc., and may not be used without permission.

Warner Books, Inc., 1271 Avenue of the Americas, New York, NY 10020

Visit our Web site at www.twbookmark.com.

 An AOL Time Warner Company

Printed in the United States of America
Originally published in hardcover by Warner Books, Inc.

First Trade Printing: January 2003
10 9 8 7 6 5 4 3 2 1

The Library of Congress has cataloged the hardcover edition as follows:

Lee, John R., M.D.
    What your doctor may not tell you about breast cancer : how hormone balance can help save your life / John R. Lee, David Zava, and Virginia Hopkins.
        p. cm.
    Includes bibliographical references and index.
    ISBN 0-446-52686-X
    1. Breast—Cancer—Endocrine aspects.   2. Carcinogenesis.   3. Breast—Cancer—Prevention.   I. Zava, David.   II. Hopkins, Virginia.   III. Title.

RC280.B8 L35 2002
616.99'449—dc21   2001045468
ISBN 0-446-67980-1 (pbk.)

Book design by Giorgetta Bell McRee
Cover design by Diane Luger

The book is dedicated to all the women who have lost their lives to breast cancer, and to all women currently fighting breast cancer.

ACKNOWLEDGMENTS

There are dozens of people to thank for helping bring this book into being, not to mention the thousands who have written and called us, sent us information, asked great questions at talks, and challenged our thinking. It all helps us fine-tune the information that much better.

Of course we owe thanks to our friends and families for supporting us through the sometimes heart-heavy process of delving deeply into the causes of breast cancer; the folks at PMC and ZRT Lab who patiently got the work done as best they could while we were distracted with this project; Melissa Block, who once again contributed her research and writing skills; and our patient editor Diana Baroni, who somehow knew that the book eventually would be completed, and hung in there with us.

In the scientific field we would like to thank Dr. Ercole Cavalieri for his brilliant, pioneering work with estrogens and breast cancer and his patience in explaining it; Dr. Jose Russo for doggedly following the hCG trail and giving us insights into when and why breast tissue is vulnerable; Helene Leonetti, M.D., for daring to do progesterone research; and T. S. Wiley and Dr. Bent Formby for thinking outside the dots.

C. W. Randolph, M.D., deserves thanks for having the courage to be the busiest practicing clinician we know using natural hormones, and being willing to generously pass on his insights and experience.

Robert Gottesman, M.D., was instrumental in creating this book. He was ever-willing to share his clinical experience, read a chapter, or give his point of view on a piece of research. His moderating influence, focused inquiries, and friendship helped keep us centered on the goal.

Others we would like to personally thank for their help and inspiration include Sri Gary and Joy Olsen, Dennis Holtje, Carol Adams, and Mark Hochwender.

CONTENTS

INTRODUCTION

Your risk of surviving malignant breast cancer is just about the same as it was 50 years ago, when the only treatment was mastectomy: about one in three. In other words, despite billions of dollars in research and hugely expensive and risky treatments, the conventional medical approach to breast cancer isn't working, and talk of prevention is virtually nonexistent.

Our focus in this book is on what causes breast cancer, and how to help prevent it. We believe that the prevention strategies are useful both for helping prevent breast cancer altogether, and for helping prevent a recurrence in women who have already had breast cancer. We'll start by exploring the politics of the breast cancer industry, and what we *do* know in a general way about what causes cancer, otherwise known as risk factors.

We wrote this book because we believe it's time for conventional medical doctors to admit that breast cancer treatments aren't working, and to have the courage to step forward and try new approaches. It's time for them to stop updating their medical education with information from drug company representatives and journals funded by drug companies; to start revisiting their biochemistry textbooks; to spend regular time on Medline keeping up with current research; and to at least be open to discussing and exploring alternative methods of treatment with patients who want to choose this path. It's time for physicians to work in cooperation with alternative health care professionals (and vice versa), and for each type of healer to take advantage of the strengths and skills of the other.

It's time for oncologists to look beyond radiation and chemotherapy, and for research facilities to take risks, think outside the dots, and make healing more important than the financial bottom line. It's time for those *giving* the money to find scientists and physicians who will work outside the influences of drug companies, because the majority of current breast cancer research seems to be about making money selling drugs, and that's not where the cure for breast cancer lies.

It's also time for women to become aware that conventional medical cancer treatments aren't working, and to avoid slipping passively into the cancer industry machinery—only to be spit out at the other end, permanently damaged and still with no reasonable assurance of survival. Women with breast cancer need to be supported in demanding their right to be fully informed about the treatments they receive, and to be able to refuse treatment if they—through education or intuition—feel it's wrong for them, without being "disowned" by the medical system.

And it's long past time for the media to stop blindly spouting press releases from big drug companies touting new cures for breast cancer that are poorly researched and may do more harm than good in the end. It's long past time for journalists to have the integrity to do independent research and check out obviously biased information to see if it's accurate and truthful.

By the time you finish the chapters on the nature of cancer and breast cancer, you'll understand why breast cancer is rarely caused by one single factor or event, and likewise why there's no one drug that will turn it off. We do have a mountain of good research showing that an excess of the female hormone estrogen in one form or another is a central condition in the cause of breast cancer, and that avoiding excess estrogen can help prevent breast cancer, and we'll explain this to you in plain English.

Dr. Lee has coined the term *estrogen dominance* to describe this condition.

Having said this about estrogen, we want to say right up front that we're not bashing estrogens. They're essential for health, and the protective hormone progesterone doesn't work without some estrogen accompanying it. Estrogens do not cause breast cancer by themselves—our complex biochemistry always operates in an interrelated, weblike fashion.

We will explain how, when estrogens go down the wrong metabolic pathways in your body, they can damage your DNA and cause cancer. We'll explain what causes this to happen and give you many down-to-earth, commonsense, easy-to-implement, low-cost options for stopping this damage in its tracks. And don't worry: We're not just going to scare you about breast cancer and sign off; we're also going to give you real solutions for staying healthy.

Although we would dearly love to see more large, double-blind, placebo-controlled studies proving our points, this book is very well referenced and backed up by science and by the experience of many clinicians who have patients with breast cancer. You can find references divided by chapter at the end of the book. Every month that goes by, another major study is published that supports the premises of this book, so it's helpful to keep up with the current research if you have breast cancer. (The Resources section at the end of the book will give you ways to do this.)

A good portion of this book will focus on the conditions under which estrogens can cause cancer and how progesterone can help you prevent it, but we don't want you to skip over all the diet and exercise advice and go straight to the progesterone as if it's a cure-all. It's an amazing substance, but it's not a magic pill; it's one chemical among thousands in your body.

Estrogen, although pretty much cast as the villain in this story, is just as necessary to life and health in a woman as progesterone is. It just so happens that our reliance on petrochemical (petroleum-oil-based) products has created a world that is awash in an excess of environmental or exogenous estrogen, from the air we breathe to the food we eat and the furniture we sit on. Progesterone is what opposes, or balances, estrogen in your body, and thus it gets to play the role of the hero. Neither of these substances is inherently good or bad; both are just part of the complex orchestra of biochemistry that keeps your body going.

Balancing your estrogen and progesterone levels isn't a cure-all either—especially if you're still spraying your roses with pesticides, microwaving your food in plastic wrap, bingeing on french fries and snack chips, and regularly stressing yourself out to the point of exhaustion. If this describes you, you need to take better care of yourself and change your lifestyle, starting now. We'll provide you with information on how to do this. The good news is that in the process of taking steps to prevent breast cancer, you'll also be preventing other types of cancer, heart disease, stroke, diabetes, arthritis, allergies, and many other chronic diseases.

The information in this book about hormones and cancer is very controversial, and you'll clearly understand why within the first few chapters. Women can opt for alternative treatments to radiation, chemotherapy, and tamoxifen but should be prepared to take these treatments very seriously, to make dramatic lifestyle changes, and to devote a lot of time and energy to maintaining these changes. Treating any kind of cancer is a life-and-death battle that demands focused attention and the willingness to change the conditions that created the disease in the first place.

There's a bizarre, almost surreal refusal in American medicine to admit that we pretty much know what causes cancer and how to prevent it. Cancer specialists, called oncologists, continue to "slash, poison, and burn" (as breast surgeon and author Susan Love, M.D., so aptly termed surgery, chemotherapy, and radiation treatments for breast cancer), even though they know that, in the end, the treatments are unlikely to make much positive difference in the lives of their patients.

Perhaps this blindness has to do with the fact that a physician can lose his or her medical license by deviating from the so-called standard of care in medicine. This is particularly true in the area of cancer. Physicians who try unapproved treatments for cancer face swift and decisive action from local medical boards and are labeled quacks by their colleagues.

Other than the possibility of healing a patient facing expensive and harmful medical treatments, there's no advantage or benefit for a physician to go outside the established norms in treating cancer of any kind. In fact, punishment is severe and could mean lawsuits, as well as the permanent loss of a job and/or a license. No wonder physicians are afraid of new approaches to healing cancer. There's legislation pending in California giving patients and doctors the legal right to try alternative approaches to treating cancer. Isn't it a little frightening that in the United States of America we have to fight the medical establishment by making laws that give us the freedom to get the medical treatment we feel is best for us? Shouldn't this automatically be our right in a democracy?

Women who opt not to use radiation and chemotherapy to treat their breast cancer will often face intense resistance from their medical community, who will tell them that if they don't do what the doctor tells them to, they will die. Knowing what we do about how powerful the mind–body connection is, and how strong the power of suggestion is (especially coming from a physician), this type of mistreatment should be considered malpractice. There's no excuse for such behavior coming from any health care professional. We have received many heartbreaking letters with this type of story, and they only serve to underscore how conventional medicine desperately needs to make fundamental changes in how patients are perceived and treated. You will hear more about this throughout the book.

We are also frequently told of doctors who threaten to "disown" women who don't do as they say. For example, Dr. Lee had a call from a woman who wanted just a lumpectomy, but her doctor told her that if she didn't also agree ahead of time to chemotherapy and radiation, he wouldn't do the surgery and would no longer be her doctor. Again, this type of behavior is inexcusable, and is a testimonial to how far conventional medicine has drifted from being a healing profession. We'll talk later about why many physicians behave this way, and we hope that this will make it easier to work *with* your doctor. Breast cancer is scary, and the prospect of losing the support of your doctor can make it even scarier.

This book is about the prevention and treatment of breast cancer. It's not about conventional medical treatments for breast cancer such as radiation and chemotherapy. (We will cover the topic of tamoxifen.) It won't contain an in-depth look at all the various types of breast cancer, their multiple diagnostic stages, and the considerable variety of treatment approaches—and controversy—that surrounds each one. Conventional medicine is already in a state of confusion and disagreement about these subjects, and there's no reason to add anything to the discussion except to say that the approach is definitely not working, and there is no cohesive or unified theory of breast cancer at this time. We also won't be going into the vast panoply of alternative medical treatments for cancer: We'll provide other resources for this at the end of the book.

Dr. Lee often says in his talks that doctors seem to think that *M.D.* stands for "Minor Deity," and the usual audience response is loud applause. Patients are to do as they're told and not question the physician's decision. If a woman follows her doctor's orders and then complains that she doesn't feel well as a result, she's made to feel as if it is her fault, or that it's all in her head, and she gets a prescription for a sedative or an antidepressant.

Women are rebelling against this kind of treatment. Their mothers were told that DDT and diethylstilbestrol (DES) were safe, and that Valium wasn't addictive. They watched as their older female relatives died of endometrial cancer in the 1960s because they were given unopposed estrogen—promised as the fountain of youth. New studies are coming out every day showing that conventional hormone replacement therapy (HRT), despite earlier promises and assurances, *does* increase your risk of developing breast cancer and does *not* help with heart disease. Women aren't dumping tea into Boston Harbor, they're dumping their HRT down the toilet!

It's essential that if you have breast cancer, you work with a health care professional who listens and genuinely cares. This is much more challenging and time consuming than passively accepting whatever comes along, but the long-term rewards are clearly better health and a longer life!

Once you've read the first two chapters of this book, you'll understand why your doctor is unlikely to understand or appreciate the information we're going to give you about breast cancer, and why we want you to have compassion and understanding for the difficult position physicians are in these days. If he or she at least has an open mind, you are blessed. Hang in there and offer him or her a copy of this book! If every woman who read this book gave a copy to her physician, HRT and breast cancer treatments would shift dramatically within a few years. What we're proposing here isn't the least bit radical, unreasonable, or complex, although it is radical in its simplicity and appeal to common sense. What we're proposing is simply outside the paradigm of conventional medicine. We've never met a physician who wasn't grateful and relieved to be practicing medicine with these concepts, which get back to some very solid medical basics and create much happier, healthier patients.

We would *much* prefer that women work *with* their health care professionals, in cooperation, mutual respect, and trust. It can be difficult and daunting to hold your ground when you're faced with an impatient, irritated physician in a white coat who's anxious to get to the next patient—but a life-threatening disease is even more daunting. Think of it this way: Every time you stand your ground and insist on your right to have your doctor listen to what you're saying, or on your right to try something different *with* his or her support, the aftereffect could be that you're helping yourself *and* thousands of other women who come after you, including your sisters, daughters, and great-granddaughters. The ripple effect of just one individual act of courage can last for generations.

PART I

THE HISTORY, POLITICS, AND NATURE OF BREAST CANCER

CHAPTER 1

THE HISTORY AND POLITICS OF THE BREAST CANCER INDUSTRY

Why We Can't Seem to Prevent or Cure Breast Cancer

Why is modern medicine going nowhere in its attempts to treat breast cancer? Our research has found that the answer to this question lies primarily with the politics of medicine, the cancer industry, and the industries that create the pollutants that contribute to breast cancer. We believe that the only way to truly prevent and treat breast cancer is to go outside the current way of doing things in medicine and stop the wholesale pollution of our planet with petrochemicals, but the forces that would keep things the same are very powerful and entrenched. That's why, just as they did with hormone replacement therapy (HRT), women need to educate themselves about pollutants, about breast cancer, and about alternative treatments. They need to rebel against ineffective and harmful treatments, and do what they can to teach their doctors.

Over the past few decades, conventional medicine has done very little to make any meaningful difference in what will happen to you if you get breast cancer, and virtually nothing it has done has reduced the incidence of the disease. The harsh reality is, if you get breast cancer, you'll get more treatment than you did 50 years ago, you and your insurance company will spend a lot more money, and if it's fatal you may gain a few more months of life (usually of very poor quality), but statistics clearly tell us that conventional medicines for treating breast cancer such as tamoxifen, radiation, and chemotherapy just aren't working in the long run. The way breast cancer is currently treated is a way of doing *something* in the face of not knowing what else to do. If you have an invasive or nonlocal breast cancer, your chances of dying from it are still about one in three, the same as they have been for decades.

The incidence of breast cancer (how many women are getting it) is steadily rising, and the numbers are appalling: According to the National Cancer Institute, breast cancer incidence rates increased by more than 40 percent from 1973 to 1998. In 2000 approximately 182,800 women were diagnosed with breast cancer. Some will argue that this rise is due to better and earlier detection. But even for women over 80 years of age, where this early detection issue is doubtful, the incidence of breast cancer has risen during the past 30 years from 1 in 30 women to 1 in 8 women. The American Cancer Society estimated that in 2000, 552,200 people in the United States would die of cancer, and 40,800, or just over 7 percent, of those would be women dying of breast cancer. This means that about 15 percent of women who die of cancer are dying of breast cancer. These are the annual statistics for the United States, but it's even more sobering to realize that worldwide about 1,670,000 women have breast cancer.

The mortality (death rate) from breast cancer is also staggering. If you combine mortality rates from the United States and Canada (which have the highest rates of breast cancer in the world), in North America a woman dies of breast cancer every 12 minutes.

Do Radiation, Tamoxifen, Mammograms, and Chemotherapy Help or Hurt?

How can we be so bold as to state that conventional medical treatments for breast cancer aren't working? It's very well documented. It seems as if every time we open a medical journal lately, there's an article showing that conventional breast cancer treatments are ineffective, harmful, or both. Just in the past few years, major studies published in prestigious peer-reviewed journals meeting all the conventional medical criteria for so-called evidence-based medicine have shown that:

- Mammograms don't really save lives (G. Sjonell et al., *Lakartidningen* 96 [1999]: 904–913).
- Radiation doesn't really save lives (*The Lancet,* 22 May 2000).
- Tamoxifen doesn't really save lives (Mitchell et al., *Journal of the National Cancer Institute,* November 1999).
- Chemotherapy doesn't save lives (which isn't news; we've known this for a long time).

So what's left for the conventional medical doctor to treat breast cancer patients with? Nothing but the same surgical removal of the cancer that they were doing 50 years ago. More American physicians need to face the hard, cold facts that current therapies just aren't working and open their eyes to alternatives for prevention and treatment of breast cancer. Let's take a broad look at the current treatments.

Radiation

Radiation is the most common treatment for breast cancer following surgery, and yet a recent article in the prestigious British medical journal *The Lancet* showed that this treatment is not working. In fact, while using local radiation to treat breast cancer reduces deaths from this disease by 13.2 percent, it increases death from other causes, mostly heart disease, by 21.2 percent. The obvious conclusion of this study: "The treatment was a success but the patient died."

In other words, the radiation obliterates the breast cancer tumor in a small percentage of women, but in the process it causes many of them to die from other diseases. Proponents of newer and more localized radiation procedures are claiming that it doesn't cause the damage the older radiation techniques do, but at present this is only a claim and not backed up by long-term follow-up. This means that there's no long-term benefit from using radiation to treat breast cancers, because even though the cancer may not recur at the site of the radiation, the overall chances of survival stay the same or are slightly worse. And yet despite the fact that radiation helps so few women—and eventually kills many of those whom it helped in the short term—it remains the standard of care in medicine for women who have breast cancer. How can this be? It's because conventional medicine has little else to offer that reduces death even by 13.2 percent. If you were starving and someone handed you a bowl of moldy old rice, you'd gratefully eat it up because it's better than nothing.

Despite this study, published in one of the most prestigious medical journals in the world, if you have breast cancer your doctor will most likely *insist* that you undergo radiation treatments rather than exploring possibly safer alternatives not popular among conventional doctors.

Treating women with radiation who later die of heart disease caused by radiation damage also affects breast cancer statistics. It means that the diagnosed cause of death was shifted from breast cancer to cardiovascular disease. As more and more breast cancer patients are subjected to radiotherapy, fewer will be said to die from breast cancer, but more will be said to die of radiation-induced heart disease. These deaths aren't counted in breast cancer statistics, but they should be if we are to have a truthful picture of what's happening to women who get this disease.

Tamoxifen

In the same issue of *The Lancet* as the above study on radiation was a curious letter from Oxford professor Sir Richard Peto, with a graph showing that breast cancer deaths rose about 20 percent from 1960 to 1985. From 1985 to 1997 breast cancer deaths were said to have decreased about 20 percent. Without speculating on the cause of the 1985 rise in breast cancer mortality, or citing the sources of his information, Sir Peto instead addressed only the matter of the recent decline.

An aside: The probable cause of the rise in breast cancer deaths was the prescription of unopposed estrogen (not balanced with progesterone) to menopausal women, a common practice from the early 1950s to the mid-1970s. While the medical community acknowledged that this practice caused endometrial (uterine) cancer, it never admitted that it also caused breast cancer. From the mid-1970s, doctors were instructed to prescribe synthetic progestins along with the estrogen to prevent the endometrial cancer. This is also when the incidence of hysterectomy skyrocketed: Women felt so terrible on progestins that they refused to take them, so doctors offered them a hysterectomy so they would no longer have to take the progestins, and could take estrogen only. To add insult to injury (literally), it was common practice (and still is in some places) to remove a woman's ovaries along with her uterus as a preventive for ovarian cancer. This misguided practice leads to many other health problems, including osteoporosis, heart disease, fatigue, and a diminished quality of life due to low libido, hot flashes, and other symptoms of "instant menopause."

Back to the supposed decline in breast cancer deaths: Because of the "suddenness" of the decline, Sir Richard felt it was not due to fewer breast cancers but more likely to "changes in the way breast cancer is diagnosed and treated." He speculated that it was "not from a single research breakthrough" but from "the adoption of many interventions," whatever that means. He was later quoted in other news articles as giving credit for the fall in breast cancer deaths to the anti-estrogen drug tamoxifen.

We hope that those promoting tamoxifen remember to mention how many women taking it suffer from blood clots, deterioration of vision, and diminished quality of life (hot flashes, night sweats). Also, how many women have been forced to have a hysterectomy due to a particularly aggressive form of tamoxifen-caused uterine cancer? It's rarely mentioned that women actually die of tamoxifen-induced uterine cancer. When these women die of uterine cancer instead of breast cancer, it improves the breast cancer statistics. This makes tamoxifen look good, but it's a moot issue to the women in question.

If the side effects of tamoxifen are this bad, why is it being used at all, and why is it being trumpeted so loudly as the great cure-all, to the extent that the Food and Drug Administration (FDA) even approved its use as a preventive? It's the moldy rice problem again. It's the lesser of many evils; it's better than nothing. Very few other FDA-approved pharmaceuticals have been made available to oncologists treating breast cancer. Theoretically—on paper, in test tubes, and in laboratory animals used as models for human breast cancer—tamoxifen looks promising, and the rationale for using it is based on a solid scientific foundation: Estrogens increase the rate that breast cancer cells proliferate, and tamoxifen slows the rate of cell proliferation by acting as an anti-estrogen.

Unfortunately, breast cancer cells in a test tube and laboratory animals can't really explain to us how they feel, and don't live long enough to give us a genuine appreciation for long-term health risks. Research investigating the effects of tamoxifen on hormone-dependent cancers looks good in the short term. However, in reality, tamoxifen is unnatural to the human body, and these side effects are the body's warning signals that something is terribly wrong.

Tamoxifen has been available for 25 years and its effect on breast cancer prevention is still being debated: This in and of itself should tell us something. Two studies, a five-year placebo-controlled one from England in 1992, and a nine-year placebo-controlled one from Italy in 1998, showed no difference in cancer incidence between tamoxifen-treated women and controls. The only large study in the United States was cut short, supposedly because the incidence of breast cancer dropped so much in the tamoxifen group that they couldn't justify withholding this treatment from the placebo group. It's worth noting, however, that the trial was stopped at about the same time that breast cancer began to reappear, despite the tamoxifen, in the two European studies.

The lessons we learned from those studies are that in some women tamoxifen may put a breast cancer to sleep for a few years, and in women who have breast cancer it may slow the rate of recurrence for a few years. But in the long term it tends to do more harm than good. Again, the only reason this is such a popular treatment right now is that it seems to oncologists to be better than doing nothing, which many of them believe is the only other viable option open to them. But as you'll discover, it's definitely not the only option available.

For the most part, it's only in the United States that doctors still believe tamoxifen significantly prevents or reverses breast cancer. In fact, now even the National Cancer Institute (NCI) has come out with a statement that in all but a very narrow group of women under the age of 60, tamoxifen may do more harm than good in terms of preventing cancer. Despite this, the FDA just approved the use of tamoxifen to treat a form of breast cancer known as ductal carcinoma in situ (DCIS). You'll understand later in the book why we believe this is an outrageous move.

Mammography

Like tamoxifen, radiation, and chemotherapy, mammography is big business these days. Mammography is also conventional medicine's only real answer to breast cancer "prevention," although it isn't preventing cancer at all, it's simply detecting it.

Countless advertisements and physicians are telling women to have mammograms. But the value of this procedure is far from clear. We all know women diagnosed with breast cancer that wasn't detected by mammography, and we all know that mammograms present a real risk of false positive and false negative findings. The test procedure is unpleasant and the radiation is potentially harmful. Both tissue damage and radiation are known risk factors for breast cancer, so it may even be logical to assume that mammography can *contribute* to breast cancer.

A summer 2000 study published in the journal *Spine,* and looking at data collected over 40 years, showed that women with scoliosis who received many diagnostic X rays during childhood and adolescence have a 70 percent higher risk of breast cancer than women in the general population. The more X rays a woman was exposed to, and the higher the dose of radiation, the greater her risk of breast cancer. Although the dose of radiation in a typical X ray is now much lower than it was when these women were being x-rayed, the point is still valid: Radiation is a potent risk factor for breast cancer, its effect is cumulative, and mammography involves forcefully squashing the breast and then shooting radiation through it.

It has been claimed that mammography lowers the risk of dying from breast cancer. Proponents argue that mammography can detect breast tumors a year or so earlier than simple palpation such as breast self-exams. This early detection, so the argument goes, leads to earlier treatment and a lower risk of breast cancer mortality. Statistics, it is claimed, have validated this argument.

Many statisticians, however, disagree. Statistics are not immune from biases, which include mechanical factors (use of different measuring instruments in different subjects), study methodology, conscious or unconscious assumptions, age of subjects, socioeconomic factors, faulty randomization of subjects and controls, duration of observation, and other confounding factors.

More than 15 years ago Dr. John C. Bailar III observed that counting survival time after treatment creates a bias in most mammography studies because mammography detects breast tumors a year before they would have been found by palpation. He pointed out that subjects with breast tumors found by palpation have lived at least a year prior to the time when they would have been found by mammography. When this year is added to the survival time of the control women (those who did not use mammography), their survival results match those of subject women whose tumors were found by mammography.

This means that the apparent difference in survival after treatment was due not to earlier treatment, as a result of mammography, but merely to starting the counting of survival time one year earlier among mammography subjects. When this factor is included in the statistical analysis, the so-called benefit of mammography and earlier treatment disappears. Dr. Bailar, now professor of epidemiology and biostatistics at McGill University and senior scientist in the Office of Disease Prevention and Health Promotion, U.S. Department of Health and Human Services, called this the lead-time bias.

This should not be surprising. For a breast cancer cell to become large enough to be detected by palpation, the cancer has usually been growing for about ten years. If found one year earlier by mammography, the cancer has been growing for about nine years, which is plenty of time to spawn metastases if the cancer is prone to do that. The one-year difference between palpation and mammography detection is ultimately of little importance.

Does mammography truly save lives? If you read the numerous ads for it, you might think the case is closed—of course it does. If you read the studies themselves, the answer isn't so clear. For example, a 1999 epidemiological study found no decrease in breast cancer mortality in Sweden, where mammography screening has been recommended since 1985.

As a result, two Swedish scientists reviewed all published mammography trials to evaluate their methodological quality. Their purpose was to ascertain whether mammography truly saved lives. Their findings are worth a close look.

In their analysis of eight different clinical studies on mammography, the authors found six of them seriously flawed by baseline imbalances and/or inconsistencies of randomization. The flaws were sufficient to nullify the studies' claims of a benefit from mammography. The two adequately randomized trials found no effect of mammography screening on breast cancer mortality.

The metanalysis conclusion is clear. Since there is no reliable evidence that mammography screening decreases breast cancer mortality, mammography screening for breast cancer is unjustified. This means that physicians should not order routine mammography screening.

However, mammograms have become a substitute for breast self-exams. If you stop having mammograms, it becomes essential that you examine your own breasts thoroughly at least once a month. If you're premenopausal, you should examine them shortly after your period, when hormone levels are low, so that premenopausal lumps aren't confused with a cancerous lump. You should also examine your breasts in the mirror and look for any unusual skin abnormalities or dimpling. After a few months you'll become very familiar with how your breasts feel, and you'll be able to detect very small abnormalities.

Chemotherapy

It's difficult to make generalizations about chemotherapy these days, because there are so many different kinds, most of them extremely poorly studied: The women who agree to try new chemotherapies are guinea pigs for a type of treatment with a notoriously poor track record. Like most other aspects of the breast cancer industry, there's little agreement about what constitutes chemotherapy. We'll make the generalization that chemotherapy is an attempt to poison the body just short of death in the hope of killing the cancer before the entire body is killed. Most of the time it doesn't work. There are new chemotherapies that target specific parts of the cancer process, but none have proven themselves truly effective in stopping the entire process.

Some chemotherapy does prolong life for a few months, but generally at the high price of devastating side effects, and if a woman does happen to get lucky and survive that bout of cancer, her body is permanently damaged; recurrence rates are high. The use of chemotherapy is purely a gamble, and we don't think it's worth taking. Sometimes it works, and sometimes it doesn't, and sometimes it makes things worse. Precious little is known about why it works or doesn't, and it seems much smarter to find an alternative therapy with a good track record that will both support your body in fighting off the cancer and promote health.

There are some chemotherapy-like approaches to fighting metastatic cancer, including inducing a high fever for a number of days and insulin potentiation therapy (see the Resources section at the end of the book), that hold much promise with less potential damage done to the body. They are much more widely used in Europe than the United States. They may never be widely available in the United States, because there's no patent medicine to sell. Europe is decades ahead of the US in its approach to treating cancer.

The Breast Cancer Numbers

It's important for women to understand how much breast cancer numbers are misused and abused, juggled, twiddled, and tweaked, depending upon who wants you to believe what. So let's keep it simple:

Breast cancer is the most common cause of death from cancer among women between the ages of 18 and 54, and it's the most common cause of death period among women aged 45 to 50.

Women younger than 45 years old have a 26 percent higher risk of a recurrence of breast cancer compared to older women. The types of cancer that these middle-aged women are dying from are *not* the mostly benign, "99 percent curable" DCIS "cancers" that have been detected since the early 1980s with mammograms (thus increasing the rate of detection); they're deadly metastatic cancers that kill quickly once they start to spread.

According to the Centers for Disease Control, cancer ranks higher than heart disease in terms of age-adjusted death rates among people under age 65 in the United States. While heart disease has declined, cancer has not.

Breast cancer is the second most common form of cancer in women after lung cancer, which is almost always due to smoking cigarettes.

Statistical Shell Games

The breast cancer industry has been playing a statistical shell game with the disease by including ductal carcinoma in situ (DCIS) as a breast cancer diagnosis when in fact it's rarely fatal, with or without treatment. Many oncologists like to say that DCIS is "99 percent curable." (Since DCIS wasn't detectable—and thus not diagnosed or treated—until the advent of mammograms, we don't even really know the true nature or course of untreated DCIS, because it has always been treated if diagnosed.) We'll go into this in more detail later in the book, but for now, we want to focus on the fact that some 30 percent of breast cancers are DCIS.

Given that DCIS is rarely fatal, let's make some gross generalizations to illustrate a point. If we simply eliminate DCIS from breast cancer statistics, and thus subtract 30 percent of those who have survived breast cancer from the statistics, we would then not have a recent drop of 20 percent (as claimed by some) but rather a rise of 10 percent in breast cancer mortality rates. This is a crude way of making the point, but it's important to consider when a doctor is using these types of statistics to justify a treatment. For example, let's say a doctor justifies putting you on tamoxifen to prevent breast cancer based on the now much-quoted "fact" that breast cancer deaths have dropped by 20 percent thanks to tamoxifen (see chapter 12 for details). If you know going into the doctor's office that this is a highly questionable statistic, you'll be more empowered to make the right decisions for yourself. In fact, we suspect that if women with low-grade DCIS weren't subjected to tamoxifen, chemo, and radiation, their survival rate would stay the same—but the women wouldn't be damaged for life by the treatments.

A Word about Prevention

Of course the key to reducing the incidence of breast cancer is prevention, but *prevention* is a dirty word in the breast cancer industry unless you're referring to tamoxifen or mammograms, neither of which is really remotely like prevention. TV personality and author Bob Arnot, M.D., wrote a book called *The Breast Cancer Prevention Diet*, which contained mostly good, solid, practical dietary advice associated with reducing the known risk factors for breast cancer. Sadly, he was terribly trashed by the American media for using the word *prevention*, as if he were suggesting that diet was a cure-all (he wasn't), and as if he were somehow hurting women by suggesting that a healthy diet could fend off breast cancer (it can only help). Arnot was an unfortunate victim of the intense breast cancer political establishment, which savagely attacks those who stray outside conventional medical boundaries and dare to suggest that something besides surgery, chemotherapy, radiation, and tamoxifen might be helpful.

It may shock you to know that despite breast cancer being the leading cause of death among middle-aged women in the United States, only 5 percent of the National Cancer Institute's budget is allocated to research on cancer *prevention*. And just in case you thought some other branch of the U.S. government was going to pitch in with some unbiased, nondrug, prevention-oriented research, the enormously expensive, taxpayer-financed Women's Breast Cancer Initiative will be researching only pharmaceutical drugs (Premarin plus various synthetic estrogens and progestins) in relationship to breast cancer. We believe this is like subsidizing the drug companies—which already make billions of dollars in profits *after* spending billions on advertising, public relations, and lobbying money to influence congressional decisions. Drug testing should be the responsibility of the drug companies, not taxpayers. To add insult to injury, this is research that should have been done by the drug companies decades ago, before the drugs were approved.

The prevention picture is equally dreary in other big cancer organizations. When you log onto the Web site for the American Cancer Society (ACS) and access the area about cancer prevention, it says, "At this time, there is no way to prevent breast cancer." This is true only in that we can't point to one cause and make it the culprit. The reality is that we know so much about what causes breast cancer that of course we know what we can do to help prevent it, in the same sense that we know how to help prevent heart disease or diabetes.

For example, there's no question that you can significantly reduce your risk of these diseases by eating a wholesome diet, getting regular moderate exercise, maintaining a healthy weight, and managing stress effectively. This same approach will also help you lower your risk of breast cancer by creating better overall health. The factors that dictate which women get breast cancer and which don't *include* all of the practical commonsense solutions listed above. Yes, we all know of a health-food nut who has gotten breast cancer, but all the tofu and vegetables in the world may not make up for a devastating insult to breast tissue such as years of estrogen dominance or heavy exposure to pesticides or solvents. And then again they might make a difference, depending on your genetics and a dozen other factors. There is no one right formula for preventing breast cancer in every woman. The key to prevention of breast cancer is being aware of the various factors that cause the disease and avoiding them as much as possible, while at the same time being aware of what discourages cancerous growth in breast tissue and promoting that kind of lifestyle.

Preventive medicine is a multidimensional approach that takes the entire human—the physical, emotional, mental, and spiritual aspects—into account, and optimizes health for that particular individual. Conventional medicine, which is narrowly focused on diagnosing disease and then prescribing a drug to kill it, is a failure when it comes to treating cancer and chronic diseases such as diabetes and arthritis, because it ignores most of the human it's purporting to heal. And this is also why, in 2000, patient visits to alternative health care professionals exceeded visits to conventional physicians—despite the fact that insurance doesn't cover most alternative health care. Take a middle-aged woman with breast cancer who is terribly depressed and emotionally devastated because of a major trauma or loss in her life: All the drugs in the world aren't going to help her unless her emotional and spiritual needs are also addressed.

Prevention is also a dirty word during the richly endowed, much-hyped and -touted Breast Cancer Awareness Month that occurs every October, because it's largely sponsored and funded by the drug company that makes tamoxifen. Ironically, this firm also manufactures some of the toxic chemicals that help cause breast cancer. Breast Cancer Awareness Month is about being aware of cancer establishment treatments; there is little focus on preventing breast cancer or raising funds for independent research. It really should be called Breast Cancer Unawareness Month.

The Politics of the Breast Cancer Industry

To get to the bottom of why progress isn't being made in preventing or treating breast cancer, it's important to consider the breast cancer industry and what makes it tick. The detection and treatment of breast cancer is hugely profitable in the United States, generating billions of dollars a year. All those mammograms, biopsies, lumpectomies, and mastectomies, and all that chemotherapy, radiation, and tamoxifen, create a substantial income stream for hospitals, physicians, their support staff, those who make all the equipment, and especially those who make the drugs. And that doesn't even take into consideration all the research being done that's funded by the hundreds of millions of dollars donated to nonprofit breast cancer organizations. Where's the financial incentive to go outside this framework?

If just a fraction of the research money now going into perpetuating the above industries were honestly put into prevention and effective treatment, the mortality rate from breast cancer would very likely drop precipitously within a few years. But doctors keep squishing and radiating women's breasts with mammograms, and possibly increasing their chances of getting breast cancer in the process, perhaps because it's lucrative and it's the standard of care. (Thanks to new technology using the—hopefully—safer techniques of thermography and ultrasound, mammograms are becoming obsolete anyway, but it will probably take decades to phase out all those expensive machines.) Doctors keep doing unneeded biopsies because they could get sued if they don't. They keep removing women's breasts and giving them toxic drugs because they don't know what else to do, and they feel they have to do *something*.

In its zeal to find a magic drug to stop breast cancer, the industry has forgotten about healing. It doesn't have time. It has to run the patients through the HMO mill, get them out of the hospital faster, cut costs, avoid lawsuits, keep positions and funding, and make the drug companies happy by promoting and prescribing their products so that they'll keep funding the universities and hospitals.

Where does this leave the woman with breast cancer? She's terribly afraid and confused, but she's also pretty much crushed by the cog wheels of the medical machinery. Granted, she's what keeps the machinery going, but she certainly isn't the center of attention; she's a supporting player in a much larger drama. She'll be shuffled off to this operating table or that radiation clinic not because it's necessarily best for her as an individual, and not because that's what's going to truly help and heal her, but because she fits into that slot, that's how the breast cancer industry machine works, and there's no other choice. What conventional medicine presents her with is that she's going to die if she doesn't do it. But if she sorts out the statistics accurately, she's going to realize that if she has a nonlocal (non-DCIS) cancer, even if she does everything the doctors tell her to do there's still a one in three chance that she's going to die, from the cancer or as a result of its treatment. These aren't great odds, and the path to possible recovery is paved with treatments that can do permanent damage.

An aside: In contrast, Dr. Zava recently had contact with a woman who was given three to six months to live in 1993 because she had a very large, node-positive breast cancer tumor. She opted against conventional chemoradiation therapy and began juicing and progesterone therapy as an alternative. She called Dr. Zava (in 2001) to update him on her progress and to get a saliva test! Granted, this is just one story, but we hear them on a regular basis.

To make matters even more confusing for the average woman with breast cancer who wants to do some research on whatever course of treatment her doctor is suggesting, a great deal of medical research needs to be interpreted in light of the context in which it was conceived and/or carried out. Unfortunately, much of it is sponsored by drug companies, so it's no surprise that thousands of small studies come out every year advocating some point that the companies want to pay a scientist to support. You can come up with all kinds of medical theories and support them with perfectly reputable references from peer-reviewed journals found on Medline, the National Library of Medicine's huge research database.

The Politics of Medical Research and Media Information on Breast Cancer

The politics of physician attitudes that don't support healing, medical research, and media information on breast cancer are disheartening, because they're largely controlled by large drug companies with one agenda: Sell more drugs.

At the root of physician beliefs and attitudes about breast cancer treatment is the fact that the pharmaceutical industry now powerfully influences both medical education and research. A recent *Journal of the American Medical Association (JAMA)* reported that 31 percent of medical school funding comes from governmental and pharmaceutical grants; we think this is a gross underestimate. As a consequence, drug company money has a profound influence on the medical research that's chosen. For example, if a drug that has the potential to be patented is competing for funding with a drug that can't be patented because it's found in nature, there's no contest. The patent drug wins, even if the drug found in nature might be the biggest breakthrough since penicillin.

You don't hear much that's positive about non-drug alternative health treatments in the national media, yet millions of people visit the Internet daily looking for information on alternative health. Would they be flocking to the Web in such large numbers if they were getting what they need from their doctors, or from print media and TV? We think not. Drug company money is a primary source of advertising revenue for the media, especially for TV and magazines, so unless you're Bill Moyers you're unlikely to expose drug company and medical politics or talk about alternative health in positive terms and still keep your job.

How about the FDA—aren't they looking out for the consumer? On the contrary, endorsement of a drug or treatment by the FDA should not necessarily give you confidence that it's a safe and effective treatment. According to the prestigious *Jour-*

nal of the American Medical Association and *New England Journal of Medicine*, the side effects of *properly prescribed* prescription drugs are the fourth- or fifth-leading cause of death in the United States. This doesn't even include deaths from improperly prescribed drugs, deaths from in-hospital errors, and unreported drug deaths; if these were thrown into the statistics, drug treatments in general would easily be in the top three causes of death in the nation. All the drugs that are killing so many people are approved by the FDA and considered part of the standard of medical care.

A recent scathing editorial in *The Lancet* took the FDA to task for its inappropriately close association with pharmaceutical companies. The title of the article was "Lotronex and the FDA: a fatal erosion of integrity," and it described the process by which the drug Lotronex, developed for irritable bowel syndrome (IBS), was approved by the FDA and subsequently was reported by the FDA to have killed five people and resulted in the hospitalization of many others. The drug was voluntarily withdrawn from the market by the manufacturer, but then the company requested that it be reinstated after a change to the warning label. *The Lancet* editorial concluded that ". . . private communications appear to have subverted official procedures, while suppressed scientific debate has superseded a full and open review process. . . . The Lotronex episode may show in microcosm a serious erosion of integrity within the FDA, and in particular CDER [Center for Drug Evaluation and Research], whose operating budget now depends on industry money." Buyer beware.

The original intent of the FDA was to protect consumers from dangerous products, but the agency appears to have lost its way, and to be heavily influenced in its decisions by the drug industry. A recent survey conducted by the newspaper *USA Today* found that 54 percent of the time, experts hired to advise the FDA on which medicines should be approved for sale have a direct financial interest in the drug or topic they're asked to evaluate. In turn, it's very common for FDA employees to retire to well-paid positions on the advisory boards of large drug companies.

So what's a woman to believe? You need to find medical authorities whose opinions you trust: people who have been successful in their practice and proven right in their viewpoints over and over again for decades. People whose opinions are not based on how large a grant they're getting from the drug industry, or the soy industry, or the dairy industry, or a vitamin company, but people who are objectively and intelligently looking at the facts, interpreting experience, and evaluating studies. Put your trust in a physician who's willing to take the time to talk with you; after all, this is a life-and-death matter.

How about doctors who would like to try treatments for cancer that are outside the mainstream? They can't: They're forced to use medications (even if they know they aren't working well), because there are no large-scale studies to prove the effectiveness of alternatives and thus the FDA will not approve them. (The evidence proving the effectiveness of conventional medical treatments is scant, but that's politics.) If an alternative treatment doesn't have FDA approval, a doctor can be fined, be reprimanded, or even lose his or her medical license for using it. If you find the rare and courageous physician willing to guide and support you through an alternative treatment, be grateful!

The Implications of Being Honest

The political and financial implications of admitting that conventional hormone replacement therapy, plastics, pesticides, and other environmental toxins disrupt the body's ability to manufacture normal levels of hormones and consequently contribute to causing breast cancer are enormous. (We'll explain how and why these things can cause breast cancer later in the book.) Just think what would happen to the drug company giants if they were forced to admit that their products had contributed to the deaths of tens of thousands of women. The tobacco companies would have to move over in the litigation courts. However, the largest drug companies alone (never mind the pesticide and plastics companies) spent $74.4 million in 1997–1998 to influence congressional thinking via their lobbying efforts. That's one powerful influence. The only potentially stronger influence is your vote.

Thanks to an undeniably steep rise in the incidence of prostate and testicular cancer, Congress has taken some action to find out more about how chemicals that mimic hormones affect humans. A 1996 mandate from Congress charged the Environmental Protection Agency (EPA) with examining the hormonal effects of the top 100 selling chemicals in the United States. As the first studies trickle out, the evidence is clear: We are awash in a sea of chemicals, many of them estrogenic in nature, that profoundly affect every aspect of our health. Because estrogens oppose or negate the actions of testosterone, our little boys—and eventually men—are as profoundly affected as women are.

As it becomes clear to our political representatives that these chemicals are affecting their own families, perhaps they'll be inspired to take action to protect their constituents. It's also incumbent upon each individual to maintain a lifestyle that's protective—this alone would dramatically change the economics, because millions of people would stop spraying their homes, lawns, and gardens with pesticides; start buying organic produce; and stop eating hormone-laden meat. (Did you know that U.S. beef is banned in Europe because of the hormones it contains?)

The Bottom Line

The bottom line is that a woman with breast cancer is left with few viable options from the medical community. She can't completely trust breast cancer research or recommendations about medical treatments, and she lives in a culture that's averting its gaze from the real causes of her disease. Thus, it takes enormous courage and fortitude to stand up and take charge of your health, to question your physician and ask for clear answers, and to carefully examine alternatives. We hope that through this book we can inspire you to do just that. Perhaps this excerpt from a letter to Dr. Lee will be inspiring:

> My deepest appreciation to you for being gutsy enough to tell me your opinion concerning tamoxifen. You advised me against it, giving me the courage to buck my very pushy oncologist who wanted me to take it. I have been thriving without tamoxifen. I've had several follow-up mammograms and was told the opposite breast looked "textbook perfect," and the breast that had the lumpectomy looked normal and benign.
>
> I am 56, postmenopausal, and am using progesterone cream. You reassured me it was safe even for a woman like me with high estrogen and progesterone receptors, explaining this means progesterone can get in and do its job of stopping the cancer when the receptors are present.
>
> When I heard the flap about the "hazards of progesterone" I knew before even checking further that it was probably a botched reporting job that really referred to the synthetic progestins.
>
> Thanks to you my life has been quite serene despite my diagnosis of cancer. I think progesterone is a mood elevator, also. I have blessed you silently many times since you replied to my letter asking about tamoxifen.
>
> Blessings on you and your work,
> MH

CHAPTER 2

RISK FACTORS
FOR BREAST CANCER

Why It All Points to Estrogen

As you learned in the last chapter, conventional medicine doesn't like to talk about prevention when it comes to breast cancer, but it's more than willing to talk about risk factors. It's important for you to know what your risk factors are and how to put them into context for yourself, both if you're concerned about preventing breast cancer and if you have it. For example, if your doctor insists that you take the drug tamoxifen to prevent breast cancer because your risk factors are high, you should know what this means.

A risk factor is something that statistically correlates with the incidence of a disease, but is not necessarily a true or direct cause of the disease. Known risk factors for breast cancer are fairly well laid out by researchers at this point, but within the narrow boundaries of what conventional medicine considers a risk factor, only 25 to 30 percent of the women who get the disease have acknowledged risk factors. This number has likely increased significantly in the past year or so, as more studies have proven that HRT and use of oral contraceptives at a young age increase breast cancer risk. If exposure to xenohormones and toxic chemicals was included as an official risk factor, the number would rise even higher.

As you'll soon understand, almost all risk factors associated with breast cancer are directly or indirectly related to excess estrogen or estrogen that isn't balanced with progesterone. We believe that correcting this imbalance, which Dr. Lee has termed *estrogen dominance,* is the essence of preventing and treating breast cancer.

Risk factors are calculated by epidemiologists, or scientists who study health trends in large groups. This type of statistical information is not infallible, but when more than one study shows the same trend, it's an indication that the information is pretty good. One way to help prevent breast cancer, and to help prevent a recurrence, is to reduce your risk factors.

There are many myths, as we like to call them, about risk factors for breast cancer, and new ones seem to come out every month. Many of these myths are created with data that have been tweaked by companies that stand to profit from the information. For example, Japanese women have less breast cancer than U.S. women, and the soy industry uses this statistic to claim that the reason is because the Japanese eat a lot of soy. However, there is no scientific evidence to back up this claim— it is an epidemiological guess. There *is* evidence that Japanese women have a genetic predisposition to process hormones differently than Caucasian women, and this may account for the difference in the rate of breast cancer. It's also true that when Japanese women move to the United States, their granddaughters' rate of breast cancer matches that of U.S. women. Does this prove a dietary connection? Probably, but not necessarily. If it is a dietary connection, it could have more to do with eating more hormone-contaminated meat than with eating less soy. If it's not a dietary connection, it could be that pollution of our environment with xenohormones is much higher than that in Japan, or that when Japanese women come to the United States they use oral contraceptives and HRT more than they do in Japan, or that their stress levels are increased here. In other words, there are many factors that can increase or decrease the risk of breast cancer.

Current thinking is that the increase in breast cancer and the chronic diseases so common in the United States among Japanese immigrants is created because they consume more calories, and more of the wrong kind of calories from highly processed foods laden with fake fats (trans–fatty acids such as partially hydrogenated oils), refined carbohydrates, and sugar.

For a while it was reported that higher fat intake correlated with higher breast cancer risk, but bigger, better, and more objective studies have shown this correlation to be inaccurate. Since it's been nutritionally politically correct to make fat the bad guy since the 1970s, this quickly became a popular risk factor, even though evidence for it was scant. It's likely that, again, the correlations that were found were due to eating more calories. The point is that we need to be very careful about believing generalizations made about risk factors.

Much of the information about risk factors for breast cancer comes from data collected from women who have breast cancer. This is called retrospective data, or data that looks back at a woman's life history. This type of data has yielded valuable information about what protects women from breast cancer, such as early pregnancy and late onset of menstruation, and what increases the risk of breast cancer, such as early onset of menstruation and not having children. We'll delve into these in more detail later in this chapter.

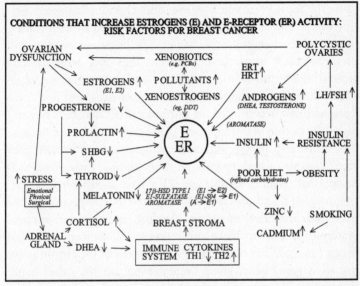

Many factors in breast cancer point to estrogen. By the time you finish reading this book, each of these factors will make sense to you.

Known Risk Factors for Breast Cancer

Age

Women who are in their mid-thirties to their mid-forties have the highest escalating risk of breast cancer. In other words, your risk of having breast cancer increases the most steeply in these years. The most common age for the initial stages of breast cancer to be detected is five years or more *before* menopause. This is well before estrogen levels fall, but coincides with a drop in progesterone and the associated problems of estrogen dominance.

After menopause, the rate of increase in the risk for breast cancer drops dramatically. This means that although the odds of getting breast cancer are higher in an 80-year-old woman—because the more years you live, the more chance you have of getting breast cancer—there are more middle-aged women getting breast cancer than any other age group. These are what we call premenopausal women, and they're the ones who, usually around their mid-thirties, start to have menstrual cycles in which they don't ovulate, or in which they ovulate but don't produce adequate amounts of the hormone progesterone. They still make the hormone estrogen and bleed each month, but because they don't "pop an egg" and create progesterone, or because they aren't capable of making enough progesterone, their estrogen is unopposed. Women of this age often have a difficult time getting pregnant, and they're often subjected to hysterectomies due to fibroids and heavy menstrual bleeding. Estrogen without progesterone is a setup for many reproductive cancers—not just breast cancer. What estrogen says to the cells of the reproductive organs is *grow! grow! grow!* Progesterone, on the other hand, counteracts the estrogen stimulation, instead encouraging the cells to mature (differentiate) and die on time (apoptosis), to be replaced by the new cells that are continually developing.

In women whose breast tissue has been damaged in some way—from exposure to radiation or toxic chemicals, for example—excessive stimulation by estrogen is an invitation for that tissue to start to go bad, so to speak. Let's say there's a small area of cells whose DNA has been damaged by radiation, and this has escaped the detection systems in the body that normally would have repaired it. Thanks to a healthy young immune system and monthly doses of progesterone made by the ovaries, however, the damaged tissue stays self-contained. If you suddenly take the progesterone away for a few months (you don't ovulate, a common occurrence in premenopausal women) and expose these cells to unopposed estrogen, they (along with the normal breast cells) will be getting powerful signals to multiply and grow, allowing the genetically flawed cells to flourish. If these aberrant cells have reprogrammed their genetic information in favor of survival and unregulated growth, they could eventually express themselves as a new colony, or cancer. If the DNA of these cells has been damaged, the cells can become cancerous and infiltrate the tissue around them.

Chronological age is a risk factor for breast cancer simply because as you age your body's immune defense systems wear down and become less effective, and because gene mutations accumulate over time. The fat in your breast tissue can also be more dangerous at age 60 than at age 20, because you've had more time to accumulate and retain toxins within the fat tissues of the breast.

However, in some countries the risk of breast cancer after menopause is very low. This may be due to less exposure to environmental estrogens and HRT; it may be due to diet; and it may be due to more exercise: Risk factors tell us they all play a role.

Geography, Race, and Genetics

Women of non- or less-industrialized countries have less breast cancer than women of industrialized countries. Dr. Peter Ellison of Harvard, author of *On Fertile Ground* (Harvard University Press, 2001), has documented markedly higher hormone levels among women of industrialized countries. Dr. Ellison is convinced that something in industrialized countries causes elevated hormone levels and, therefore, a higher risk of breast cancer. He believes the elevated hormone levels may be due to excess calorie intake and lower expenditure of physical energy among women of industrialized countries (more junk food and less exercise). Regardless of cause, the fact remains that higher hormone levels correlate with higher incidence of breast cancer. Although progesterone levels are also higher in women of industrialized countries, studies done in France show that women with breast cancer have *lower* progesterone levels during the luteal phase, or the middle of the menstrual cycle. Simultaneously their estrogen levels are high, and here again we have a setup for estrogen dominance.

The incidence of breast cancer varies widely by country, and it's difficult to say in some cases whether these differences are due to geography, culture, genetics, or diet. The different races are known to process prescription drugs differently, and we're now learning that they also process hormones differently, so some of the differences are surely in our genes. As a whole, Asians, whether industrialized or not, have lower rates of breast cancer than Europeans and North Americans, by as much as five times. However, as we mentioned earlier, the breast cancer rate of Asian women who move to North America rises to match that of North Americans within two generations, indicating that whatever's happening in the environment in North America outweighs any protection conferred by genetics.

The fact that the mortality (death) rate for breast cancer is only 3.4 per 100,000 women in Gambia and 20 per 100,000 in India may be due to the genetics of race, or it may be due to diet, culture, or the water! These distinctions are even more difficult to make when you compare seemingly similar countries such as Poland, which has a mortality rate of 38.7, with the nearby Netherlands, whose rate is 72.7 per 100,000. White women in the United States have the highest mortality rate from breast cancer on the planet—89.2 per 100,000 women.

Israel once had one of the highest breast cancer mortality rates in the world. Within a few years of banning three organochlorine pesticides (DDT, BHC, and lindane) in the early 1970s, however, breast cancer deaths dropped 8 percent, while they were rising everywhere else in the world. We'll discuss pesticides and other environmental toxins that can cause breast cancer in chapter 18.

Geography *is* a risk factor for breast cancer if you live in an area polluted with industrial waste. According to a 1989 Environmental Protection Agency (EPA) study, breast cancer rates are higher in the 339 U.S. counties with hazardous waste sites and groundwater contamination.

Only about 10 percent of breast cancer in Western industrialized countries can be attributed to genetic mutations that are passed down through generations. The type of breast cancer that most often runs in families is caused by a mutation in genes known as the BRCA genes. These mutations tend to be passed down from either parent (who may or may not have the disease), and are found most often in women of Ashkenazi Jewish descent, and also in women in Iceland.

In general, women with a genetic predisposition to get breast cancer tend to get it before the age of 50. In general, women with a first-degree relative (mother, sister, or daughter) who had breast cancer before the age of 65 have at least twice the risk of getting breast cancer, and the younger the relative was when she got the breast cancer, the greater the chance that it's inherited. If two first-degree relatives have breast cancer, the risk of getting the disease is four to six times higher.

Pregnancy

Women who become pregnant before the age of 24 have as much as five times less risk of breast cancer later in life as women who have a child after the age of 30. This is probably because the hormones of pregnancy and lactation develop and differentiate the breast tissue in ways that are highly protective. Researcher Jose Russo, M.D., of the Fox Chase Cancer Center in Philadelphia, believes that it is specifically human chorionic gonadotropin (hCG) that sends the very specific genetic signals to breast tissues that then confer protection. The hCG is normally one of the first substances released by a woman's body in response to conception, and it stimulates the formation of more progesterone by the corpus luteum. (More about this later.)

Progesterone is a dominant hormone during pregnancy. Only

the first full-term early pregnancy conveys protection. Interrupted pregnancies (miscarriages and abortions) do not afford protection, and research is accumulating that indicates they can actually increase the risk of breast cancer. This may be because the tissue begins to differentiate and then is stopped partway through the process.

Women who never had children are at a higher risk for breast cancer than those who had one or more children at any age. This again is probably due to the differentiation of breast tissue that occurs during pregnancy and lactation.

Removal of Ovaries

A woman's ovaries are her primary source of hormones (including estrogens, progesterone, testosterone). Removal of the ovaries is "instant menopause" and results in a precipitous drop overnight in hormones. This reduces hormone levels and the associated risks of breast cancer, but at the same time predisposes a woman to serious health problems such as heart disease and osteoporosis. In women subjected to oophorectomy (removal of both ovaries) prior to age 40, the risk of breast cancer is significantly reduced, probably because their estradiol (a type of estrogen) levels are significantly reduced. However, the protective effects of early oophorectomy are negated by administration of estrogen with or without progestins (synthetic progesterones). Because women who have their ovaries removed prior to age 40 are at a much higher risk for heart disease, arthritis, and osteoporosis, this should not be considered a viable type of preventive treatment for breast cancer.

Radiation

Radiation is one of the most potent risk factors for breast cancer, and its effects are cumulative. This means that the damage done to the breast tissue doesn't disappear with time: Each dose of radiation to the breast adds to the last one.

Most women in the United States are exposed to radiation through chest X rays. As mentioned in chapter 1, women who have had scoliosis and received many diagnostic X rays during childhood and adolescence have a 70 percent higher risk of breast cancer than women in the general population. The more X rays a woman was exposed to, and the higher the dose of radiation, the greater her risk of breast cancer. Radiation does the most damage in girls and teens with undeveloped breast tissue. Girls who were exposed to radiation in the bombing of Hiroshima during World War II have double the risk of breast cancer.

Lumpy and Painful Breasts

This is a controversial area in the study of risk factors, with little agreement among a wide variety of studies. It is clear that women who have a biopsy report that reads "severe atypical epithelial hyperplasia" (*hyperplasia* means that cells are dividing very rapidly, which is one of the signals that cancerous changes are taking place) have an increased risk of breast cancer, and therefore this is considered a precancerous condition. This finding should be interpreted as a serious warning sign from the body that the underlying metabolic abnormality (most likely estrogen dominance) causing the condition has progressed to the point that cancer may ensue if it's not corrected.

However, the risks are less clear for women who have premenstrually painful and lumpy breasts, and for women who have benign cysts and chronically lumpy breasts, sometimes called fibrocystic breast disease (even though it's not, strictly speaking, a disease). It's become clear to us that painful and lumpy breasts of almost every description are caused by estrogen dominance and can be helped with the use of transdermal natural progesterone (not synthetic progestins, which often make them worse). The French recognized in the mid-1970s that application of progesterone topically to the breasts helped clear up problems with fibrocysts. Dr. Lee receives mail every week from women telling him how grateful they are that their breasts became smooth and painless after one, two, or three cycles of progesterone cream. This is also one of the most consistent reports we receive from clinicians who use progesterone cream in their practices. It's a well-established fact that postmenopausal women on conventional HRT (such as Premarin and Provera, a progestin) have denser breast tissue, which makes it more difficult to detect abnormalities in mammograms.

We believe that estrogen dominance is an unrecognized risk factor for breast cancer, and in this context it makes sense that chronically lumpy and painful breasts would also be a risk factor. The good news is that the underlying metabolic imbalance causing the estrogen dominance is fairly easy to correct with small doses of progesterone cream that mimic what the body would be making if it were ovulating. (See chapter 13 for details.)

Oral Contraceptives Given to Teenagers

Use of oral contraceptives by teens is now an established risk factor for breast cancer. The younger the girl, the higher her risk of breast cancer. In general, girls under the age of 18 who use oral contraceptives triple their lifetime risk of breast cancer. The younger a woman begins using oral contraceptives, the greater is her increased risk of premenopausal breast cancer. Again, this is most likely due to the progestins (synthetic progesterone) in the birth control pills (or shots) blocking the beneficial actions of real progesterone, and also blocking ovulation and thus the production of a woman's own hormones.

In women older than 20, taking oral contraceptives long term, and for ten years afterward, confers a slightly higher risk of breast cancer. In women in their thirties, however, birth control pills that are testosterone-derived, such as norgestrel, appear to confer some protection against breast cancer. This may be because testosterone is a major antagonist of estrogen, combined with the fact that birth control pills create a lower overall hormonal milieu.

Conventional Hormone Replacement Therapy (HRT)

For years conventional medicine has been in a state of denial about the potential for HRT to cause breast cancer. At one point virtually every woman aged 50 or older who walked into a doctor's office was ordered to take estrogen or, if she had a uterus, estrogen and a progestin. These commands were usually given without measuring hormone levels to see if the HRT was actually needed, and without regard to symptoms. Women who complained of common side effects such as weight gain, insomnia, anxiety, and depression were given antidepressants, anti-anxiety drugs, and sleeping pills.

Thanks to some major new studies clearly showing that conventional HRT does *not* protect against heart disease and that it *does* increase the risk of breast cancer, doctors are starting to be a little more cautious about prescribing it.

Almost all the family doctors and gynecologists in the United States who are paying attention to their patients will affirm that they've seen many women begin taking high doses of conventional HRT, only to return six months later with breast lumps and/or breast cancer. We've received hundreds of letters and e-mails telling this story, and have confirmed it with numerous clinicians. This effect may be due both to the excessive doses of estrogen prescribed to many menopausal women and to the poisonous effects of the progestins on breast tissue.

Breast cancer does not spread like a sphere that gradually grows bigger; it spreads tentacles into the surrounding tissue, and these are gradually filled in, creating an ever-larger lump. It may be that giving excessive doses of estrogen causes the rapid filling in of smallish tumors, giving the impression that a lump has just suddenly appeared.

Diet

This is a controversial and unclear area of breast cancer research. Countries in which people eat more fat have higher rates of breast cancer, but this isn't necessarily a direct correlation. Current thinking is that this is due to a higher calorie intake:

More calories = a greater number of free radicals in body = greater damage to tissue = higher incidence of cancer

However, the types of fat that you eat are important. Unsaturated fats such as corn oil that quickly go rancid are particularly dangerous. What this means is simply that fats that easily oxidize have potential to do harm because they more easily generate free radicals. A study in Italy, where most of the population eats monounsaturated olive oil, found that carbohydrates, not fats, are a bigger risk factor, which is likely due to the effects of refined carbohydrates on insulin and insulin resistance. Insulin is a growth factor, and we'll talk about its connection to breast cancer later in the book.

The weak correlation between fat intake and breast cancer found in some studies could mean that the hormones and pesticides found in the fat of meat are what's causing the higher rate of breast cancer, and not the fat itself. Unfortunately, dietary studies have not made good distinctions about the types of fat eaten, other than saturated fat. Studies based in Greece, Italy, and Spain have shown that women who consume olive oil at more than one meal a day have a 25 percent lower risk of breast cancer. We think there's a good chance that a high intake of the trans–fatty acids called hydrogenated and partially hydrogenated oils, which are found in most processed foods, could contribute to breast cancer risk, and we'll cover this topic in more detail later in the book.

It could also be, as Dr. Peter Ellison of Harvard postulates, that a higher calorie intake and lower rate of exercise create a higher hormonal milieu, which increases the risk of reproductive cancers. For possibly similar reasons, obesity is correlated with a higher risk of dying from breast cancer. This could be due to the fact that women who are obese tend to have less healthy lifestyles (more calories, less exercise, for example), and also that fat cells produce estrogen. Thus, the more fat a woman has, the more estrogen she'll make, even after menopause.

Although this has not been well studied epidemiologically, it's clear that a diet high in sugar, refined carbohydrates, and trans–fatty acids creates many imbalances in the body, including in the sex steroids and in insulin, which all play a role in breast cancer.

It's also clear from dozens of studies done around the world that, in general, people from all countries, of all races, and in all cultures are healthier and have less of all types of cancer when they eat more fresh vegetables and fruits, and more whole foods. Some studies have shown as much as a 46 percent reduced risk of breast cancer in women who eat lots of fresh vegetables. We'll explain later in the book why broccoli and its cruciferous cousins have direct cancer-protective properties.

Drinking milk from cows given the milk-production stimulant called recombinant bovine growth hormone (rBGH) may increase the risk of breast cancer. According to cancer risk specialist Samuel Epstein, M.D., this biotech hormone induces a marked increase in levels of insulin-like growth factor 1 (IGF-1) in cows' milk. There's little doubt that if you have too much IGF-1, it can play a role in causing breast cancer. The bottom line is that if you feel you must drink milk (we don't recommend it), it's probably wise to drink hormone-free or organic milk.

A handful of studies are indicating that how you cook meat affects your breast cancer risk, and that all those studies that correlated eating red meat and saturated fat with breast cancer may have had more to do with how the meat was cooked than with the meat itself. Charring, frying, flame broiling, or barbecuing meat at temperatures between 300 and 500 degrees Fahrenheit produces compounds called heterocyclic amines (HCAs), some of which resemble—you guessed it—estrogen. The moral of this story is to cook your meat at lower heats or by roasting or stewing.

Alcohol

Women who have more than one drink of alcohol per day have a higher risk of breast cancer. This is probably because alcohol keeps the liver working overtime, and thus it is less able to process estrogens out of the body, so the body has chronically higher levels of estrogen than it would otherwise. A study done in Finland showed that women with moderate alcohol intake who also used oral contraceptives had increased estradiol and decreased progesterone levels. Women not using oral contraceptives had only decreased progesterone levels. Decreased progesterone would put a woman at higher risk for estrogen dominance and therefore at higher risk for breast cancer. But before you give up that glass of red wine with dinner, which is good for your heart and possibly for your state of mind, remember that according to the same study, at most 4 percent of breast cancers are linked to alcohol.

If you like to have an alcoholic beverage in the evening, one way to put less stress on your liver is to make sure that you consume the alcohol with food. Drinking on an empty stomach dramatically increases stress on the liver.

Exercise

Many studies point to the fact that moderate exercise reduces cancer risk, and breast cancer is no exception. Recent research done as part of the Harvard Nurses' Health Study, which analyzed data from 166,388 women, found that those who engaged in moderate or vigorous exercise for seven or more hours per week had, when compared to women who exercised for less than one hour per week, a nearly 20 percent lower risk of breast cancer.

It's important to note, however, that this benefit applies to *moderate* exercise. Highly strenuous exercise actually suppresses the immune system and greatly increases oxidation in the body. In the long term this could put a woman at higher risk for breast cancer. Even though it's great PR for some companies, we don't recommend that women who have recently had breast cancer try to climb a high mountain or run a triathalon; your body needs all the balance it can get to completely heal and protect itself and return to a balanced state, and training to scale a mountain peak or run a marathon probably isn't going to help your body stay physically balanced, it's going to add enormous stress. The Harvard Nurses' study cited above found that frequency of exercise was more important than how vigorous it was.

Workplace Hazards

Because employers are loath to admit it when they discover a higher-than-normal risk of cancer in the workplace, it's very difficult to prove or even to track breast cancer incidence by occupation. However, Sweden conducted a huge study that followed well over a million women for almost 20 years to assess which occupations had the highest rates of breast cancer. The high-risk occupations include physicians, pharmacists, teachers, systems analysts and programmers, telephone operators, office switchboard operators, telegraph and radio operators, metal platers and coaters, and hairdressers and beauticians. Risk was also greater among women living in urban areas than it was among those in rural areas. Swedish researchers theorize that the increased risk in some occupations is due to their sedentary nature, exposure to electromagnetic fields (EMFs), and, among production workers and beauticians, exposure to toxins such as heavy metals, solvents, and hair dyes.

Electromagnetic Fields

EMFs are emitted from almost any type of device that runs on electricity, to a greater or lesser degree. Although the research is very controversial, we think it's prudent to avoid strong EMF fields. Microwave ovens—when turned on—are among the worst offenders, and other household appliances from toaster ovens to coffeemakers also emit strong EMFs when they're on. However, the fields drop off very quickly with distance, and most appliances are safe just a few feet away. This makes it smart not to stand right in front of the microwave and watch your food cook. Another major source of EMFs, especially for office workers, is computers. Do not put a computer right next to your body; put it a few feet away. Other sources of EMFs are fuse boxes, electric meters, clock radios, TVs, and hair dryers. You can purchase a simple handheld gauss meter for around $40 to measure the EMFs in your house.

Bras and Underarm Antiperspirants

Although research has not proven that underwire bras or underarm antiperspirants cause breast cancer, common sense says that if you don't block lymph gland circulation from under your breasts with an underwire bra, it's going to be better for your breast health. We're not telling you not to don something special if you're going out on the town, but there's no reason to wear an underwire or even a very tight bra every day. Girls in their teens and twenties have all but made going braless a fashion statement, which is probably a good thing for that generation's breast health. Not wearing a bra will *not* make your breasts sag more than they do naturally.

Sweating through the skin is one of the primary ways that your body releases toxins, and your underarms are your most active sweating areas. Again, just plain common sense would tell you to avoid putting something under your arms every day that stops sweating altogether, as antiperspirants do, and that also contains myriad chemicals, which both antiperspirants and deodorants do. Showering daily is the best way to keep body odor under control; the crystal deodorants found at your health food store contain a minimum of objectionable ingredients and are effective at stopping odor.

The Bottom Line

Some of the risk factors for breast cancer, such as race, age, and family history, are out of your control, so the bottom line in minimizing your risk of breast cancer is to lead a healthy lifestyle, use your common sense, and avoid excess estrogen, whether it be from pesticides (throw your ant spray away), HRT, or oral contraceptives. The only risk factor for breast cancer that we're aware of that's not directly or indirectly associated with estrogen is radiation—stay away from chest X rays as much as possible.

CHAPTER 3

THE NATURE OF CANCER

Normal Cells That Refuse to Grow Up

Despite what your doctor might tell you, thanks to thousands of studies on cancer done all over the world, right down to the genetic level, we do know a great deal about when, where, how, and why cancer begins and progresses. Although there are still some details we still don't entirely understand, cancer is *not* a complete mystery.

If we know so much, then why are we being badly beaten in the war on cancer? Aside from the difficulty of changing prevailing medical dogma and treatment, preventing and healing cancer in a big way would entail vast and dramatic changes in lifestyle for Westernized countries. We would have to severely reduce or give up our pesticides. We would need much better control of industrial pollution. We would need to reduce our reliance on plastics that shed estrogen-like chemicals, as well as other petrochemical products that emit harmful chemicals, such as carpets, furniture, and the particleboard used to build houses. We would need to drastically reduce our use of prescription drugs and change the way HRT is prescribed. The use of hormones to fatten livestock and fowl for market and to stimulate milk production in dairy cows would need to be banned. We would need to cut way back on the amount of processed foods and sugars we eat and adopt a balanced whole-foods diet. We would need to sacrifice some monetary gain to reduce stress levels in our lives. That's the big picture. Now let's move down to the cellular level and fill you in on the basics of what we know about cancer.

When Does Cancer Occur?

Cancer occurs when normal cells multiply (proliferate) faster than normal, lose their ability to differentiate (remain immature), and have diminished apoptosis (cell death) rates. Don't worry, we'll explain all of this.

Cancer cells are primitive in that they haven't grown up and become skin, or bone, or liver, or uterus—in medical terms they are *undifferentiated*. At the stage where they would normally keep developing into a specific type of cell, they divide instead into another primitive cell. This is because something in the genetics of the cells that gives instructions on how to differentiate, or mature, is broken; communications have become faulty.

This miscommunication is usually caused by damage or some sort of toxic environment within the cell sufficient to affect the cell's chromosomes (genes). Such damage can result from estrogens, viruses, radiation, genetic predisposition, exposure to toxic chemicals, or injury to the tissue.

Most tissues of the human body are not necessarily more susceptible to cancer after being injured, but breast tissue is unique in its combination of vulnerability (it's not safely tucked away inside the belly like the uterus and ovaries) and ability to change in response to hormones. Women are well acquainted with how quickly their breasts can grow larger (and become tender) premenstrually. Once pregnancy is under way, breasts change dramatically. This ability to undergo rapid growth is one reason breast cells have greater susceptibility to DNA damage through tissue damage. Cancer biologists are well aware that when a tissue replicates rapidly, its genetic code (DNA) is more vulnerable to damage by chemicals, viruses, and radiation that may express itself some years later as cancer.

Injury to tissue can include anything from a puncture to a blow to the breast. For example, early in his practice Dr. Lee had a patient whose dog bit her in the breast. Years later she found a lump in the same spot that turned out to be a malignant cancer. Dr. Lee encourages women who have had a breast injury to put progesterone cream directly on that breast for at least three months after the injury. Injuries leading to breast cancer are why biopsies are so questionable in terms of their value: The breast is either being cut into in a surgery or punctured by a needle, and both constitute injury to the breast. Thus, it's questionable whether a biopsy could ultimately *cause* a breast cancer. We're not suggesting that if you have a suspicious lump, you shouldn't have a biopsy, but we are suggesting that physicians need to be concerned about this possible effect on the breast and be more conservative in their use of biopsies.

Some breast specialists will argue that the research doesn't show that injury to the breast contributes to breast cancer, but most doctors who have been in practice for a few decades, seeing the same women year after year, will tell you it definitely does have an effect: They see it in their practices.

The same type of questions we're asking about biopsies could be asked in regard to mammography, since both radiation and tissue damage can contribute to breast cancer. In mammography the breast is squashed quite forcefully and radiation shot through it. Does this sound healthy for the breast? We think not! Again, if you have a suspicious lump in your breast, by all means get a mammogram, but we question the wisdom of routine annual mammograms.

Eventually, when there are enough of them, cancer cells often take on a life of their own. They set up their own blood supply for nourishment, invade adjacent tissue, and force out normal cells.

The cells of the breast are usually protected against cancer by a variety of defenses, all relying on proper nutrition, proper hormone balance, and proper enzyme function. Lacking these, the cell can't neutralize and/or excrete toxic products and can't repair itself well enough to counter the damage of the factors above. When sufficient gene damage occurs, the cell reverts to a more primitive life-form (undifferentiated) and becomes a cancer cell. Since the chance of irreparable genetic damage increases over time, the chance of developing cancer increases with age.

How Does Cancer Get Started?

The first stage of cancer is known as *initiation*. This is when the initial damage, or modification of the genetic material of a normal cell, occurs. This damage is caused by a carcinogen, which could be a hormone, a chemical, a virus, radiation, trauma, or a combination of these factors. The result is a permanently altered cell with defective growth controls. Scientists now believe that it usually takes more than one "insult" by carcinogens to DNA before a normal cell is transformed into a cancerous cell.

For example, as a teenager you might have been exposed to pesticides or birth control pills during the time when your breasts were developing. In your early twenties you might have used oral contraceptives. A few years later you might paint the inside of your house without adequate ventilation and be exposed to xenoestrogens in the form of solvents. Throughout your life you get chest X rays that expose your breast cells to radiation. In your thirties you fall and hit your breast hard. In your forties you get a mammogram, both squashing the tissue and exposing it to radiation, and then you follow it up every few years with another one. In your fifties you are given an excessive dose of estrogen along with synthetic progestins. This is quite an accumulation of insults, but it's very typical of most postmenopausal women, and most could add a dozen or more incidents to this list.

The final insult to the breast cell that transforms it into a full-blown cancer cell probably occurs at least 10 to 20 years (depending upon the individual) before the tumor can be recognized by palpation (by hand) or by mammography.

Meanwhile, the body has many protective factors in place for stopping DNA damage before it begins, including sophisticated detoxification and excretion mechanisms; specialized cells that remove dead and damaged cells from the breasts; antioxidants and other nutrients that help the cell protect and repair DNA; and hormones such as progesterone, which encourages cells to differentiate and to die when they're supposed to.

Cancer arises when the DNA in a cell is permanently damaged, and this escapes the body's normal detection systems. The damage is passed on from one generation of cells to the next, resulting in an accumulation of DNA-damaged cells without the proper controls needed to keep them normal.

The Growth Process

The second stage of cancer, called *promotion,* involves the expansion of the tumor cell population to the point where it begins to interfere with the normal workings of the body. This stage occurs over an extended period of time, as long as 10 to 20 years, and varies depending on many factors. For example, tumor growth rate will depend on whether there's a good blood supply around it for delivering nutrients to its cells, and on growth factors such as estrogens, the hormone prolactin, and the substances called insulin-like growth factors that trigger breast cell division. We'll give you more details on these factors later in the book. Tumor growth will also depend on substances that inhibit growth such as progesterone, thyroid hormone, melatonin, dehydroepiandrosterone (DHEA), and phytochemicals from fruits and vegetables.

Let's put the growth rate of a breast cancer in a different kind of perspective. The human body contains approximately 64 trillion cells. A drop of blood contains about 3,000 to 5,000 white blood cells and 5 million red blood cells. If a single healthy cell in a breast becomes a cancer cell, it usually takes 8 to 12 years for this cell to multiply into a detectable tumor. Another way of understanding the rate at which breast cancer tumors grow is that on average, they double in size every two to four months.

Assuming 100 days as the doubling rate for the average breast cancer cell, there would only be about 4 to 5 tumor cells the first year, 30 to 50 tumor cells the second year, and so on. Finding a tumor this small would be more challenging than finding a needle in a haystack. Not until the seventh year would there be about a million tumor cells. This may seem like a lot of tumor cells, but if you packaged them into a perfect ball it would measure only about a millimeter across—not much bigger than an average pencil dot. Tumors these sizes are not detectable by mammography. Only after the tumor grows for another three to four more years, or for a total of 10 to 12 years, and contains 1 billion to 10 billion cells is it large enough (about 1 centimeter in diameter; 1 inch equals just about 2.5 centimeters) to be detected by mammography.

Of course tumor growth patterns are never this simple. The in situ tumors, or those tumors whose growth is confined to the breast ducts from which they originated, tend to grow more as spheres or tubes because their growth is confined to the inside of the ducts. Invasive tumors, in contrast, don't generally grow as perfect spheres but radiate out in a clawlike pattern—hence the term *crab,* or cancer—as they invade normal tissue and seek nutrients for growth. This type of spread can make them even more difficult to detect within the confines of the normal breast tissue.

When a cancer is first detectable by mammogram, it takes only a year or two more for it to increase in size to be detectable by palpation (hand). This two-year time interval, statistics have shown, has little effect on the likelihood of a breast cancer to metastasize (spread through the lymph or blood system to other parts of the body). This is why routine mammography for low-risk patients has little effect on ultimate mortality from breast cancer. Recent studies have clearly shown that mammography is of dubious value, and that women can probably achieve the same benefit by carefully examining their own breasts once a month.

As we discussed in chapter 1, surgery, radiation, and chemotherapy may be less than satisfactory in treating breast cancer. If we are to minimize the scourge of breast cancer, we must learn to identify and limit the causative or cancer-promoting factors and maximize the protective or cancer-preventive factors.

Programmed Cell Death Gives Us New Life

In any given breast cancer tumor, not all cells are identical; they have obvious differences. Present anticancer treatments may destroy or negate some but not all of the cancer cells. Just imagine, if chemotherapy kills 99.99 percent of all cancer cells in a tumor, and an average tumor contains a billion cells, this means that 100,000 tumor cells still remain. This is one of the reasons that it's unlikely our present treatments will improve our cure rates.

Like all cancers, breast cancer cells are not foreign invaders like bacteria, viruses, and allergens, but, as British researcher A. B. Astrow aptly put it, "essentially normal cells in which proportionately small changes in their genes lead to large changes in behavior."

One of the most important new findings in what causes breast cancer has to do with apoptosis, or programmed cell death. *Apoptosis* (ah-po-TOE-sis) literally means "falling away"—like leaves from a tree in autumn. It's often explained as "programmed cell suicide." It's now well understood by cancer specialists that delayed apoptosis of older cells increases their risk of becoming cancer cells.

With the exception of neural (nerve) and muscle cells, all the cells of the body are constantly being replaced with newly made cells. (And now we're learning that even nerve cells can change.) This requires that cells live for a specified period of time, and then die as new cells come along to replace them. The death of old cells is necessary for continued good health. Old skin cells are shed, as are the lining cells of the lungs and digestive system. In the breast, however, the old cells that undergo apoptosis are consumed by macrophages (special white blood cells).

Cell Differentiation and Proliferation

Most breast cancer originates as a change in milk duct epithelial cells and, as with other types of cancers, in addition to a slowing of apoptosis, these cells show a *loss of differentiation* and *increased proliferation rate* compared to normal breast cells. As cells grow, they differentiate into the special type of tissue they were meant to be. Usually, those that are proliferating or multiplying faster will also be less differentiated. In contrast, the more differentiated the cell, the slower it will proliferate and the more it will be like a normal cell, and therefore less threatening.

We know a great deal about factors that promote the growth of cancer cells once they come into existence. This is important, since the faster the growth rate, the more quickly a cancer can become life-threatening. A comparison of breast cancer with prostate cancer is enlightening. In a man over 65 years of age, prostate cancer has a doubling time of five years, whereas in a woman with breast cancer, the doubling time may be as short as three months. Obviously, slowing the proliferation rate would be advantageous to a person's survival time. In this regard we find that estrogen increases the proliferation rate of breast epithelial cells, while progesterone slows it down considerably. We'll discuss this in more detail shortly.

One way that oncologists have of assessing a breast cancer tumor is by looking at the presence of receptors on the cells for estrogen and progesterone. When comparing hormone receptors of breast cancer cells with their state of differentiation (remember, the more differentiated, the better), it's found that the tumors with the highest estrogen receptor (ER) and progesterone receptor (PR) content are the most differentiated. Tumors that have lost their capacity to express ER and PR are the most undifferentiated and aggressive. The presence of ER, however, also makes it possible for excessive estrogen exposure (as with conventional HRT) to lead to accelerated growth and allow more aggressive cancer cells to emerge from this population with faster growth potential. Normal cells also respond to excess estrogen with accelerated growth, resulting in more dense and lumpy breasts, and fibrocystic changes. On the other hand, the presence of progesterone receptors correlates with cancer cells that are more differentiated and less dangerous. In fact, Dr. Zava has seen samples of breast cancer tumors taken from women who were using progesterone that were technically malignant; upon examination he found that the majority of the cells in the tumor were well differentiated and quiescent, meaning they weren't replicating. The same quiescent pattern has been observed in normal breast ductal cells in women treated with topical progesterone in a study by K. J. Chang.

Estrogen also activates an oncogene (cancer-promoting gene) called Bcl-2 that slows apoptosis. Progesterone, in contrast, activates gene p53, which restores proper apoptosis. Thus, by considering apoptosis, cell differentiation, and cell proliferation, we see that estrogen is a potent promoter of breast cancer while progesterone protects against breast cancer by countering the growth-promoting actions of estrogens.

To review the cancer basics, we know that there are three characteristics by which cancer cells differ from normal cells.

They multiply or proliferate more rapidly, they are less differentiated (immature) than normal cells, and they don't die (apoptosis) when they're supposed to. In contrast, a healthy cell multiplies at normal rate, differentiates into a specific type of cell, and dies on a genetically predetermined schedule to make room for new cells.

It should not be surprising that sex hormones have a role in all three of these processes in breast cells. This is what we will explain in more detail in coming chapters.

Getting Down to the Gene Level

This next section is a bit dense with information and technical terms, but if you have breast cancer and want to research it further, you'll run across these words and concepts. We feel it's important that you have a reference point for understanding them.

If genes are damaged—for example, by radiation, toxins, or viruses—normal cells can develop into cancer cells. Certain genes called proto-oncogenes are normal to cells but may mutate into oncogenes, which create products that allow excessive proliferation (cell growth) or delayed apoptosis (cell death), resulting in the change of the cell into a cancer cell. Other genes, known to be tumor suppressor genes, inhibit cell division or stimulate apoptosis, thus preventing cancer. A person's risk of cancer depends in large part on the relative activity of oncogenes versus tumor suppressor genes. Several groups of molecular biologists have been investigating the actions of two genes in these categories named Bcl-2 and p53.

Bcl-2 is a proto-oncogene, and by now it's well known that it plays a pivotal role in the progression of cancer. Bcl-2 production inhibits apoptosis and thereby promotes breast, ovary, endometrial, and prostate cancer, as well as follicular B cell lymphoma.

Gene p53 is a tumor suppressor gene. Up-regulation of p53

will inhibit Bcl-2 action, halt cell proliferation, and induce apoptosis, thus helping prevent cancer.

In cancer cell cultures, researchers B. Formby and T. S. Wiley found that when the human estrogen estradiol (in concentrations similar to what the human body makes) is added to the culture, Bcl-2 is activated and cancer growth promoted. But the addition of progesterone (again in concentrations consistent with normal bodily levels) down-regulates Bcl-2 and up-regulates p53, thereby stopping cancer growth. This may sound simple, but it's actually a very profound and important piece of the cancer puzzle, because it involves a major anti-cancer substance that's made naturally in the human body. Their work has now been duplicated in a number of laboratories worldwide.

Thus, we now know at least one gene-related mechanism of action that connects estrogen to cancer promotion. Corroboration of these findings comes from research showing that one of the pathways some estrogens take as they are processed by the body leads to a by-product called estrogen-3,4-quinone, which causes gene mutation and cancer. We'll look at this more closely in chapter 7.

The Deadly Stage of Cancer

The third stage of cancer, known as the *progressive* stage, is the final stage of the disease. In this stage a distinct tumor grows in size; invades surrounding tissues, blood vessels, and lymphatics; and migrates to (metastasizes) and grows in other tissues of the body.

Once a cancer has invaded other parts of the body, stopping its growth becomes much more complicated, but it can be done. The good news is that breast cancer is a disease of long duration, and we have daily opportunities over a lifetime to make decisions that will encourage the body to get rid of a cancer. The interval between the initial transformation of a normal cell to a cancer cell and the full-blown clinical detection of a tumor the size of a pea, containing as many as a billion cells, may take decades.

As we emphasized in the beginning of this chapter, we do know a lot about what causes cancer, and there's a lot you can do to help prevent it. We'll be giving you lots of specifics on helping prevent cancer throughout this book.

Why Pregnancy Confers Protection: The Differentiation Power of hCG

As we mentioned in chapter 2, having a full-term pregnancy before the age of 24 can reduce a woman's risk of breast cancer by more than half. The reasons behind this have been thoroughly investigated by Jose Russo, M.D., a senior member of the Fox Chase Cancer Center in Philadelphia, adjunct professor of pathology and cell biology at Jefferson Medical School, and adjunct professor of pathology and laboratory medicine at the University of Pennsylvania Medical School. Dr. Russo has received several research awards from the National Cancer Institute of the National Institute for Health (NIH) for his original work in breast cancer.

We interviewed Dr. Russo for the *John R. Lee, M.D., Medical Letter*. This is an excerpt from what he had to say about pregnancy hormones and differentiation of breast tissue:

> Humans have areas of breast tissue that are highly proliferative [have a tendency to grow] and are much more vulnerable to damage by any given carcinogenic agent (something that causes breast cancer), such as those found in the environment, estrogen and radiation. During pregnancy, hormones cause changes in the breast, called differentiation. These changes appear to protect breast tissue

against carcinogens. The immature breasts of young girls contain structures called lobules type 1 that have a high proliferative activity, and those are the areas that are more susceptible to damage from a given carcinogen. For example in the atomic bombing of Hiroshima and Nagasaki, in Japan, a lot of radiation was created. Girls who were between 10 to 14 years old at the time, and who were exposed to the radiation, later developed breast cancer at a much higher rate than the general population. The reason is because their breasts contained a lot of these undifferentiated, more vulnerable lobules type 1 at the time of the bombing.

When the breast is stimulated by the sequential cascade of the hormones released during pregnancy the [breast] gland differentiates and with that process specific genes are activated that make the tissue more resistant to cancer. Cells that are differentiated have a better ability to repair the damage induced in the DNA (genetic material). These have allowed us to postulate a biological law that is "The differentiation of the mammary gland determines its susceptibility to carcinogenesis." We are using this concept to develop strategies for preventing breast cancer.

Even though Mother Nature set it up so that young girls could get pregnant and be protected against breast cancer, that doesn't happen often in Western countries. So how do we protect the breasts in women who may not be getting pregnant until their mid-twenties to their mid-thirties? We started looking for a way to stimulate differentiation in the breast without pregnancy. In experiments with rats, we found the best protection using human chorionic gonadotropin (hCG). When administered to non-pregnant animals, it induces the same level of differentiation as pregnancy. The remarkable effect that this produces is a resistance to the development of cancer when these animals are challenged with a chemical carcinogen.

The hormone hCG has two pathways of action. One is through the ovary by increasing the levels of estrogen and progesterone, which creates differentiation in the mammary glands. We found out that hCG also has a direct effect on the mammary tissue. It binds to a specific receptor and elicits a cascade of events that include the activation of a nonsteroidal glycoprotein called inhibin. Inhibin regulates cell proliferation and induces the activation of genes that control programmed cell death and differentiation.

We also have found that when we use this hormone in patients with primary breast cancer, the proliferative activity of the cancer tissue is significantly reduced after seven doses of this hormone in a two-week period. These data are important because they also indicate that the differentiation of the mammary tissue could be achieved in cells that are already cancerous.

We believe Dr. Russo's work is highly significant and could represent a major step toward protecting women—especially women who have children late or don't have them at all—from breast cancer, as well as a major step toward treating breast cancer itself. This is exactly the type of research that can be difficult to find funding for, because it is for a natural substance (hCG) and not a drug.

The late Dr. Henry Lemon studied the role of estriol in mammary cancer prevention and found that when young susceptible rats were treated first with estriol to induce breast ductal differentiation, the incidence of mammary tumors induced by chemicals or radiation was reduced by 80 percent. Estriol, in addition to hCG and progesterone, is high during pregnancy, and Lemon postulated that the estriol was playing a role in causing differentiation of the breast stem cells.

Ductal Carcinoma in Situ (DCIS)

While it isn't within the scope of this book to comment on all of the dozens of types and variations of breast cancer, we do feel that it's important to comment on a breast abnormality called ductal carcinoma in situ.

Prior to the advent of routine mammographic screenings in the early 1980s, the diagnosis of DCIS was a rarity. Less than 1 percent of newly diagnosed cases of breast cancer were found to be DCIS, because it rarely progressed to the point where there was any type of a mass to palpate. When it was diagnosed, it was generally because it had become palpable, or a nipple discharge had developed. Later (after 1983 or so), when screening mammograms became routine, radiologists were able to find areas of calcification (which look like scattered grains of salt on the film) that represent DCIS, and subsequently to diagnose it fairly commonly.

But even experts debate whether DCIS is really a cancer. The name—*ductal carcinoma in situ,* meaning "a cancer within the duct"—is ambiguous. The *in situ* means the pathologists saw abnormal cells scattered here and there throughout a field of normal cells: Think of dandelions here and there in your lawn. Literally the phrase means "in place," indicating no penetration of the deeper layers of cells. But invasive or infiltrating carcinoma, by its very definition, invades the deeper tissue, while DCIS is contained within the duct. If DCIS becomes even the tiniest bit invasive, then it's automatically no longer considered DCIS.

A few years ago there was an editorial in the medical journal *The Lancet* discussing this misuse of words in DCIS. Titled "Have Our Pathologists Gone Amok?" it basically made the above points in a witty fashion. The English do have a sense of humor, but the politics of calling this marginally malignant tissue a cancer are also of interest, and the women who receive mastectomies, radiation, and chemotherapy for a "cancer" that is "99 percent curable" (as many DCIS experts like to say) may not find it amusing.

What makes the DCIS diagnosis even more confusing is that there are many different grades of DCIS, most of which are virtually benign, but a few of which have a slightly higher risk than normal of leading to invasive breast cancer.

The calcium deposits and scatterings of abnormal cells found in most DCIS are probably the result of some underlying metabolic dysfunction—the debris of a battle and not a real cancer. If they occur in one breast, they're likely to show up in both breasts. This is another sign that the problem is a systemic metabolic dysfunction and not a random local incident.

The politics of DCIS are created when it's included as a breast cancer diagnosis, and thus made part of breast cancer statistics. DCIS diagnoses have accounted for 17 to 40 percent of breast cancer diagnoses (depending on the year) over the past two decades, but since only a small fraction of them ever go on to become actual cancer, it makes the "cure" rate statistics look much better. If DCIS weren't included as a breast cancer diagnosis, the cure rate for breast cancer would look significantly worse and the billion-dollar breast cancer establishment, with its surgery, radiation, and chemotherapy treatments, would look incompetent. Thus do politics and money dictate medical diagnosis.

Another aspect of DCIS politics is the recurrence statistics, which are used to justify treatments such as mastectomy, radiation, and chemotherapy. It makes sense that if DCIS is the result of an underlying metabolic imbalance, and the imbalance isn't corrected, it will come back. Statistics clearly show that when DCIS is treated with a lumpectomy and radiation, the recurrence rate is lower than if it is treated only with lumpectomy. However, recurrence isn't a real issue with most cases of DCIS—which is essentially a benign condition—and therefore to risk permanently damaging the body with radiation may be a grievous overtreatment. A recent meta-analysis of studies of radiation for breast cancer clearly demonstrated increased risks of dying from the radiation compared to the breast cancer itself—in good part due to the negative effects of radiation on the blood vessels and heart.

What's unknown is what percentage of women with DCIS go on to have invasive breast cancer—a real malignancy. If having DCIS signaled an imminent danger of a malignant cancer, then it would make sense to treat it fairly aggressively. Unfortunately, since conventional medicine never used an evidence-based approach to justify treating DCIS with surgery, radiation, and chemotherapy back in the early 1980s, we really have little idea what the natural course of DCIS is if it's left alone. One restrospective study (Welch et al.) showed that on autopsy, between 5 and 7.5 percent of women had DCIS, indicating a "reservoir" of undiagnosed DCIS cases that never turned into malignant breast cancer.

Statistics on how much of treated DCIS goes on to become invasive breast cancer are mixed, but for all except the severe, inflammatory types of DCIS, they show either a normal risk of breast cancer (the same as if a woman didn't have DCIS) or, in some cases, even a reduced risk. One study published in the *Journal of the American Medical Association* in 1996 took all women diagnosed with DCIS between 1983 and 1991, regardless of treatment (or no treatment), and found that their survival rates were ranged from 100 to 104 percent. This meant that these women were less likely than the general population to die of breast cancer *or* other causes.

Tragically, because DCIS calcifications tend to be scattered around in the breast tissue, in the 1980s women were often prescribed a mastectomy for treatment of this non-cancer, because it's so difficult to remove all of the breast tissue with microcalcifications. This is a brutal form of overtreatment that leaves women psychologically and physically scarred for life. It has become much less common, but it's still done with women who have a lot of calcifications.

DCIS is also detected more frequently in younger women than in older women. According to an analysis of breast cancer data collected by the National Cancer Institute and published in *JAMA* in 1996, "Among women with no report of a palpable mass in one mammography screening program, 43 percent of breast cancers detected in women age 40 to 49 years and 92 percent of those detected in women age 30 to 39 years between 1985 and 1995 were DCIS."

Ultimately, how you choose to treat DCIS should be based on a thorough analysis of its severity, which can be done with a biopsy. DCIS that is low grade, small celled, and without necrosis (dead and dying tissue) is less likely to become invasive, especially if you correct the underlying imbalance that caused the problem in the first place. On the other hand, the more aggressive types of DCIS, which are high nuclear grade, large celled, and with comedo-type necrosis, have more potential to become invasive, and you should have them removed. These types of analyses can only be done in partnership with a trusted physician or onocologist, and preferably with a second opinion.

What Causes DCIS?

We believe the underlying metabolic disorder that leads to the cell changes and calcifications that create DCIS is likely to be estrogen dominance and progesterone deficiency, and that when balance is restored by progesterone supplementation, the cells will return to normal. The calcifications are often permanent, but they aren't the disease, merely the result of past imbalance.

If DCIS lesions are found to be low grade, we recommend using progesterone cream, following an overall hormone-balancing lifestyle as outlined in *What Your Doctor May* Not *Tell You about Premenopause,* and following the breast condition with mammograms (or some of the newer types of diagnostic test such as ultrasound) every six months or so for the next few years. If there's no change, then it makes sense to continue with progesterone. If, for some reason, there is a change indicating more lesions, then it may be time to consider surgery. Optimally, women need to participate in their treatment decision and become as fully informed as they can about the nature of their disease. Again, it's important to consult with a physician whose judgment you trust.

CHAPTER 4

OTHER FACTORS THAT AFFECT SUSCEPTIBILITY TO BREAST CANCER

Insulin Resistance, Birth Control Pills, Early Puberty, DHEA, Prolactin, Melatonin, Thyroid

Although excessive estrogen in its many forms, unopposed by progesterone, is at the heart of what causes breast cancer, there are other factors that can tip the scale for or against cancer. When teenagers take birth control pills, they increase their risk of breast cancer. Imbalances in the hormones DHEA, prolactin, melatonin, and thyroid can all push the body toward cancer. Chronic, unremitting stress, with its high cortisol and adrenaline levels, can eventually suppress the immune system to the point that it can no longer effectively protect the body. A lifetime of poor eating choices and yoyo dieting can undermine a sound foundation of health by creating chronic nutritional deficiencies, which are detailed in chapter 17. Among the poor nutritional choices that can increase the risk of breast cancer, none is more dangerous and destructive than excessive sugar, so we'll begin with that.

Insulin Resistance Increases Breast Cancer Risk: Sugar Is the Sweet but Dangerous Treat

Women who have a syndrome called insulin resistance, which is virtually epidemic in Western countries, have a higher risk of developing breast cancer. Like estrogen, insulin, a blood-sugar-balancing hormone released by the pancreas, is a two-edged sword that on the one side is essential for life, but on the other can be debilitating and ultimately deadly when there's too much or too little of it.

Because insulin is released in response to sugars in the bloodstream, what you eat has a direct effect on your insulin balance. When you eat simple sugars such as white sugar, they go quickly and directly from your digestive system into your bloodstream and increase your blood sugar levels in a big surge, which in turn releases a big surge of insulin from your pancreas. This is definitely not how Mother Nature intended you to get your sugars, or how your pancreas was intended to release insulin.

The big rush of insulin escorts the sugar out of your bloodstream and into your cells, where it's used for energy or stored as fat. That's insulin's primary job: to take sugar out of the bloodstream and into your cells. However, the big rush of insulin caused by simple sugars takes too much sugar out of the blood, which causes a big drop in blood sugar levels. Low blood sugar, or hypoglycemia, causes many people to become tired, sleepy, foggy, moody, and dizzy. In response they eat a candy bar or a doughnut to get their blood sugar up again quickly so they'll feel better, and they're back on the same roller coaster, their blood sugar levels surging up and back down again.

Carbohydrate foods are also broken down into sugars. Carbohydrates are found in their most concentrated (complex) forms in grains such as wheat, millet, corn, and rice, but are also found in beans, vegetables, fruits, nuts, and seeds. Carbohydrates from most whole foods break down into their sugar components in the digestive system more slowly than simple sugars do. This slow breakdown is good for insulin balance, because the pancreas releases the insulin more gradually, over a longer period of time.

However, the type of carbohydrate that you eat is everything to your pancreas: a bagel, some pasta, or a piece of white bread made of refined white flour—known as simple or refined carbohydrates—breaks down into sugars almost as fast as table sugar does. In contrast, the carbohydrates found in whole grains, vegetables, and beans—known as complex or unrefined carbohydrates—must undergo breakdown by enzymes in the small intestines and be converted primarily to smaller sugars before they enter the bloodstream. (When sugars enter the bloodstream, they are called glucose.) The fiber, vitamins, minerals, and other nutrients found in complex carbohydrates make them break down into sugar more slowly. Refined carbohydrates have the fiber and most of the vitamins and minerals removed, so they're broken down quickly by the enzymes in the intestines and flood the body with excess sugar, causing a quick release of insulin from the pancreas to balance the sugar overload.

It's much easier on your body to have sugars released into the bloodstream gradually, followed by a gradual release of insulin, followed by a gradual ushering of glucose into your cells. With this scenario, the glucose that's taken into cells is more likely to be burned as energy than stored as fat.

Insulin resistance occurs when your insulin is no longer able to get the glucose into the cells effectively. In response, the body keeps pumping out more and more insulin, but since it's unable to do its job, you end up with chronically high levels of insulin *and* glucose in your blood. Both high insulin and high glucose in the bloodstream lead to a long list of chronic health problems, from diabetes and heart disease to blindness and breast cancer. Insulin resistance is almost always caused by eating too much sugar, combined with obesity, a sedentary lifestyle, and, to some extent, genetics. Other factors such as smoking and synthetic hormone replacement therapy can also increase the tendency to insulin resistance. Insulin resistance is often a precursor to type 2 diabetes, in which your insulin stops working to the extent that it eventually becomes life-threatening.

Gerald Reaven, M.D., coined the term *Syndrome X* to describe the group of symptoms that mark insulin resistance. One of the strongest blood markers for individuals with insulin resistance is a high level of triglycerides. Knowing your triglyceride level may help you determine if insulin resistance, and predisposition to diabetes, is a problem. Most doctors will include triglycerides when they order a basic blood test for you, called a chem panel. In type 1 diabetes, which usually begins in childhood or adolescence, the pancreas is unable to produce enough insulin. This is now thought to be an autoimmune disease.

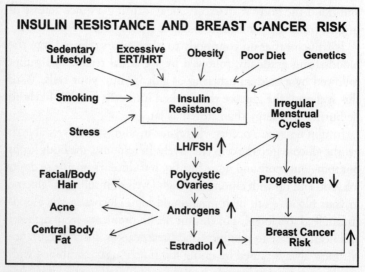

Many lifestyle factors contribute to insulin resistance, which in turn contributes to breast cancer risk.

How Too Much Sugar Affects Your Ovaries

While insulin's primary job is to escort sugar into your cells, it indirectly affects many other systems in your body. For example, chronically high insulin levels alter the brain's normal cyclic production of follicle-stimulating hormone (FSH) and luteinizing hormone (LH), which regulate the cyclic production of estrogens and progesterone by the ovaries with each menstrual cycle. When insulin levels remain high due to insulin resistance, the pituitary gland in the brain produces too much LH relative to FSH. Ordinarily, FSH is produced early in a woman's menstrual cycle, allowing proper maturation of eggs in the ovaries. Once a dominant follicle (egg) forms, LH is then produced about mid-cycle to hasten the maturation and release of the dominant egg and to stimulate the production of progesterone. However, when FSH is low, a dominant follicle never develops. Multiple follicles form, resulting in cysts on the ovaries, known as polycystic ovaries. These underdeveloped follicles respond to the excessive LH and produce excessive amounts of testosterone, just as the testes in males respond to LH and produce testosterone.

When insulin levels are persistently elevated, as with insulin resistance syndrome, polycystic ovary syndrome (PCOS) can occur. PCOS causes the ovaries to become anovulatory, meaning that the normal cyclic production of estrogen, followed by progesterone, ceases or becomes dysfunctional. Insulin stimulates the ovaries to produce predominantly androgens (male hormones)—which, in combination with the higher insulin and glucose, result in more weight gain around the waist (the apple body type, which is a risk factor for breast cancer). Signs that the body is being exposed to higher levels of the male hormones include acne, loss of hair on the head, and an increase in body hair (face, arms, and legs).

The Path to Breast Cancer: Early Insulin Resistance and PCOS

PCOS has become a near epidemic among young women who subsist on junk food and suffer from low-level insulin resistance starting in their teens. They complain of acne, terrible PMS, and excessive hair growth on their face and arms. Eventually they also begin complaining of estrogen dominance symptoms. The typical physician will ignore issues of diet and exercise and put these girls on birth control pills and/or oral diabetes drugs that lower insulin levels. This is a gross error in approach; simple lifestyle changes—less sugar, a more wholesome diet, and regular exercise—will often solve the problem within a couple of menstrual cycles. Medicating these young women with birth control pills that can increase their risk of breast cancer, and oral diabetes drugs that all too often damage the liver should not be an easy option.

IN A NUTSHELL:
HOW OVEREATING JUNK FOOD EARLY IN LIFE CAN INCREASE BREAST CANCER RISK

Overeating junk food makes you fat. Increased body fat and lack of exercise lead to insulin resistance. (Smoking makes it happen faster.) Insulin resistance leads to further craving of sugary carbohydrates to generate energy for the body. More insulin is released in response to increased carbohydrate intake, leading to more weight gain. More fat leads to more estrogens, which, in turn, lead to earlier breast development and menstruation. Earlier onset of menstruation leads to more ovulatory cycles and a greater lifetime exposure to estrogens without adequate progesterone. A greater lifetime exposure to estrogens increases breast cancer risk.

Simultaneously, increased consumption of simple carbohydrates, coupled with insulin resistance, leads to polycystic ovaries and lack of ovulation during menstrual cycles, resulting in excess production of androgens and estrogens, along with inadequate production of progesterone. Excessive estrogen production in the absence of progesterone production leads to estrogen dominance and increased breast cancer risk. Use of contraceptive hormones increases insulin resistance, exacerbating all the above problems.

If you have a preteen or teenage daughter who is a junk-food-eating couch potato, it's essential to get her involved in some type of exercise. Team sports such as basketball, soccer, and volleyball are ideal, but for those girls who don't have good eye–hand coordination, or who don't enjoy competition or team sports, there are plenty of other types of vigorous exercise, from running and in-line skating to horseback riding and swimming.

Getting plenty of exercise will delay puberty, decrease the flow of estrogens, and narrow the window of vulnerability to breast cancer. We know from clinical studies that young women who are involved in regular and vigorous aerobic exercise programs begin puberty later and have nearly a twofold *decreased* risk of developing breast cancer later in life.

While you can generally be assured that your child eats well at breakfast and dinner, lunch may be out of your control, and that can be a problem. It's high time that parents became activists in seeing that schools provide a wholesome lunch. Purveyors of junk food have invaded American schools, which should be perceived as a national scandal and a national health crisis. Pizza and soda, or a double cheeseburger and a shake, is a recipe for insulin resistance and a world of health problems later in life. (Chapter 17 gives you detailed yet easy-to-use information on creating a healthy diet.)

The Double Whammy: Insulin Resistance Combined with Menopause

Symptoms of PCOS, high androgens, and insulin resistance can also be symptoms of approaching menopause. Higher androgens and an increased waist-to-hip ratio (fat around the middle) are significant risk factors for breast cancer, because the increased fat around the waist results in a greater capacity to form estrogens from androgens, further increasing breast cancer risk. In fact, it may not be the increase in androgens per se that increases breast cancer risk, but rather the enhanced capacity, caused by insulin resistance, to convert them to estrogens in fat tissue adjacent to the breast cells. At the same time, the drop in the cyclic production of estrogen and progesterone, as well as in androgens such as DHEA, can also increase the chances of developing insulin resistance, and the lowered progesterone contributes to estrogen dominance.

Proper supplementation with the right types (natural) and amounts (physiologic) of estrogens, progesterone, and DHEA have been shown to decrease the symptoms associated with insulin resistance. Synthetic progestins such as Provera and those found in some birth control pills have been shown to *increase* insulin resistance.

It's intriguing, and we believe more than coincidental, that many of the risk factors for insulin resistance are also risk factors for breast cancer. These include rapid weight gain at menopause, increased circulating androgens, lack of ovulation, physical inactivity, smoking, and, particularly, overeating a refined carbohydrate diet (junk food).

Adrenal Androgen Deficiency Increases Breast Cancer Risk

Numerous clinical studies have shown that *pre*menopausal breast cancer patients have depressed levels of adrenal androgens, specifically DHEA and its sulfated conjugate DHEA sulfate (DHEAS). This correlation does not appear to hold true for postmenopausal women; in this case high DHEA appears to be associated with an increased risk.

In premenopausal women, low blood levels of DHEA and DHEAS precede the onset of breast cancer by as much as ten years. Research studies on mice highly susceptible to breast cancer revealed that DHEA effectively prevented the spontaneous development of the disease.

These studies led researchers to conjecture that DHEA supplementation in women who are deficient might reduce the incidence of breast cancer in susceptible premenopausal women. To our knowledge, no clinical studies have been carried out to determine if DHEA supplementation in DHEA-deficient premenopausal women protects them against breast cancer. We believe that the link between low DHEA and breast cancer in premenopausal women is likely related to the very important role DHEA plays in maintaining a healthy immune system. Low DHEA and high cortisol—a situation that occurs under various stress situations—can lead to a defective immune system that can actually stimulate, rather than inhibit, the growth of breast cancer cells. We will discuss this further in later chapters (see Immune System and Cancer).

For more detailed information on when and how to use DHEA supplements, please read chapter 14.

Hypothyroidism Increases Breast Cancer Risk

Early studies dating back to the 1950s indicate that low thyroid function (hypothyroidism) predisposes women to breast cancer. When thyroid hormone is low, estrogens are unable to activate proper amounts of the estrogen-binding protein called sex hormone binding globulin (SHBG) in the liver. SHBG in the bloodstream binds tightly to estradiol, keeping too much from entering cells and stimulating the growth of tissues in areas such as the breast and uterus. The result of low SHBG in hypothyroid women would be more "free" or bioavailable (available to the body for use) estrogen in the bloodstream, which in effect causes higher estrogen activity. Because thyroid balance is so important to your health, we'd like you to have a better understanding of how it works.

What Your Doctor May Not Tell You about Thyroid

Thyroid hormone is now the most common of all drug prescriptions, though estrogen sales may still be the most profitable. The premise of thyroid is simple—the thyroid gland makes thyroid hormone, which sets the metabolic rate (the rate at which energy is used) for all the cells of the body. Thyroid hormone is said to be the throttle, or gas pedal, or governor for all metabolic activity. All first-year medical students get this right. Then they learn that there's a computer in the hypothalamus gland in the brain that monitors and modulates thyroid hormone levels to control metabolic activity. This computer makes a hormone called thyrotropin-releasing hormone (TRH), which signals the pituitary gland in the brain to make another hormone, thyroid-stimulating hormone (TSH, also called thyrotropin), which in turn instructs the thyroid gland to make more or less thyroid hormone for circulation throughout the body. This sets the body's metabolic rate. If the hypothalamic computer detects a lagging metabolic rate, it signals the pituitary to make more TSH, which activates the thyroid gland to make more thyroid hormone. If the metabolic rate is too high, it reduces TSH to slow the production of thyroid hormone. What a beautiful system! A low TSH reading may indicate high thyroid levels, while a high reading may indicate low thyroid levels.

But then things get a bit more complicated. You'd think that by measuring the thyroid level in the bloodstream, or the level of TSH, or TRH (a more difficult test), you could easily determine whether thyroid hormone supplementation was necessary. As it turns out, the "normal" range is broad. Having a thyroid level that's in the lab's normal range doesn't necessarily mean that all's well with your thyroid or metabolic regulation. What's normal for one individual may not be normal for another. If someone is lacking energy, or cold all the time, or depressed, sluggish, and achy in the morning (all symptoms of hypothyroidism—low levels of thyroid hormone), perhaps the cause is merely lack of sleep, the need for a vacation, bad diet, stress, or some nutrient deficiency. If we succumb to the erroneous belief that normal thyroid tests rule out thyroid problems, there are plenty of other suspects to consider, and the potential thyroid problem is ignored.

The Basics on T_3 and T_4

Here's a closer look at how thyroid hormone really works. Thyroid hormone is a remarkably simple compound, made of a single amino acid (protein building blocks) called tyrosine plus the addition of some iodine atoms. Actually, the thyroid gland makes two thyroid hormones, thyroxine (with four iodines) and triiodothyronine (with three iodines). In medical parlance, thyroxine is called T_4, and thyronine is called T_3, indicating the number of iodines in each molecule.

T_4 blood levels are higher than those of T_3, but T_3 is four times more potent. Normally the body converts T_4 to T_3 as needed. The total thyroid effect is a combination of both T_4 and T_3. Though not common in conventional medicine, ideal thyroid replacement therapy should consider the use of both T_4 and T_3. The most commonly prescribed thyroid medication is Synthroid, which is only T_4. Armour Thyroid is derived from cows, sheep, and/or pigs and contains whole ground-up thyroid gland; it's standardized to deliver both types of thyroid hormone in the same ratio found in human thyroid.

What Thyroid Hormone Does

Thyroid hormone increases the number and activity of mitochondria, those little intracellular inclusions (they exist separately from the cell but are found inside the cell) that convert food we eat (particularly carbohydrates) into energy for the body. Mitochondria can also be thought of as small organelles within each cell of the body that act as furnaces which burn the food we eat to release heat and energy, which is stored for later use. Thyroid increases the efficiency of these intracellular furnaces, allowing them to burn the nutrients we consume more efficiently, thus creating heat and energy. When thyroid isn't operating properly, the mitochondrial furnaces don't burn fuel properly, and we suffer from lower body temperature and lack of energy. Cold intolerance and fatigue are two of the most common symptoms doctors use to diagnose low thyroid.

Thyroid increases protein synthesis (for growth and repair), excites the nervous system (for alertness and quicker reflexes), and stimulates the endocrine (hormone) system in general. Thyroid deficiency can cause an amazing variety of symptoms. A brief list includes general fatigue, feeling more chilly than most people, difficulty in losing weight, muscle aches and pains, mental sluggishness, dry skin, dry hair and hair loss, waking up tired, anxieties and/or depression, increased menopausal symptoms, slow pulse, and digestive problems. Each of these symptoms might well be caused by something else, but when enough of the whole set is present, it's wise to think of hypothyroidism. People with underactive thyroids also show an increased tendency toward autoimmune disorders.

Low thyroid can intensify the ill effects of other diseases, because all metabolic actions require energy, and thyroid hormone sets the energy level. If thyroid is low, your energy is low and your body is less able to deal with other conditions such as chronic stress, poor sleep, colds and other viral or bacterial infections, malnutrition, anemia, injuries, or surgery. Without good thyroid levels, recovery is delayed.

Other Potential Causes of Hypothyroidism

Why should thyroid deficiency be so common now? Historically, iodine deficiency was the most common cause of hypothyroidism and goiter (enlarged thyroid gland). Without sufficient iodine, thyroid hormone production results in thyroxine being stored in the gland rather than being released into the circulation. This leads to engorgement of the gland, causing goiters. The condition was most prevalent in populations that didn't live near the sea, because all ocean fish, crustaceans, and seaweed contain iodine. Now that iodine is added to salt and seafood is widely available, iodine deficiency isn't as common. Our present epidemic of thyroid problems is not due to iodine deficiency. We must look elsewhere.

The Estrogen-Dominance Factor

No hormone works in isolation from other hormones; they all function within a complex, subtle web of interconnectedness. If thyroid is low, cortisol and sex hormone production lag. Estrogen inhibits thyroid hormone activity and thus exacerbates thyroid deficiency. In contrast, progesterone, cortisol, and testosterone are thyroid allies. Hypothyroidism occurs predominantly in women, especially during the perimenopausal period (around the time of menopause) when estrogens dominate and progesterone is low. Persistent estrogen dominance, which is most likely to occur during the perimenopausal period, creates a cycle of lowered thyroid function, decreased SHBG, and further increases in the bioavailable levels of estrogens. Breast cancer incidence begins to rise sharply during this period. Progesterone therapy often restores normal thyroid activity, perhaps by its anti-estrogenic actions. Here again, estrogen dominance, unopposed by progesterone, underlies the link between thyroid dysfunction and breast cancer.

Dr. Zava often sees what he describes as thyroid resistance, in which thyroid parameters measured in blood are normal (normal TSH, T_4, and T_3), but symptoms characteristic of low thyroid are present. These individuals nearly always suffer from severe imbalances in their steroid hormones. In monitoring salivary hormones and symptoms, Dr. Zava finds that estrogen dominance (usually associated with normal or high estrogen, but always low progesterone) and adrenal dysfunction (low or high cortisol) correlate closely with symptoms common to low thyroid. If your doctor is telling you that your thyroid hormones are normal, but you have most of the classic thyroid symptoms, you may want to test your steroid hormones in saliva. (See chapter 15 for more on saliva testing.)

The Autoimmune Factor

The immune system is also a major factor in hypothyroidism. In particular, anti-thyroid antibody disease (Hashimoto's thyroiditis), once considered rare, is now a common finding, especially among women. The antibody attack on the thyroid causes chaos in the hormone cycle. It may provoke hyperthyroidism (elevated T_4 levels or excess thyroid) or classic hypothyroidism (low T_4 levels). Since the cause is usually unknown, conventional treatment consists of thyroid supplementation sufficient to drive TSH to very low levels, thus effectively stopping endogenous (made-in-the-body) thyroid hormone synthesis.

The Fluoride Factor

The thyroid molecule is simply a thyronine molecule with some iodines attached. Thyroid works only if iodine is attached. Iodine is a halogen, one of a group of nonmetallic elements that also includes fluorine, chlorine, and bromine. If you look at the periodic table of elements, you note that they all are short by one electron of having a complete outer ring of electrons. They all seek to acquire an extra electron. In chemical reactions, a more reactive halogen will replace a less reactive halogen. Iodine is the largest of the four common halogens, and its chemical activity is the least among them, whereas fluorine is the smallest of the halogens and is the most chemically active.

In the past two generations fluoride exposure has increased greatly due to fluoridated water and toothpaste. Prior to fluoridation, the common daily intake of fluoride was about 0.1 mg per day. Now fluoride intake even in unfluoridated communities is 30 to 40 times greater. If fluorine (elemental fluoride) replaces iodine in the structure of thyroxine, it would make it unsuitable for thyroid hormone effect. Years ago, fluoride was used to treat hyperthyroidism. Why is this fluoride poisoning now ignored? Not only is fluoridated tyrosine unsuitable for thyroxine construction, but it may stimulate antibody formation, leading to thyroiditis.

The Xenohormone Factor

Many petrochemical toxins are also known as endocrine disrupters or xenohormones (see chapter 18 for details), and thyroid is among the endocrine systems disrupted by these pollutants. In the case of thyroid, a plausible mechanism for damage is known. The thyroxine molecule has a remarkably similar structure to that of polychlorinated biphenyls (PCBs), widespread industrial pollutants that are not only estrogenic but also toxic to the thyroid gland itself. The development of the inner ear in human embryos requires thyroid hormone. If exposed to PCBs, cochlear development is inhibited, causing low-tone hearing loss. Animals exposed to PCBs develop thyroid tumors—now common in cats, for instance. It's entirely possible that chlorinated biphenyls are perceived by the immune system as abnormal thyroxine. In the process, a person's antibodies attack the thyroid gland. Thus PCBs or other similar petrochemical endocrine (hormone) blockers may be a major cause of hypothyroidism caused by thyroiditis.

Low Melatonin Increases Breast Cancer Risk

The pineal gland is a pea-sized organ located in the center of the brain. It's responsible for the production of melatonin, a hormone that regulates sleep cycles. It also plays a role in regulating ovarian hormones and the immune system, and is an antioxidant. Melatonin levels are very high in adolescence but drop dramatically after puberty and then continue to fall steadily as we age. In the early 1980s an American researcher discovered that melatonin prevents rats from developing breast tumors induced by the chemical carcinogen dimethylbenzanthracene (DMBA). Further studies with human breast cancer cells in culture flasks (in vitro) showed similar results: Growth of the breast cancer cells was suppressed by 75 percent with melatonin. These test tube and animal studies support clinical studies (those involving humans) demonstrating that nighttime melatonin levels in urine are much lower in women with breast cancer than in healthy women.

Another interesting observation that neurosurgeons have been making for many years is that the pineal gland in breast cancer patients is more likely to be calcified, which means it's less likely to produce melatonin. Other studies verify that women with early breast cancer have lower circulating levels of melatonin. It's difficult to know if the low melatonin levels are a cause or consequence of breast cancer, or some other unrelated health problem.

High melatonin levels reduce the ovarian production of estrogens and progesterone, and it is this feedback that's thought to be protective against breast cancer. Such studies, although not directly designed to investigate the role of melatonin in breast cancer prevention, may eventually shed light on this important topic.

Melatonin is readily available at your local pharmacy or health food store, and is used by millions of people to help them sleep. It works particularly well for older people who have very low melatonin levels and frequently have trouble getting a good night's sleep. If you're under the age of 50, however, it's probably best not to use melatonin unless you're having trouble sleeping and can't attribute it to any other cause such as estrogen dominance, too much caffeine, or stress-caused anxiety. Like all the body's hormones, more is not better when it comes to melatonin. If you do use it, you need only 1 mg or less sublingually just before bedtime.

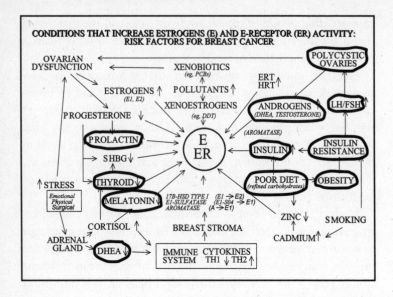

CONDITIONS THAT INCREASE ESTROGENS (E) AND E-RECEPTOR (ER) ACTIVITY: RISK FACTORS FOR BREAST CANCER

Note the circled items pointing to estrogen and breast cancer that have been included in this chapter.

High Prolactin Increases Breast Cancer Risk

The link between prolactin and estrogens is a strong one. Prolactin is a hormone produced by the brain's pituitary gland, which is best known for its role in stimulating lactation (milk production) and breast cell division. However, it has well over 300 other effects on the body. Estrogens stimulate prolactin secretion and increase the formation of prolactin receptors in breast tissue, further enhancing the sensitivity of the breast to prolactin. Prolactin, in turn, stimulates the synthesis of estrogen receptors as well as its own receptors, thus providing a positive feedback system to perpetuate the growth-promoting actions of estrogens on the breast. Recent research shows that some breast cancer tumors begin to produce their own prolactin, which in turn stimulates tumor growth.

Progesterone acts to inhibit all actions of estrogens and prolactin by down-regulating the receptors for these hormones. Clinical studies carried out by Dr. Patrick Walsh and coworkers found elevated estradiol and prolactin levels during the last few days of the luteal (mid-cycle) phase in premenopausal women with benign breast disease (BBD), but not in women with no history of breast disease. Curiously, the elevated blood levels of estradiol and prolactin were observed only when samples were collected in the evening, not in the morning. The authors of this study concluded that "an increased concentration of prolactin may simply be a marker for increased underlying estrogenic activity." Estriol, unlike estradiol, does not increase prolactin synthesis, which may underlie one of the protective actions of estriol in breast cancer prevention.

Women with high prolactin levels often find relief when they use progesterone cream, which seems to reduce prolactin levels.

Teens Taking Birth Control Pills Increases Breast Cancer Risk

When teenage girls take birth control pills, it increases their risk of breast cancer. It has been well established that when girls between the ages of 13 and 18—and to a lesser but still significant effect, women up to the age of 21—use birth control pills, their risk of breast cancer can increase by as much as 600 percent. The younger a girl begins to use contraceptive hormones, the greater her risk of breast cancer. Because girls are reaching maturity much earlier today than even 10 or 20 years ago, and are more freely using contraceptive hormones, we have to ask whether this scenario is going to lead to a significant increase in breast cancer, particularly premenopausal breast cancer—which tends to be more aggressive.

Even though we know that contraceptive use in teens increases the risk of breast cancer, the FDA tragically allows the advertising of birth control pills in teen magazines for the treatment of acne.

Why do birth control pills increase breast cancer risk? Some scientists point to the type of synthetic estrogens and progestins that contraceptives contain. Because the natural hormones used to make the synthetic hormones have been warped by the addition of other molecules to make them patentable and more easily assimilated in pill form, the resultant "Frankenstein" or synthetic progestin often becomes a more promiscuous molecule, interacting with other hormone receptors. For example, some of the synthetic progestins can have estrogenic activity, causing persistent stimulation of the breast tissues. Furthermore, the younger a girl is, the more stem cells (undeveloped cells more vulnerable to damage by cancer-causing agents) she has in her breast tissue. With time, these breast cells mature and are less susceptible to insults by excessive hormones in birth control pills. As we discussed earlier, pregnancy, with its increases in protective hormones (progesterone, estriol, hcg), helps these stem cells mature to forms less susceptible to cancer-causing insults. Instead of allowing the breast tissue to mature, this constant stimulation by contraceptive estrogens would further open the breast cells' window of vulnerability to carcinogens.

Another problem with contraceptive hormones is that they create a state of anovulation (lack of ovulation), which blocks the ovaries' natural production of hormones, including progesterone, with all of its protective properties. The synthetic progestins that are in all birth control pills are no substitute for progesterone; they lack many of progesterone's benefits and have many of their own unique negative side effects.

Birth control pills are also known to deplete a number of vitamins, including vitamin B_6 and folic acid. Folic acid is essential for protecting DNA from damage, which is more likely when excessive amounts of synthetic hormones are present. A deficiency of these vitamins is also known to contribute to cervical hyperplasia, and it's reasonable to expect that their deficiency may also contribute to excessive proliferation of breast cells.

Thus, the birth control pills used to treat acne act as a double-edged sword: They not only potentially damage DNA but also reduce the body's capacity to protect and repair it.

Early Puberty Increases Breast Cancer Risk

Girls are reaching puberty earlier and earlier, which increases their risk of breast cancer. The medical community does not want to face the implications of what is causing this, so rather than search for a cause, it has adjusted the "normal" age of puberty down to reflect current trends.

Early puberty is a well-established risk for breast cancer. The earlier a woman reaches puberty, the longer her breast tissues will be exposed to potentially harmful cancer-causing agents (chemicals, radiation, estrogens). Early puberty combined with having children later, or not having them at all, is yet another factor that increases a woman's susceptibility to breast cancer. In the not-too-distant past our ancestors reached sexual maturity much later and were getting pregnant at a much earlier age. These factors alone would have significantly narrowed their window of vulnerability to breast cancer.

CHAPTER 5

THE NATURE OF BREAST CANCER

Nurturing Gone Awry

There are many types of cancer, and although they each have some basic traits in common, each one also has its own unique profile. Breast cancer has its own ways of beginning and progressing. It has its own subtypes, stages, and grades, as well as its own mixes of genes that have to be damaged in order for it to be created and grow. Breast cancer also differs from other cancers in that it can be promoted and stimulated by specific hormones, and its growth can also be slowed or stopped by specific hormones.

The breasts of mammals, and of human females in particular, have a unique structure and function that predetermine how they respond to hormonal signals as well as to toxins that accumulate in the fatty tissue. For example, early pregnancy is protective against developing breast cancer because of specific changes that take place in breast tissue during gestation, and taking birth control pills before the age of 20 increases the risk of breast cancer, probably because of developmental factors in breast tissue that are permanently blocked by the synthetic hormones in oral contraceptives.

How the Breasts Develop

Women's breasts and nipples are as varied in appearance as women's faces—they come in a nearly infinite variety of shapes, sizes, colors, and textures. It's very common for one of a woman's breasts to be somewhat different in size and shape than the other—in fact, they are rarely perfectly symmetrical. According to the cultural programming that sends thousands of women out to plastic surgeons to get breast implants each year, only Barbie dolls have truly normal breasts. But according to Mother Nature, a breast is normal if it's capable of producing milk for a woman's offspring, regardless of its size and shape.

Human female breasts are milk glands that develop from a line of sweat glands that run down the front of the torso. In some mammals these sweat glands evolved to multiple nipples—the kind we see on our cats and dogs. These glands first appear when the human fetus is only six weeks old, and then disappear by the end of the third month. Thus, you can understand that a woman's breast tissue can be influenced by hormonal factors while she's in the womb.

Breasts begin to grow in response to a rise in estrogen and progesterone levels. The usual age for the beginnings of breast growth used to be age 11 or 12, but now—thanks primarily, we believe, to the hormonal influences of pervasive pollution—girls can begin growing breast tissue as early as eight years old. The rise in hormones signaled by these changes can elicit feelings of sexuality in girls that they're entirely unequipped to deal with emotionally. They're still playing with dolls! This should be reason enough to feed your children hormone-free meat and dairy products and pesticide-free fruits and vegetables. The effects on little boys are less obvious but surely equally profound.

The Effects of Toxins on Breast Tissue

In most girls the nonfatty breast tissue is fully developed by age 15 or 16. Fat makes up about one-third of breast tissue, and the breasts can grow or shrink with weight gain or loss. Fatty tissue is one of the factors that comes into play in breast cancer, because toxins such as the pesticide DDT and other pesticides, industrial wastes such as PCBs and dioxins, and heavy metals that aren't secreted immediately from the body tend to be stored in fat, and especially in breast fat. As long as a toxin is sitting in fatty tissue, it creates a risk for genetic damage to nearby lobule and duct cells, which creates a risk for breast cancer. To add insult to injury, many of these toxins are estrogenic in nature and so deliver a potent message of proliferation to breast tissue. Corporate polluters like to point out that the amount of toxins they're exposing us to is small, but in the fatty tissue of women's breasts the toxins can accumulate over time, and combinations of them may be dangerously synergistic.

Breast Tissue

Breast tissue is made up of *lobules,* which make milk, and *ducts,* which deliver it to the nipple, all sandwiched in with fat, connective tissue, blood vessels, and nerves. The ducts tend to be more concentrated in the front of the breast, and the lobules tend to be more concentrated in the back and sides of the breast and even up into the armpits. Although there are muscles underneath and on the sides of the breasts, the only muscles in the breast itself are tiny ones in the areola, the pigmented area around the nipple.

Nipples

Nipples are as varied as breasts are, in size, shape, positioning, and color, but their ability to deliver milk isn't necessarily dependent on how they look. Nipples tend to be larger after pregnancy, and thanks to its muscles, the areola can contract and cause the nipples to become erect in response to cold or sexual arousal. Your breast tissue doesn't change much after puberty, although pregnancy does bring on important changes, which we'll discuss shortly.

Breasts and Monthly Cycles

The monthly cycles of menstruation also bring on changes in the breast. During the first part of the cycle when estrogen is highest, the ducts swell; during the luteal phase or the middle of the cycle when progesterone is high, the lobules become larger. According to Jerilynn Prior, M.D., a Canadian clinician, researcher, and professor of endocrinology at the University of British Columbia, premenstrual breast tenderness that occurs at the sides of the breast under the armpits suggests that ovulation has occurred during that cycle. If the breasts are sore up front and over the nipples, it tends to suggest high estrogen, or estrogen dominance, which can indicate a lack of ovulation. Soreness on the sides *and* the front may indicate that ovulation occurred but that not much progesterone was produced three or four days after ovulation, and thus estrogen dominance is occurring.

Breasts and nipples can be extremely sensitive, especially premenstrually and when a woman is first nursing and all her lobules, ducts, and connective tissue are stretched to the maximum. Breast sensitivity varies enormously among individual women, but generally if you have chronically lumpy breasts they're going to be more sensitive overall. Healthy breasts can also be exquisitely sensitive sexual organs; some women can achieve orgasm with nipple and breast stimulation alone. When the nipples are stimulated, prolactin—the hormone that rises with milk production—rises. Prolactin can also cause uterine contraction.

Lumpy and Painful Breasts

You now know that painful breasts can be a result of hormonal imbalance, but what about the condition that so often goes along with painful breasts, which is lumpy breasts? Lumpy breasts are often diagnosed by doctors as "fibrocystic breast disease," but this is not a disease. It can be a symptom of an underlying metabolic imbalance in a woman's hormones. These breast lumps are frequently tender but benign (harmless). They're composed of dense, fibrous tissue and variably sized cysts that arise from fluid engorgement of either breast duct segments or lobes. If the cyst is large enough, an experienced physician can usually tell by squeezing a lump whether it's solid or fluid filled.

Most cysts go away at the end of your cycle, within a few days of when bleeding begins. If a lump stays around for a few months, even if you're using progesterone cream, then you should see a doctor. If he or she says that the lump is fluid-filled, then it can be drained with a needle in the doctor's office. If the lump is solid, then you should have it biopsied. Cancerous lumps generally feel solid and hard and are not usually painful.

Using progesterone cream per Dr. Lee's instructions (see chapter 13) will frequently clear up lumpy, painful breasts within a few menstrual cycles.

The Psyche of Breast Cancer

We encourage you not to use this section of this chapter to beat yourself up and blame yourself if you have breast cancer. All too often we use the fact that our minds and emotions can affect our bodies to play the blame game, and feel guilty that we've helped create a disease. Breast cancer is a multifactorial disease that is created on many levels, perhaps beginning when *your* mother was in the womb and what she was exposed to there that she passed on to you. This doesn't mean that you're helpless to do anything about it, because there's a lot you can do. It just means, don't use this type of awareness to be hard on yourself. That is completely counterproductive to healing.

In addition to having its own unique biochemical profile, breast cancer has its own unique psychological profile. Dozens of studies have been done on the emotional and mental attitudes of women who get breast cancer, and a very clear picture has emerged: In short, women who get breast cancer tend to take care of everyone but themselves. This is part of why the subtitle of this chapter is Nurturing Gone Awry. Something has gone fundamentally wrong when we stop taking care of ourselves. And ironically, if you get breast cancer, you certainly won't be able to take care of your family in the way you used to. This may sound a little harsh, but sometimes it takes a little shock to the system to jolt us awake enough to inspire real changes in ourselves.

Two Australian studies found that women with breast cancer were slightly more likely to report an "acute stressor," such as the death of a loved one, loss of employment, or divorce, within two years before their breast cancer diagnosis. The more significant information, however, showed up when researchers compared women who had "intimate emotional support" as they went through their acutely stressful situation with women who had none: Those without support had nearly ten times the rate of breast cancer compared to those who rated themselves as having good emotional support. What does this mean to you if you're a stressed-out woman (and who isn't these days)? If you don't have family or friends who can help you through a crisis in a way that's supportive for *you*, find a support group or a therapist.

The symbolism of this psychological profile for breast cancer is inescapable. Although our culture has made a woman's breasts sexual icons, at a much deeper and more fundamental level they are our ultimate human symbol of nurturing. They're a built-in, ready-made source of nourishment and sustenance in the early months when an infant is completely helpless and vulnerable. That your own breasts can, in effect, turn around and attack you with a cancer when you aren't nurturing yourself (or receiving nurturing from others) is a valuable lesson that should not be lost on any woman of childbearing age.

Christiane Northrup, M.D., in her classic book, *Our Bodies, Ourselves* (which we recommend every woman have on her bookshelf), says, "Much breast cancer is related to our need to be self-contained and self-nurturing. Caroline Myss notes, 'The major emotion behind breast lumps and breast cancer is hurt, sorrow, and unfinished business. . . . An important 1995 study found that breast cancer increased by almost 12 times if a woman had suffered from bereavment, job loss, or divorce in the previous five years. . . . Women with breast cancer frequently have a tendency toward self-sacrifice, inhibited sexuality, an inability to see themselves as supported by others, an inability to discharge anger or hostility, a tendency to hide anger and hostility behind a facade of pleasantness, and unresolved hostile conflict with their mothers.'" In this context it's interesting that the support groups for women with breast cancer, which tend to create a very self-nurturing and self-supportive atmosphere, can double life expectancy.

Remember that most of us have the above crises and tendencies in our lives at some time or another. Your predisposition to breast cancer is going to have as much to do with *how* you cope with stress as it does with how much stress you have. Your personality and life's tragedies and stresses are not necessarily your destiny. Education and awareness can protect women from self-destructive behaviors that predispose them to breast cancer. If you go to the grocery store and find yourself putting everyone's favorite food in the shopping cart except your own (and you can't even remember what your own is), then you might want to pay a little more attention to your own needs. Next time you're making a shopping list, be sure to write down your favorite food for yourself.

If your kids are always outfitted with the latest shoes and sporting the latest haircuts while you're wearing the same running shoes you wore in college and cut your own hair, it might just be time for an attitude readjustment. If you don't take care of yourself, who will? This is not a call for self-indulgence and selfishness, it's a suggestion that balance in nurturing is as important as balanced hormones. It's not going to help anyone if you sacrifice yourself on the altar of unselfishness. It's quite okay to take care yourself while you also take care of others.

This type of profile doesn't apply only to mothers. In fact, women who don't have children are more at risk for breast cancer than those who do. We all know women who don't have children who have a tendency to sacrifice their own well-being for others: Nursing and social work are professions that come immediately to mind. How about the many women who form the tireless support groups behind politicians (mostly male) running for office? Or the executive secretary who devotes herself to the boss to the exclusion of all else? Teachers of all sorts come to mind, including coaches. And how about nuns?

In addition, the young women in Gen X and Y frequently postpone having children to throw themselves completely into a career. If this isn't balanced with self-nurture, they may be at increased risk. We are culturally biased to believe that women who nurture themselves are selfish. It's time to wake up, think clearly, and throw out that destructive old point of view. Take a vacation, take a walk in a beautiful place, or even just take a bubble bath—with candles! And while you're doing it, contemplate how you can better listen to yourself, tend to yourself, and support yourself.

Medical Attitudes toward Breast Cancer

Attitudes in conventional medicine toward breast cancer tend to be equally destructive, and while these attitudes have admittedly improved in the past decade, the fact that women with DCIS breast cancer (which is very rarely fatal, and some of which is debatably even a true cancer) are still subjected to mastectomy, sometimes even chemotherapy and radiation, and most recently tamoxifen, is evidence of a medical attitude that may care more about liability and lawsuits than quality of life.

Medicine has become so frenzied in its determination to treat breast cancer with an arsenal of weapons that it's completely lost sight of what's really working and what's not. For example, because DCIS wasn't even detectable prior to mammograms, and thus wasn't treated very often, we don't really know what the mortality rate is for this type of cancer if it's *not* treated with surgery, chemotherapy, and radiation. What if DCIS were treated by correcting the obvious underlying metabolic imbalance that's occurring? What if the woman with DCIS were supported in creating a better diet, taking the right supplements, boosting her immune system, balancing her hormones, managing stress, and supporting herself emotionally? Because surgery, radiation, chemotherapy, and tamoxifen each have side effects that are harmful at the very least, and can be deadly, we believe that more women would be alive and healthy today if their DCIS wasn't treated the way "nonlocal" cancers are treated.

Get an Attitude!

While it's important for a woman to work in partnership and cooperation with the health care professionals in her life, it's also important that she be actively and intelligently involved in her treatment. The days of passively submitting to the almighty doctor are done and gone. If you want to be more than a cog in the medical machine, you need to participate fully in your own treatment. You need to get an attitude and *know* that you have a right to individualized, personal medical attention! Remember, *you* are paying all these doctors, nurses, and other health care professionals to treat you—*you* are the client, and it's *their* privilege to serve *you*, not the other way around.

How can you get an attitude? Ask a lot of questions and don't take a condescending pat on the head for an answer. If you're not getting the answers you need, it's time to visit more doctors and spend some time on the Internet, which is a wonderful source of chat groups and forums on breast cancer where women share their experience and what they've learned. (Beware of drug-company-funded chat rooms and forums that are there to push a particular drug or treatment.) Granted, there's a lot of junky and hyped-up information out there, but you can use your own powers of discernment and discrimination to sift out the gold for your own use. We will give you some great Internet resources at the end of the book. You may even want to visit a medical library. If you invest in a paperback medical dictionary, you'll be surprised how much you can understand.

Part of the problem for a woman who strikes out on her own is information overload. If you've been told that you have a malignant cancer that may have spread, your doctors will be pressuring you to have treatment very quickly, leaving you little time to educate yourself and contemplate how you want to go about taking care of yourself. When you go into a bookstore, what you face is dozens of books on cancer and breast cancer, and hundreds of alternative treatments to sort through. If you have a malignant lump in your breast, you justifiably want it out as quickly and thoroughly as possible—you don't have six months to leave your life and educate yourself.

In the back of this book, under Resources, we will point you to what we feel are some reliable sources of information about treating breast cancer, both conventional and alternative. This will help reduce your search for good information considerably. Reading the rest of this book will also help, because you'll have a deeper understanding of just what gets a breast cancer started, and what stops it.

In part I we have laid the foundation for your understanding and awareness of some important aspects of breast cancer by examining the politics of the breast cancer industry, your risk factors for breast cancer, how breast cancer gets started at the gene level, the physiology of the breast, and what we know about how attitudes, emotions, and stress can play a role in breast cancer. In part II we'll give you detailed information on how some hormones can affect breast tissue, and what this means to you.

PART II

THE SEX HORMONES AND HOW THEY AFFECT BREAST CANCER

CHAPTER 6

THE NATURE
OF ESTROGENS

Angels of Life, Angels of Death

Because of their tremendous range of effects—both beneficial and harmful—the hormones known as estrogens were dubbed "the Angels of Life and the Angels of Death" by Dr. Ercole Cavalieri, a scientist who has spent the last three decades studying their effects. We'll talk about his work in some detail in this book, and particularly in the next chapter.

Dr. Cavalieri's phrase is telling. An excess or a deficiency of estrogens can make a world of difference in a woman's outlook on life and in her overall health and well-being. For example, too much estrogen and you're likely to feel bloated and oversensitive, have insomnia, and gain excessive weight around the hips and buttocks. Too little and you may feel mentally lethargic and fuzzy, have memory problems, and feel depressed. One of the keys to achieving and maintaining hormone balance is learning how to recognize when your estrogen levels are out of balance.

The word *estrogen* is not the name of any specific hormone but is a class name for a large group of compounds with estrogenic properties. These include human estrogens, animal estrogens, synthetic (not-found-in-nature) estrogens, phytoestrogens (plant estrogens), and xenoestrogens (environmental estrogens, usually from toxins). The three major human estrogens produced naturally in the body are estradiol, estrone, and estriol.

A rise in estrogen at puberty is responsible for the development and maintenance of female sex organs and secondary sex characteristics such as breasts, as well as for menstrual cycles and pregnancy. A primary role of estrogen is to control the growth and function of the uterus: Specifically, estrogens create the proliferative endometrium or blood-rich lining of the uterus, preparing it for pregnancy in monthly cycles.

Estrogen effects are also seen on the ovaries, cervix, fallopian tubes, vagina, external genitalia, and breasts. Vocal cord changes and fat deposition in the breasts and hip area are also attributable to estrogen. The emergence of estrogen at puberty stops the growth of long bones in both males and females. Just prior to puberty there is a spurt in height, but after puberty, when estrogen is higher, height does not increase.

As a general rule, estrogen promotes cell growth, primarily of the tissues responsible for reproduction. It's responsible for giving the female body the signals to promote the growth of the blood-rich tissue in the uterus in the first part of the menstrual cycle, and it's part of the hormonal signaling that stimulates the maturation of an egg-containing follicle in the ovary.

It is estrogen's tendency to promote cell growth that makes its excess such a dangerous promoter of cancer. This is also why it's so important to use progesterone if you have the symptoms of estrogen dominance (see the list, following), or if you're taking estrogen for hormone replacement. Progesterone gives your body the ability to keep estrogen's growth-promoting properties in check.

Estrogen's stimulatory effect on cell growth makes it useful in wound healing. A study in the journal *Nature Medicine* showed that wounds healed more slowly in older women, though with less scarring. When they were given estrogen, their wound healing time was improved. Young female rats with their ovaries removed took significantly longer to heal wounds, but when topical estrogen was applied to the wound it healed very quickly. Both estradiol and estriol increase the production of type III collagen (which helps the skin heal faster) and hyaluronic acid (which helps retain moisture and keeps skin plump).

Excess estrogen, on the other hand, tends to create deficiencies of zinc, magnesium, and the B vitamins, all important to the maintenance of hormone balance. Magnesium, sometimes called the antispasm nutrient, is especially important in the prevention of heart attacks.

Estrogen dominance is a term coined by Dr. Lee in his first book on natural progesterone. It describes a condition in which a woman can have deficient, normal, or excessive estrogen, but has little or no progesterone to balance its effects in the body. Even a woman with low estrogen levels can have estrogen dominance symptoms if she doesn't have any progesterone. The symptoms and conditions associated with estrogen dominance are:

- Acceleration of the aging process
- Allergies, including asthma, hives, rashes, sinus congestion
- Anxiety, often with depression
- Autoimmune disorders such as lupus erythematosus and Hashimoto's thyroiditis, and possibly Sjögren's syndrome (dry mouth)
- Breast cancer
- Breast tenderness
- Cervical dysplasia
- Cold hands and feet as a symptom of thyroid dysfunction
- Copper excess and zinc deficiency
- Decreased sex drive
- Depression with anxiety or agitation
- Dry eyes
- Early onset of menstruation
- Endometrial (uterine) cancer
- Fat gain, especially around the hips and thighs
- Fatigue
- Fibrocystic breasts
- Gallbladder disease

- Headaches
- Hypoglycemia
- Increased blood clotting (increasing risk of strokes)
- Infertility
- Irregular menstrual periods
- Irritability
- Insomnia
- Magnesium deficiency
- Mood swings
- Osteoporosis
- Polycystic ovaries
- Premenopausal bone loss
- PMS
- Prostate cancer
- Sluggish metabolism
- Thyroid dysfunction mimicking hypothyroidism
- Uterine cancer
- Uterine fibroids
- Water retention, bloating

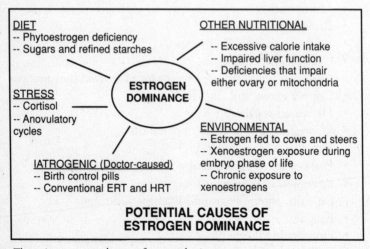

The various sources and causes of estrogen dominance.

The Causes of Estrogen Dominance

Strictly speaking, it's possible that we are all—men, women and children—suffering a little from estrogen dominance, because there is so much of it in our environment. You'd have to live virtually in a bubble to escape the excess estrogens we're exposed to through pesticides, plastics, industrial waste products, car exhaust, meat, soaps, and much of the carpeting, furniture, and paneling that we live with indoors every day. You may have on-and-off sinus problems, headaches, dry eyes, asthma, or cold hands and feet, for example, and not know to attribute them to your exposure to xenoestrogens. Over time the exposure may cause more chronic problems such as arthritis and gallbladder disease, and may be a direct or indirect cause of cancer, including breast cancer. In fact, we believe that estrogen dominance is at the very heart of what promotes breast cancer.

Estrogen Dominance in a
Premenopausal Woman

What makes estrogen dominance most noticeable in a *pre-*menopausal woman is a lack of ovulation (anovulation) or luteal insufficiency, in which not enough progesterone is made after ovulation.

Anovulation is usually associated with low estrogen and low progesterone. During her teen years, and then starting again in her mid-thirties to early forties, a woman may not ovulate during some of her monthly menstrual cycles. Ovulation is the time when an ovarian follicle releases an ovum (egg) that travels down the fallopian tube toward the uterus. After releasing the ovum, the emptied follicle becomes the corpus luteum, which makes progesterone. This is the primary way that a premenopausal woman makes progesterone. If you don't ovulate, you won't make progesterone in any significant amount. You can still have a seemingly normal menstrual cycle even if you haven't ovulated, but the lack of progesterone may cause you to experience PMS symptoms such as swollen and tender breasts, weight gain, mood swings, and cramps.

Luteal insufficiency may be even more common than anovulation. This occurs when an egg is produced but the corpus luteum doesn't produce adequate progesterone. Dr. Zava, who has seen thousands of saliva test results combined with a detailed questionnaire about symptoms, doesn't see many premenopausal women with low estrogen (which may occur with anovulation), but does see a lot of women with normal to high estrogen and low progesterone (which would occur with luteal insufficiency). These women are having normal menstrual cycles but produce very little progesterone and have typical symptoms of estrogen dominance. These same women are likely to have problems getting pregnant. Dr. Zava has hypothesized that the low progesterone these women produce, if they do get pregnant, may lead to children with attention deficit disorders due to improper brain development, because progesterone during the first trimester of pregnancy is essential for development of regions of the brain necessary for shuttling information, or memory. The alarming rise in children with attention deficit disorder, Dr. Zava believes, may lie in the harmful effects of endocrine disruptors (petrochemicals) on thyroid (see chapter 4) and the inability of the ovaries to produce adequate progesterone during the first trimester of pregnancy.

British physician Katherina Dalton, a pioneer in progesterone research who spent decades treating pregnant women with progesterone, observed that those she treated had children with higher IQs and calmer dispositions.

Low progesterone production tends to occur during two phases of a woman's life—at puberty and again at perimenopause (the time around the beginning of menopause). During both of these times of transition in a woman's life her risk of breast cancer is higher. Teenagers have undeveloped breast tissue that's more susceptible to the growth-promoting effects of estrogen, and perimenopausal women may have many cycles in a row in which they're still making plenty of estrogen but are making little to no progesterone, due to either anovulation or luteal insufficiency. Without the balancing effect of progesterone, estrogen has the potential to initiate or promote cancer.

Xenohormone exposure during embryo life damages ovarian follicles and leads to follicle failure later in life. This is probably a primary cause of cycles of luteal failure in premenopausal women. Again, these women may be making an egg, but they can't nourish it because of the lack of progesterone. The near epidemic of infertility among young women today is most likely due to damage sustained by the ovaries from pollutants, while they were in the womb. This type of exposure and its effect on a woman's reproductive organs (which are well documented in animal studies and covered later in the book) causes not only infertility but also chronic estrogen dominance. Over time this will create a cycle of what we call premenopause syndrome, which may include PMS, fibrocystic breasts, fibroids, irregular periods, and endometriosis. (Although PMS can't be attributed entirely to estrogen dominance, it's certainly one factor, and the symptoms of estrogen dominance are very similar to the symptoms of PMS.) These conditions also provide a fertile environment for estrogens to damage the breast cells, which can eventually lead to breast cancer.

There are many causes of anovulatory cycles. Stress is a common one. The wisdom of the human body evolving over time dictates that a female body under stress may not be the best environment for a pregnancy; if you don't ovulate, you won't get pregnant. The types of stress most likely to induce anovulatory cycles are heavy exercise and extremely low calorie intake such as dieting, but any type of stress will do it, including emotional stress. Women who combine careers with raising a family and women who have extremely competitive and demanding corporate jobs also tend to have more anovulatory cycles.

The combination of estrogen dominance and stress can create a self-perpetuating cycle in which stress causes estrogen dominance, which then causes insomnia and anxiety, which taxes the adrenal glands, which then creates more estrogen dominance. A woman who has been caught in this type of cycle for a few years will find herself in a constant state of "wired but tired" (or "tired but wired"), which will eventually result in dysfunctional adrenal glands, blood sugar imbalances, and debilitating fatigue that may be diagnosed as chronic fatigue syndrome. If this describes you, we highly recommend that you read the book *What Your Doctor May* Not *Tell You about Premenopause.*

Another common cause of estrogen dominance and much misery is hysterectomy or removal of the uterus, which creates surgically induced menopause, followed by estrogen replacement therapy without progesterone. Even when the ovaries are left intact, their blood supply can be severely compromised by hysterectomy, and they frequently stop functioning altogether within two years of the removal of the uterus. But these women get a double whammy from conventional medicine, thanks to the common and extremely misguided practice of prescribing only estrogen and no progesterone to women with hysterectomies. Between estrogen-only hormone replacement therapy, estrogen made in fat cells, and environmental estrogens, estrogen dominance is almost guaranteed. Supplemental estrogen in a woman who doesn't need it, or who has no progesterone to balance it, can lead to water retention, breast swelling, fibrocysts in the breasts, headaches, depression, fat storage, gallbladder problems, and, in women who still have their uteruses, heavier periods. It also leads to more opportunities for estrogen-induced changes in your DNA, which can set the stage for breast cancer. Through saliva testing and symptom monitoring, Dr. Zava finds that women on unopposed estrogens nearly always have symptoms of estrogen dominance, the most prevalent being fibrocystic breasts and weight gain in the hips.

Women without ovarian function (such as following a full or partial hysterectomy) also tend to suffer from low androgen levels, specifically testosterone and dehydroepiandrosterone (DHEA). Thus, if they've been on only estrogen replacement therapy (ERT), they frequently suffer not only from symptoms of estrogen dominance but also from symptoms of androgen deficiency (low libido, fatigue, loss of sensation in sexual organs, depression, vaginal dryness, incontinence, thinning skin, bone loss, decreased pubic hair). This failure to supplement women without ovarian function with the full range of hormones is one of the more bizarre and harmful consequences of conventional medicine's myopic view of hormone replacement that considers only estrogen to be an important hormone.

In part III we'll give you detailed guidelines for determining which, if any, hormone imbalances you may have, along with suggestions for creating and maintaining hormone balance.

Estrogen Dominance in a Menopausal Woman

By far the biggest cause of estrogen dominance in menopausal women is the estrogen almost universally prescribed to them, and we believe that it may also be one of the biggest causes of breast cancer in women over age 50. Since the huge National Cancer Institute study published in *JAMA* in January 2000 (C. Schairer and colleagues), clearly showing that conventional HRT significantly increases your risk of breast cancer, conventional physicians have become a little less eager to insist on it, but there is still enormous pressure on women to use it. We hope that you'll resist these unreasoned efforts and make an educated decision about whether you need estrogen, and if so, in what dose.

If you believe everything you hear or read in the media, you'd think that estrogen replacement therapy is a panacea for nearly all ills, including all of the symptoms of aging, especially Alzheimer's, osteoporosis, and heart disease. However, studies have been steadily trickling out for the past few years contradicting these medical myths, which were based on an element of truth that became grossly distorted and exaggerated, thanks to aggressive advertising, marketing, and public relations campaigns to sell estrogens.

ESTROGEN, ALZHEIMER'S, AND BRAIN FUNCTION

The myths about Alzheimer's and estrogen are a good example of how small, poorly done studies that are given wide exposure by the media can take on a life of their own and become medical dogma without any real basis in fact. At the time of the first studies on the effects of estrogen on Alzheimer's, it was already well known that women of higher socioeconomic status and more education had a lower rate of Alzheimer's, and yet this was not factored into any of them. There were also no long-term, double-blind studies. Nor was there any reliable accounting of which women were also taking a progestin with their estrogen and which women had an intact uterus, all confounding factors. In fact, the first study on estrogen and Alzheimer's included only 12 women—and yet it was used as *the* proof that estrogen prevents and even reverses Alzheimer's.

The next research to come out on Alzheimer's and estrogen showed that in the long term, the women taking estrogen had *poorer* cognitive (thinking) function than women who didn't. In yet another case the media claimed a study had proved that estrogen improved cognitive function, but all that had really been found was that women taking estrogen had more brain activity—not necessarily an indication of better brain function.

There's no doubt that estrogen has an excitatory effect on the brain, which might temporarily improve the symptoms of Alzheimer's. But long-term estrogen dominance can have the opposite effect on the brain, creating chronic overexcitation that leads to cell death, an increased risk of blood clots (and therefore strokes), and imbalances in cellular fluids that can cause headaches.

The right amount of estrogen is important for many of the functions of the brain. Too much estrogen is harmful, but when a woman is deprived of estrogen her quality of life suffers too. She often complains of foggy thinking, memory lapses mostly associated with not remembering names and places, and sleep disturbances, often along with the better-known estrogen deficiency symptoms of vaginal dryness and hot flashes.

It's likely that the press releases handed out to the media by the drug companies sponsoring the above research had clever wording that led to the incorrect conclusion that conventional estrogen replacement therapy improves the symptoms of Alzheimer's. (They probably could have achieved the same results with any brain stimulant, legal or otherwise.) Had the media people taken the time and effort to actually read and analyze these studies, they would have discovered that this was not the case. As a result, most American women and their doctors now firmly believe that estrogen can save them from Alzheimer's. It will probably take a decade before the truth is fully realized.

Another cause of estrogen dominance in menopausal women is obesity. Once you've reached menopause, your ovaries pretty much stop producing estrogen and progesterone, but they keep producing the androgen (male hormone) androstenedione, which is converted to estrogen in your fat cells. Thus, a woman with a lot of fat on her body can be making quite a bit of estrogen, even if she's not ovulating. The estrogen made by fat cells can be enough to cause estrogen-dominance symptoms, and this is why so many menopausal women feel so great when they start using progesterone, which balances the estrogen effects and has many beneficial effects of its own.

Chronic exposure to xenoestrogens, usually from pesticides, solvents such as nail polish, shedding from plastics into food and water, and hormone-laden meats, can also contribute to estrogen dominance. The pesticide exposure can come from supermarket produce, lawn and garden sprays, and indoor insect sprays. Each exposure taken on its own may not amount to much, but constant small exposures over time can add up to hormone imbalance.

Excessive estrogen is processed through the liver, so if your liver function is compromised by drinking too much alcohol or using prescription drugs, for example, your estrogen levels will often be higher. This is why estrogen-dominance symptoms can sometimes be cleared up simply by making some healthy lifestyle changes that improve the function of your gastrointestinal tract and liver.

Estrogen Deficiency in a Menopausal Woman

Estrogen deficiency is rare in premenopausal women, although it can occur if ovulation stops due to overexercise or undereating. The primary symptoms of estrogen deficiency are well known among menopausal women: hot flashes, night sweats, and vaginal dryness. (Hot flashes and night sweats can also be caused by fluctuations of estrogen.) Less well known is that an estrogen deficiency can cause fatigue, memory problems, and foggy thinking, but estrogen dominance can cause the same symptoms. The bladder contains estrogen receptors and is sensitive to estrogen. An estrogen deficiency can cause or worsen bladder and urinary tract problems. Many of the hormonal contraceptives are known for causing chronic urinary tract problems, possibly because they block the action of your own natural estrogen and natural progesterone.

Estrogen-deficiency symptoms can often be relieved with lifestyle changes, such as an increase in exercise and dietary changes, or by using some natural progesterone. Herbs that have estrogenic properties work well for some women. Adrenal support is also very important, since the adrenals are a source of estrogen, via androgens, in menopausal women. We cover the above options in more detail in part III, as well as detailed recommendations on how to use estrogen if you need it.

Estrogen is an amazing and useful hormone to be used with great care only when necessary, in the right amounts, in its natural form (meaning that it's identical to the estrogens made by your body). Menopausal women who are thin are more likely to be estrogen deficient, and often benefit from a little bit of estrogen. It's less common for a woman who is of normal weight or is overweight to need estrogen, but it can happen; that's why it's best to have a saliva hormone level test to find out what your bioavailable hormone levels really are. In part III we'll explain the difference between saliva and blood hormone level tests, and give you information that will help you decide whether you have excess estrogen.

The Premarin Controversy

Premarin, also called conjugated estrogen, is the most commonly prescribed form of estrogen, and is one of the ten best-selling drugs in the United States. There are many moral and ethical objections to Premarin, however, which is made from the urine of pregnant mares that are said to be confined to narrow stalls with catheters attached. Many of the clinicians we talk to believe that the equilin or horse estrogen in Premarin may put more stress on the liver than a bio-identical or human estrogen. These objections aside, Premarin is not in and of itself a bad estrogen, and there's a lot more in Premarin than estrogen. It's more like a hormone cocktail, with more than a hundred active ingredients, many of which have not been fully studied. Premarin contains a high percentage (48 percent) of estrone, which is identical to that made by the human body, and a small amount of progesterone, which no doubt conveys some small benefit. The biggest problem with Premarin is the fact that it's prescribed to many women who don't need it, in doses that are often excessive, and it's usually prescribed without the progesterone supplementation needed to moderate and balance its effects. Because of the morally objectionable way in which Premarin is obtained, we recommend that women use estradiol (such as Estrace) or estriol.

The Relationship of Sex Hormones to Breast Cancer

Much confusion reigns in the understanding (or misunderstanding) of the relationship of sex hormones to breast cancer. Most experienced clinicians understand very well that estrogen is a promoter of breast cancer, and they also understand that progesterone balances or opposes undesirable side effects of estrogen. For reasons that aren't entirely clear, conventional medicine has ignored the cancer-protective effects of progesterone in treating breast cancer despite many studies that offer solid evidence.

Even though progestins (synthetic progesterone) are used in hormone replacement therapy to offset or oppose the cancer-promoting role of estrogen in endometrial cancer, progesterone has not been widely recognized for its similar protective role in breast cancer. And yet there are studies that clearly establish this relationship. As long ago as 1966 H. P. Leis reported treating 158 menopausal women (11 percent with a strong family history of breast cancer) with both estrogen and progesterone therapy for up to 14 years; none of the patients developed breast cancer.

In rodent studies by A. Inoh, the protective effect of progesterone or tamoxifen was investigated in estrogen-induced mammary cancer. The ovaries of the rats were removed. Rats given estradiol had a high rate of mammary cancer. However, if tamoxifen or progesterone was given simultaneously with the estradiol, fewer tumors appeared, and the ones that did were smaller and less likely to spread. Tamoxifen, a patent drug, has been introduced as a standard breast cancer treatment in conventional medicine, but progesterone has been ignored. Given the toxicity of tamoxifen, we believe it is a tragedy that progesterone has been ignored in this context.

The action of estradiol and progesterone on cell multiplication (proliferation) in breast cells was beautifully demonstrated in an important 1995 study by K. J. Chang and coworkers. It tested the effects of transdermal (via the skin) hormone applications on normal human breast duct cells, from which cancer is known to rise, in healthy young women planning to undergo minor breast surgery for benign breast disease.

In this study the women were divided into four groups and began using one of the creams on their breasts 10 to 13 days before breast surgery:

- Group A applied estradiol cream (1.5 mg) daily.
- Group B applied progesterone cream (25 mg) daily.
- Group C applied a combination of estradiol and progesterone (half doses each) daily.
- Group D applied a placebo cream.

At surgery, biopsies were obtained for measuring estradiol and progesterone concentrations, and for tests of cell proliferation rates. In addition, blood plasma hormone levels were measured. Following surgery the breast tissue, about the size of a marble, was divided in half. One part was sent to a pathology laboratory for viewing under a microscope to determine how the hormones affected the growth rate of the breast cells; the remainder was sent to an endocrinology laboratory to determine how much hormone was taken up by the tissue.

Results from the endocrinology laboratory revealed that in those women treated with just estradiol, the concentration of estradiol in the breast tissue was 200 times greater than those not treated with it (placebo gel). Breast tissue concentrations of progesterone were 100 times greater in women who used progesterone than the placebo. These findings clearly demonstrate that both hormones are well absorbed transdermally (through the skin) and accumulate in target tissues in the same manner as endogenous (made in the body) hormones. This is important because it's common for conventional doctors to claim that transdermal progesterone isn't absorbed, and, as you'll discover in chapter 9, transdermal application is preferable.

The effect of these hormones on cell proliferation rates was equally clear. Estradiol increased the cell proliferation rate by 230 percent, whereas progesterone *decreased* it by more than 400 percent. The estradiol-progesterone combination cream maintained the normal proliferation rate. Again, this is clear evidence that unopposed estradiol stimulates hyperproliferation of breast cells and progesterone protects against this.

When progesterone is used transdermally, blood tests don't show a measurable rise, and this is why so many doctors believe it isn't absorbed. We'll explain why it doesn't show up in the chapter on progesterone, but for now what's important to take from this study is the fact that progesterone levels rose dramatically in the breast cells of women using transdermal progesterone, and this proves that progesterone is well absorbed when

CELL PROLIFERATION MARKERS IN BIOPSIES OF NORMAL BREAST TISSUE FROM WOMEN TREATED TOPICALLY WITH 1.5 mg ESTRADIOL (E2) AND/OR 25 mg PROGESTERONE (Pg)

Charts adapted from: Chang et al. Fertility and Sterility 63: 785-791, 1995

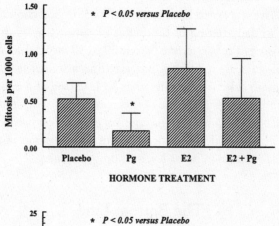

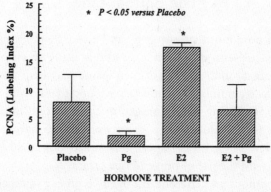

Women treated with topical (on the skin of the breast) progesterone alone prior to surgery had much lower proliferation (cell division) rates than women given nothing (placebo) and women taking estrogen alone (E2) or with progesterone (E2+Pg).

applied to the skin. The blood tests showed no measurable increase of progesterone concentration, however. This is an excellent illustration of the fact that blood testing can't be reliably used to determine the bioavailable level of progesterone when it's delivered through the skin, because very little bioavailable progesterone is carried in blood plasma, which is what's measured in a standard blood test.

Dr. Zava has noted both in carefully controlled clinical studies and in daily testing of thousands of saliva samples that this same dosing of progesterone (about 20 to 30 mg) results in a remarkable increase in salivary progesterone, as much as 10 to 50 times, more closely reflecting what K. J. Chang and colleagues found in breast tissue uptake of these hormones. Two studies recently reported from Australia confirm that topical progesterone results in very little increase in serum progesterone but a remarkable increase in saliva levels of progesterone.

The Bottom Line

There is no doubt that estrogen can be very helpful to women who are truly estrogen deficient, and that using an estrogen for a few years around the age of menopause may help slow bone loss. In fact, a number of studies have found that heavier women who are producing more estrogen in their fat cells have better bone density. Unfortunately, these women also have a higher risk of developing breast cancer, but we feel this could be ameliorated with the use of progesterone cream.

But without progesterone, estrogen becomes a significant factor in the promotion of cancer. This makes it extremely important that you always use estrogen *with* progesterone to create hormonal balance. We believe that the tendency of conventional medical doctors to indiscriminately prescribe estrogen, particularly without progesterone, for a wide range of premenopausal or menopausal symptoms is irresponsible and dangerous—and all too often has tragic consequences.

In chapter 9 you'll find out how progesterone neutralizes the dangers of estrogen, how widespread its beneficial effects are in the body, and why you want to keep your distance from the synthetic progestins, even in birth control pills.

CHAPTER 7

HOW ESTROGEN TALKS TO YOUR CELLS

The Right Communication Is Everything

As you learned in the last chapter, estrogen is an important and potent hormone. So potent, in fact, that it affects the most fundamental control center of some of your cells. This is what can make estrogen such a powerful inducer and promoter of cancer. If estrogen inflicts damage on your DNA, or sends the wrong message, the consequences can be tragic. The good news is that there's a lot you can do to encourage estrogen to send healthy messages to your cells. In this chapter we explore how the wrong messages are sent, and how you can create healthy messages.

Parts of this chapter are very technical, but as we explained in the chapter on genes, if you have breast cancer and are researching your options, you'll see these concepts and terms frequently in the literature, and it will help you tremendously to understand what they mean. This chapter may also be of some help when you're deciding on which course of treatment to use.

The estrogens we'll be focusing on are estradiol and estrone sulfate. The majority of the estradiol and estrone sulfate in your body rides around in the watery portion of your blood (called serum or plasma) bound to proteins called albumin and sex hormone binding globulin (SHBG). This estrogen is largely unavailable for use by your cells. About 2 percent of your estradiol and 10 percent of your estrone sulfate is carried in your blood on red blood cell membranes and is not protein-bound, meaning that it's available or free to enter tissues of the body. As we mentioned in the last chapter, this is why we prefer to measure hormone levels with saliva tests, since saliva measures only the amount of bioavailable hormone in your body. Blood tests, on the other hand, which are more widely used by conventional doctors, measure the largely protein-bound and unavailable estrogen found in serum.

The breast tissue contains three enzymes that are responsible for locally increasing the amounts of estrogens, particularly estrone. These are important to know if you have breast cancer and are contemplating chemotherapy, because new chemotherapy drugs are coming out all the time, some of them designed to block these enzymes.

The first of these enzymes is *aromatase*. It's present in the fatty tissues surrounding the breast ductal tissues and is responsible for converting androgens, the male hormones such as androstenedione and testosterone, to estrone. This is the primary mechanism through which menopausal women get estrogen.

A second enzyme, *17ß-hydroxysteroid dehydrongenase*, converts estrone to the more potent estrogen, estradiol.

A third enzyme, *sulfatase*, is present in relatively high amounts within the ductal breast cells and in breast tumor cells; it's what gives estrone the ability to enter breast cells. Sulfatase converts the plentiful but inactive estrone sulfate to estrone, which can then enter breast cells and stimulate proliferation.

When the estrogens enter specific estrogen-sensitive cells (such as the breast ductal cells), they're greeted by a highly specific protein we refer to as the estrogen receptor. When estrogen binds to the receptor, it's activated, in much the way the key to your car starts the engine. Once activated by estrogens, the receptor-estrogen complex then activates or unlocks specific regions of DNA containing information that sends messages to your cells. These messages may include instructions to create new cell products such as new progesterone receptors, or to create enzymes that instruct the cell to manufacture new cell components or to replicate. Estrogen-sensitive cells, like those in the breast and the lining of the uterus, contain thousands of these estrogen receptors, and when estrogens rise in the bloodstream and enter the cells, there is continuous instruction to the cells to manufacture the cellular components necessary for cell replication.

Once the estrogen-receptor complex has performed its job, the receptor is destroyed and the estrogen undergoes one of three fates (you'll find out shortly why what estrogen does when it leaves the cell is important):

1. It finds another estrogen receptor and recycles through the same system.
2. It diffuses intact out of the cell the way it entered and back into the bloodstream.
3. It's metabolized to a less potent or inactive estrogen in preparation for elimination in the urine, feces, or sweat.

Most cellular systems are organized to provide very active metabolism of estrogens once they have activated specific gene sites in DNA. In other words, estrogen is supposed to do its job and leave immediately. This is because your body, in the inherent wisdom it has gained in evolving over millions of years, knows that although estrogen is vital to the proper function of the human female body, it can be dangerous if it overstays its welcome.

When the estrogen estradiol, by far your most potent estrogen, leaves a breast cell, it's often converted to the much weaker estrone. Estrone can also be converted back into estradiol, but the opposite is much more often the case.

In this next section we are going to launch into a fairly technical description of how estrogen specifically causes cell damage to start and promote the growth of cancer. Why are we getting so technical? Up until fairly recently we knew only in a general way that estrogens were involved with reproductive cancers. Now we have much more detailed information that tells us how and why, and we have detailed information about what we can do to reduce our risk of getting breast cancer, and stop its growth. This new information also gives us hard scientific evidence that toxins such as pesticides, solvents, and industrial waste products like dioxins and PCBs are directly related to breast cancer.

"Good" and "Bad" Estrogens

Along with giving cells the instruction to replicate, estrogens also activate the production of the very enzymes that usher them out of the body, or metabolize them. Because estrogens in excess have the potential to do damage, our bodies have evolved very sophisticated ways of balancing, controlling, and excreting estrogen, complete with backup systems.

The main enzymes that carry out this function are referred to as cytochrome p450 hydroxylase enzymes, and they interact with estrogen to form by-products or metabolites called catechol estrogens. It's the function of the p450 and other enzymes to rid the cell of excess estrogens. It's also this same normal processing and elimination of estrogens that, under specific conditions, can lead to the estrogens that damage DNA, resulting in mutations and eventually cancer.

Some catechol estrogens are "good" and some are "bad," meaning some are easily and safely excreted, while others have the potential to damage the DNA of cells. The bad catechol estrogens are called 3,4-hydroxy estrogens. These are dangerous because they in turn can become an even more potent and damaging estrogen called estrogen-3,4-quinone. For simplicity's sake, we'll call these destructive end products quinone estrogens.

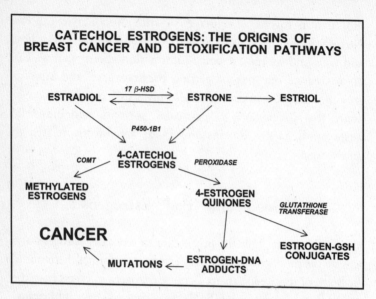

CATECHOL ESTROGENS: THE ORIGINS OF BREAST CANCER AND DETOXIFICATION PATHWAYS

The vast majority of catechol estrogens are "tagged" for safe excretion from the body through a process called methylation. Adding a methyl group, or methylation, is one of the primary ways that the body has of neutralizing toxins. Your body is constantly creating catechols and adding methyl groups to all kinds of waste products, which then leave the body without further ado: This is the primary job of the p450 pathways.

Most of the p450 activity and subsequent excretion of estrogens from the body takes place through the liver and the kidneys. There is a tremendous individual variation in how efficiently and effectively these systems work, and as a result tremendous variation in how estrogens affect individual women. The more efficient the p450 systems are, the more efficiently estrogens will be excreted. Women who have less efficient p450 systems and are given the same dose of estrogen as other women will have much higher levels of circulating estrogen, because it isn't being efficiently excreted. Virtually all prescription drugs put a tremendous burden on the p450 enzyme systems, and this can be an indirect cause of higher circulating estrogens, a factor that few doctors take into account when prescribing estrogen or, for that matter, when prescribing drugs that inhibit p450 systems.

Catechol estrogens become quinone estrogens when they are oxidized by free radicals. Free radicals are usually molecules containing an oxygen with unpaired electrons that latch onto anything they can to grab back an electron and restabilize themselves. In the process they make other cells unstable and create a chain reaction of oxidation. To understand better what oxidation is, think of how a cut apple turns brown when you leave it sitting out, or how a piece of metal left sitting in the rain gets rusty. Oxidized molecules can be used for beneficial purposes in the body, but when they're excessive they do tremendous damage.

Catechol estrogens transform to quinone estrogens when a free radical bumps into them, stripping the catechol estrogen of electrons and causing the estrogen to become highly unstable. The estrogen now goes about looking for electrons to create balance. If it finds its way to the DNA, it rips electrons from it, causing damage, or mutations. Once these oxidized catechol estrogens become quinones, the real trouble begins. While the "bad" catechol estrogens can be damaging, the "really bad" quinone estrogens are extremely reactive and unstable, and have the potential to permanently damage DNA.

Quinones form naturally in small amounts all the time, all over the body, and under normal circumstances they are rendered inactive almost instantaneously by protective enzyme systems and eliminated from the body through the bile, urine, or sweat. No harm done. But if these protective enzyme systems fail, then the quinones are less likely to be neutralized and more likely to damage DNA, causing mutations and cancer.

The enzyme systems fail when:

- Your body doesn't make enough of the enzymes (as in a genetic defect).

- Some of the nutrients used to help inactivate the estrogens are deficient.
- These systems have been overwhelmed by pollution, excess estrogens, poor nutrition, stress, or viruses, for example.
- A combination of the above.

How Estrogen Talks to Your Genes

When quinone estrogens bind to DNA, this can lead to minor changes (mutations) in the genetic blueprint that directs any number of different cell processes. If it permanently damages that part of the DNA that tells a cell when it should and should not divide, this can lead to an expanded clone, or a family of rogue cells with unregulated growth, or cancer.

It's the job of normal estrogens, through their activation of estrogen receptors, to activate cell replication. Tissues that don't contain estrogen receptors, and whose replication is not regulated by estrogens (for example, the stomach, muscles, and skin), don't form these kinds of tumors no matter how much estrogen they're exposed to.

Estrogens and the presence of cellular receptors contained within select tissues such as the breast and uterus are what render these tissues uniquely susceptible to the cancer-causing actions of the quinone estrogens.

Although it hasn't been scientifically proven, it appears to be the estrogen receptor that provides the quinone estrogens access to otherwise "protected" DNA sites governing cell proliferation. Without the receptor, the likelihood that the quinone estrogen would find the DNA site regulating cell division would be as remote as finding a book in a library without a card catalog. Scientific research has clearly shown that quinone estrogen causes damage to DNA, can bind to the estrogen receptor, and has a half life in the cell of about ten seconds, ample time to get a

piggyback ride on the receptor to gene sites regulating cell proliferation.

It's a relatively unusual occurrence when quinone estrogens
react with and damage DNA, and even then, DNA repair mechanisms usually fix the damage. But in the rare event that an
aberrant cell does happen to form as a result of damage to DNA
and mutations to the genetic blueprint, your immune system's
defenses usually recognize the rogue cell as foreign and destroy
it. This is why the full-blown expression of a colony of cancer
cells we call a tumor is so rare, given the unrelenting damage to
and repair of DNA that occurs in the trillions of cells in our
body throughout our lifetime. But cancers do occur, and it's this
rare series of events that lead to mutations, a primordial cancer
cell, and eventually a clinically detectable tumor.

The quinone estrogens mutate critical genes in the DNA
known as oncogenes and tumor suppressor genes. Dr. Ercole Cavalieri and his associates at the Eppley Institute for Research in
Cancer, University of Nebraska Medical Center, have been working for 30 years on finding how exactly these types of estrogen
form and how they do their damage. Through meticulous and extremely complex biochemical sleuthing, Dr. Cavalieri has tracked
the transformation of good estrogens to bad estrogens through
several pathways. He found that most estrogen pathways lead to
harmless products that are then disposed of.

As we explained above, it's when an estrogen heads down the
wrong catechol pathway that problems can begin, but not all catechol estrogens are bad. It has become an increasingly common
misconception that all catechol molecules are dangerous, and this
is just not the case. Some researchers believe that specific catechol
estrogens play an important role in mediating catecholamines,
which include dopamine, epinephrine, and norepinephrine, all
hormones that regulate mood and create a feeling of well-being or
an "up" feeling. This may be part of the reason that hormone replacement with estrogen—in the correct dosage—can alleviate depression in some women. On the other hand, too much estrogen

without progesterone can create a combination of insomnia and an anxious depression.

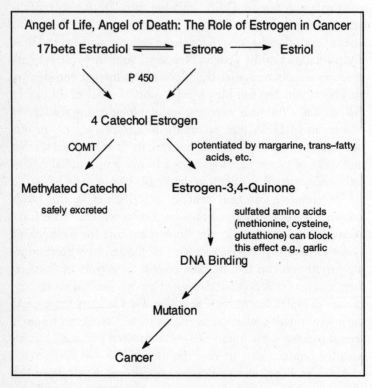

Dr. Cavalieri, recalling that estrogen is necessary for the earliest critical stages of embryo life, and now recognizing the fatal consequences of estrogen metabolism following this pathway, refers to estrogen as the Angel of Life, and the Angel of Death. COMT refers to catechol ortho-methyltransferase, the enzyme that transforms estrogen into a product that's safely excreted from the body.

The Smoking Gun: Quinone Estrogens

According to Dr. Cavalieri, not even all the quinone estrogens are bad. Both the 2 and 4 quinone estrogens bind tightly to the DNA backbone, but only the 4-hydroxyquinone estrogen causes a permanent mutation in the DNA that could lead to cancer. The 2 estrogen quinones also bind DNA, but in a stable form that can eventually be repaired. We can think of these 2 estrogen quinones as the body's last-ditch attempt to neutralize a harmful substance.

This means that the 2-hydroxy estrogens, which are increased with consumption of vegetables like onions, garlic, broccoli, and cauliflower, would not cause an increase in breast cancer. In fact, they can help prevent breast cancer by providing the raw material to encourage estrogen down the safer 2-hydroxy pathways. We have known for some time that these types of foods are associated with a lower cancer incidence, and now we know why.

The 4 estrogen quinones cause permanent damage to DNA and are associated with an increased incidence of breast and other cancers. For some time scientists thought a catechol estrogen called 16α-hydroxyestrone was the culprit in breast cancer, but the research done by Cavalieri and others points much more directly to the 4-hydroxyquinone estrogens. The amounts of 4-hydroxy estrogens are much higher than 2- or 16α-hydroxylated estrogens in breast cancer tissue compared to normal breast tissue. Moreover, scientists are finding that environmental pollutants such as PCBs and dioxins, which are known carcinogens, selectively activate the enzyme that favors 4 over 2 hydroxylation of estradiol.

The Safety Net of COMT

Under ordinary circumstances, your body has two primary ways of neutralizing catechol and quinone estrogens. As we mentioned above, the methylation process immediately takes care of probably 99 percent of the catechol estrogens with an enzyme called catechol ortho-methyltransferase (COMT). Red blood cells have some of the highest levels of this enzyme, and every tissue of the body is lined with it to protect it from the formation of catechols within or from incoming catechols. If this weren't so, the catechols such as quercetin that are found abundantly in many foods would be toxic. Methylation by COMT effectively renders the estrogens inert and targets them for elimination through bile (feces), urine, or sweat.

This methylation pathway can become overwhelmed under certain conditions in the body, allowing some of the 2- and 4-hydroxy estrogens to slip through the cracks and survive intact. Some of the conditions that can block the methylation pathway include:

- A genetic flaw in the production of COMT
- Nutritional deficiencies that result in limited availability of methyl groups for the enzyme
- Excess production of estrogens

Scientists have shown in animals that certain chemicals, when oxidized, will more readily strip the catechol of electrons and transform it into a quinone. For example, a combination of a peroxidase enzyme (which happens to be induced by estrogens) and rancid fats or oils will activate the bad estrogens. These unstable lipids often come from the polyunsaturated oils such as corn and safflower oil. Flax oil is one of the most unstable and unsaturated oils we know of, which is why we are not keen on over-using it as a nutritional supplement. (It's okay to grind the seeds and use those in moderation.) Mother Nature put these oils in our foods in small amounts for good reason! Saturated fats such as those found in meat and coconut oil do not oxidize this way. So much for the nutritional wisdom doled out by the government and the processed foods industry for the past four decades.

The Safety Net of Glutathione

If the catechol estrogens aren't caught and methylated, and become the oxidized quinone estrogens, a substance called glutathione will go to work sopping them up. Again, this probably takes care of 99 percent of the quinone estrogens.

The antioxidant glutathione is one of the most powerful and remarkable detoxification systems in the human body. It's found in every cell of your body, and its main job is to neutralize potentially damaging free radicals by stabilizing them. Once the toxin is made neutral, it's passed off to other antioxidants such as vitamins C and E, and the glutathione is then uniquely able to refresh itself, with the aid of enzymes, to go back and do the job again. Glutathione does this in each cell of the body, and also in the liver, where it's present in very high levels.

A deficiency of glutathione makes you much more susceptible to DNA damage by unstable molecules. Glutathione's primary building block is the amino acid cysteine, and if your cysteine levels are deficient, your glutathione levels are likely to be deficient. Good sources of dietary cysteine include eggs, meat, and dairy products. As long as you're eating a balanced diet, it's easy to get enough cysteine. However, substances that put your liver through a lot of work can deplete glutathione. These include excess hormones, rancid oils, overexposure to poisons such as pesticides and solvents (like those from nail polish and nail polish remover), heavy metals (mercury, cadmium, lead), and most prescription drugs. Older people who are taking two or more over-the-counter or prescription drugs are putting a tremendously heavy load on the liver. Menopausal women who are taking drugs plus conventional HRT, with its often excessive estrogen and poisonous progestins, create a double whammy. The liver will normally keep on ticking along, but the chances rise, both in the liver and in individual cells, that cells and their DNA could be damaged.

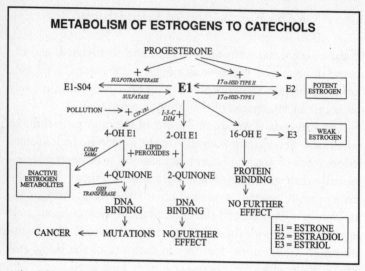

A detailed look at how estrogens go down biochemical pathways that are safe or harmful.

From DNA Damage to Cancer

What we have described above represents only the initial events that damage a normal breast cell and transform it into a breast *cancer* cell. What makes this primordial breast cancer cell different from its normal neighbors is that it has lost some of the controls that tell it when it should replicate and when it should rest and be content within the confines of its neighbors (other breast cells) and neighborhood (the breast itself). Normal cells become cancerous when they underexpress control mechanisms that suppress cell replication and when they overexpress control mechanisms that stimulate cell replication. Let's review briefly what controls the growth and development of normal breast ductal cells and then discuss how this is related to cancerous changes in breast cells.

Normal cells maintain a balance of just the right number of cells within a tissue to keep the tissue healthy and functional. In the breast ductal tissues, normal cells are replaced only as needed to maintain the ductal structures in the event of pregnancy, when the breast cells will specialize into milk-producing glands. Estradiol, progesterone, prolactin, and various other hormones are intimately involved in telling the normal breast ductal cells when to divide and when to stop dividing and mature into potential milk-producing glands.

Estradiol and prolactin induce the chemical changes within the breast cells that promote cell replication. Progesterone then induces a new set of chemicals within the breast cell that instruct it to stop dividing and mature into a cell type that is no longer capable of cell replication, but will produce milk given the signals of pregnancy. This is why we say that progesterone promotes differentiation of the cell: It instructs the cell to develop into something specific. This could be compared to the point when the leaf bud on a tree differentiates into a leaf. The difference between instructing a cell to replicate and instructing it to differentiate is at the heart of why so many physicians and even researchers misunderstand progesterone's role in breast and uterine cells. Differentiation is protective against cancer, while out-of-control replication contributes to cancer.

Progesterone will then further induce cell death, referred to as apoptosis, at the end of the menstrual cycle if pregnancy doesn't occur. This is the mechanism for shedding the uterine lining each month—menstruation—and it's governed by the waxing and waning of estrogen and progesterone produced during the menstrual cycle. This ebb and flow of estrogens and progesterone during the menstrual cycle maintains balance within the normal breast ductal cells. Estrogen dominance results in an accumulation of cells, leading to benign adenomas and fibrocysts in the breast, and endometrial hyperplasia in the uterus. While this is an overgrowth of normal cells, not cancer, the lack of shedding induced by progesterone predisposes these cells to carcinogenic insults from estrogens, chemicals, viruses, and radiation that can transform them into cancer cells. This is one of the many reasons why it is so harmful to prescribe estrogen alone to women without a uterus.

When a breast ductal cell is transformed into a cancer cell, it loses many of the control mechanisms that suppress growth. At the same time, cancer cells overexpress the chemical machinery that stimulates cell replication. Cancer cells can also invade surrounding tissues that ordinarily serve as a growth barrier to normal cells. The most aggressive breast cancer cells are those that also express growth factors that stimulate the growth of blood vessels around the tumor cells, which then furnish the tumor with nutrients. The growth of blood vessels around a tumor is called angiogenesis, and much cancer research is aimed at stopping this process.

Even in cancerous breast cells, many of the mechanisms that provide tumor cells a growth advantage over normal cells are still somewhat modulated by estrogen and progesterone through their cellular receptors. Estrogens stimulate cell replication, invasion, and blood vessel growth, whereas progesterone inhibits these mechanisms. We will talk more about how progesterone inhibits these mechanisms in chapter 9. A minority (20 to 30 percent) of breast tumors lose their estrogen and progesterone control mechanisms and divide, invade, and metastasize relentlessly.

Estrogen and the Immune System

Your immune system is normally responsible for cleaning up and removing any cells with damaged DNA, thus helping inhibit breast cancer. However, British researchers M. J. Reed and A. Purohit have clearly outlined the process by which immune surveillance systems can go awry and *promote,* rather than inhibit, the growth of breast cancer. It begins with specialized parts of immune system complexes called macrophages and tumor-infiltrating lymphocytes, which ordinarily identify and remove DNA-damaged cells and infiltrating types of tissue such as tumors. When certain signals are crossed, these complexes can stimulate the production of chemicals called cytokines, which in turn stimulate enzymes that tell normal fat and connective tissues surrounding the tumor to manufacture large amounts of estrogens. In essence, the tumor cells summon the immune system to feed them with growth-promoting estrogens.

This mechanism explains how a postmenopausal woman who's suffering from estrogen-deficiency symptoms throughout her body could be locally producing large amounts of estrogens within the microscopic confines of a newly forming breast cancer.

How Tumor Cells Attract the Immune System

Again, this information is somewhat technical, but if you have breast cancer and are researching it, this information could be invaluable in making an educated decision about what course of treatment, if any, to follow.

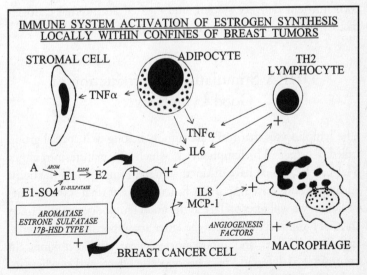

How the immune system plays a role in encouraging or discouraging breast cancer.

A breast ductal cell is surrounded by a complex matrix that includes fat, connective tissue, and blood vessels. As the cells of a breast cancer tumor begin to increase in number, they produce chemokines—chemical substances that attract the macrophages and lymphocytes to the tissue around it. Here's where the trouble begins. The normal job of the macrophages is to mop up the debris from damaged and inflamed cells, but the cancer cells trick them into sending out signals that stimulate blood vessels to grow and surround the cancer cells. Hence, the macrophages set up the necessary delivery system (blood vessels) that will assure the tumor cells a constant supply of nutrients in order to thrive.

The tumor cells also attract the lymphocytes, and these release two types of cytokines called interleukin-6 (IL-6) and tumor necrosis factor alpha (TNFα), both of which release a number of enzymes that stimulate the production of estrogen in normal cells surrounding the tumor cells, and in the tumor cells. Thus, with the help of the immune system, the tumor has set up its own nutrient delivery system, and created an internal estrogen factory that assures the ongoing proliferation of its cells.

DHEA Stimulates the Production of Good Lymphocytes

The lymphocytes that infiltrate tumors belong to a special group called T-helper (Th) lymphocytes, which can mature into either Th1 or Th2, which have distinctly different functions in the body. Although both have important functions in normal immune surveillance, we will refer to Th1 as the good lymphocytes and Th2 as the bad lymphocytes because the latter are responsible for generating IL-6, TNFα, and other estrogen-generating cytokines. In contrast, Th1 lymphocytes have opposite effects and produce interleukin-2 (IL-2) interferon, tumor necrosis factor beta (TNFβ), and other cytokines that inhibit tumor formation and suppress estrogen synthesis.

Whether the body decides to create more Th1 or Th2 lymphocytes appears to depend at least in part on its levels of the steroid hormones DHEA and cortisol. When DHEA is high, the immune system produces more of the good Th1 lymphocytes, but when cortisol is high and DHEA low, more of the bad Th2 lymphocytes are produced.

Inflammatory types of responses to injury, infection, and stress (emotional or physical) increase production of Th2 lymphocytes, the bad cytokines. This, in turn, can cause a remarkable increase in estrogens, particularly within the confines of a newly growing tumor. Some scientists are beginning to recognize one of the factors that influences Th2 production is the balance of DHEA to cortisol.

We know that DHEA levels drop steeply as we age, and that people who live longer have higher DHEA levels. In contrast, people who have persistently elevated cortisol levels have more degenerative diseases, including cancer. While DHEA production falls as we age, cortisol levels stay constant or increase. This imbalance in DHEA-to-cortisol levels sets the stage for more conversion of T-helper lymphocytes into the bad Th2 subset that tell the cytokines to invoke estrogen production.

Encouraging the Good Cytokines

As we learned above, the promotion of Th2 lymphocytes and their release of cytokines that promote estrogen synthesis would promote the growth of tumor cells. The good news is that there are ways to encourage the production of the good lymphocytes, which we'll review briefly below. Each approach is covered in more detail later in the book.

Progesterone Supplementation

Progesterone reverses the effects of the lymphocyte-induced enzymes that stimulate the production of estrogens, resulting in a lowering of estradiol production. Progesterone encourages the conversion of estradiol back to the weaker estrone. Progesterone also enhances the sulfation of estrone, which makes it less active, as well as its conversion to the "safe" estrogen, estriol. All of these events would reduce a tumor's ability to create estradiol and, hence, proliferate. Progesterone also down-regulates estrogen receptors, which helps prevent any excess estradiol from promoting tumor cell division.

Maintaining a Healthy DHEA Level

As mentioned above, a healthy level of DHEA is needed to maintain production of the good Th1 and its associated production of the good cytokines interferon, TNFβ, and IL-2. One way that healthy levels of androgens, both DHEA and testosterone, are maintained is by exercising. Meditation and stress reduction can also help encourage DHEA production. Much of the DHEA that your body produces is made in the adrenal glands, so nutritionally supporting the adrenal glands may also be helpful. This could include vitamin C, vitamin A, pantothenic acid, and herbals such as licorice. If your DHEA levels are still low, then you might consider supplementation. (See chapter 14 for details.) Keep in mind, however, that DHEA supplementation is not a good substitute for exercise, good diet, and a healthy lifestyle.

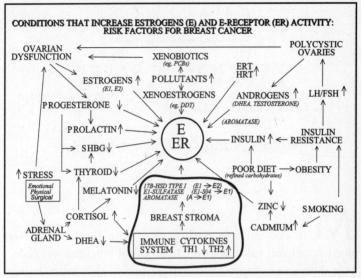

In this chapter we've explained how various parts of the immune system and enzyme systems contribute to changes in estrogen that increase breast cancer risk.

The Bottom Line

The bottom line is that estrogen is intricately woven into the initiation and promotion of breast cancer, right down to the level of your genes, your DNA, and your immune system. Exposure to excess estrogen, both from imbalances within the body and from sources outside the body (such as pesticides), increases the chances that things can go wrong at the cell level—which in turn damages the DNA, which in turn disrupts communication within the cell. You can protect yourself from these dangerous changes in your cells by avoiding excess estrogens, using supplemental progesterone if your levels are low, keeping your DHEA levels normal, and maintaining a healthy lifestyle that includes adequate rest, relaxation, exercise, stress management, and a wholesome diet that provides the building blocks of the protective systems that neutralize and safely excrete toxins from the body.

CHAPTER 8

ESTRIOL: A SAFER REPLACEMENT ESTROGEN

Mother Nature's Designer Estrogen

Most conventional medical doctors in the United States don't remember from their medical school biochemistry classes that there's an estrogen called estriol; nor do they know how to get it, how to use it, or what its benefits are. Estriol isn't even listed in the *Physician's Desk Reference (PDR),* because no pharmaceutical company in the United States sells it commercially. At the time of this writing, the only way to find estriol in the United States is through a compounding pharmacist. And yet estriol has nearly all the benefits of estradiol and estrone, but is much safer and has much fewer side effects. It has been well studied in Europe for more than 60 years, where it's commonly prescribed by physicians.

Dr. Zava has studied estriol extensively, and one of his mentors was the brilliant Professor Henry Lemon, who dedicated much of his life to the clinical use of estriol in breast cancer patients. Even though this is a book about breast cancer, we're going to give you the full story on estriol. If you're at a high risk for breast cancer, or have had breast cancer, and you're suffering from estrogen-deficiency symptoms, you can make a fully educated decision about whether to use estriol.

As we discussed in chapter 7, estrogen replacement therapy can be very helpful for some women. It can help slow bone loss, heal vaginal atrophy and chronic urinary tract infections, improve cholesterol profiles, and in some women help boost brain function. It would be great if these benefits were all that estrogens did for women. The bad news, as you already know, is that excess estradiol and estrone increase breast and endometrial cancers, and increase the likelihood that you will experience a long string of undesirable side effects, among them PMS-like symptoms, weight gain, water retention, gallbladder problems, high triglycerides, high blood pressure, breast swelling, fibrocystic breasts, and thromboembolism (blood clots). If you have or have had breast cancer, using supplemental conjugated estrogens (such as Premarin), estradiol, or estrone can be a risky business and is something even conventional doctors generally avoid.

The increased risk of cancer caused by estrogen, along with menstrual bleeding, are the two principal reasons about only 15 percent of the 37 million postmenopausal women in the United States take estrogen replacement therapy.

Can Scientists Create the Perfect Estrogen?

To get around this snag of ERT's adverse side effects, the pharmaceutical industry has been actively developing modified estrogens (often called designer estrogens), supposedly altered to promote some desirable estrogen property and avoid undesirable estrogen properties. For example, an ideal designer estrogen might improve cholesterol profiles and prevent bone loss, but not overstimulate the tissues of the breast and uterus, which can lead to cancer. These designer estrogens are referred to in the drug industry as Selective Estrogen Receptor Modulators or SERMs.

The first SERM was DES, diethylstilbestrol, introduced more than four decades ago in an attempt to prevent miscarriages. Not only did it fail in that attempt, but it also caused cancer and other serious health problems to develop in later life in babies born to DES-treated mothers. The estrogens of birth control pills are also SERMs and convey numerous potential health risks to users.

Tamoxifen is another SERM that we will cover in detail in chapter 12. During the tamoxifen clinical studies it was found that it modestly improves bone density and cholesterol profiles—increasing high-density lipoprotein (HDL) cholesterol and decreasing low-density lipoprotein (LDL) cholesterol. This is most likely what inspired the creation of the best-known SERM currently on the market, which is raloxifene (Evista). As chemical structures go, raloxifene is similar to tamoxifen, and it also improves cholesterol profiles and appears to slow bone loss, the favorable characteristics of estrogens. Raloxifene doesn't appear to have the growth-promoting effects that estrogens have on the uterus and breast, but there's some recent evidence that it increases the risk of blood clots. Although bone and heart protection, along with lack of uterine and breast stimulation, are highly desirable properties for an estrogen replacement therapy, raloxifene is missing one important component—it doesn't help eliminate hot flashes. In a recent clinical trial on 12,000 women, raloxifene increased bone density 2 to 3 percent and lowered bad LDL cholesterol, but it didn't relieve hot flashes. Since hot flashes are often no longer a problem several years after menopause, the conventional wisdom is to begin using SERMs such as raloxifene at this time to prevent osteoporosis and heart disease. However, we don't know what long-term effects these SERMs will have on the development of cancer. If raloxifene doesn't relieve hot flashes, it's likely also to aggravate cognitive dysfunction (inability to think) and thus significantly diminish quality of life.

We believe it's a form of hubris to think that a better estrogen can be created artificially than that provided by Mother Nature, particularly when we have only the most superficial understanding of how natural hormones work in the human body. So far the

SERMs have not been as successful as their manufacturers—and the women using them—have hoped. Each new SERM introduced to the marketplace in effect becomes a large experiment on tens of thousands of women.

Estriol: The Perfect Designer Estrogen

The ideal SERM the pharmaceutical industry is searching for is a drug that improves bones, cholesterol profiles, vasomotor symptoms (hot flashes), and brain function with less stimulation of breast growth or the cells lining the uterus (endometrium). Guess what? Mother Nature may have beat the pharmaceutical industry to the punch by producing the perfect SERM. It's called estriol, and it's been around for a very long time.

We were swimming in a sea of estriol in our mother's womb during the nine months of gestation. This means that, unlike the other human estrogens, estriol does not confer gender characteristics—its presence doesn't make us male or female. Estriol and progesterone are the predominant steroid hormones that we're exposed to in the womb when cells are dividing at a phenomenal rate, differentiating into hands, feet, eyeballs, brain, and myriad other functional organs. Everything that happens to our genetic machinery after birth pales in comparison to the incomprehensibly complex organizational development that occurs during our nine months of gestation. During this very critical time of our early development, when errors in the programming of our genetic blueprint are more likely to occur, we're bathed in estriol. Reason would tell us that this hormone must be highly protective of the DNA blueprint; otherwise we wouldn't be very successful as a species. The point is that estriol's purpose is obviously to *protect* our genetic machinery, not damage it. (Remember, one of the ways that the other estrogens play a role in causing breast cancer is by damaging DNA.)

Estriol has other features that distinguish it from other estrogens. Unlike estrone and estradiol, which rise and fall significantly during the menstrual cycle, estriol levels stay fairly steady throughout, with just a slight rise around the middle of the cycle.

Estriol is a much less lipotrophic, or fat-loving, molecule than estrone or estradiol. This means that when it's given in cream form, it's absorbed through the skin more slowly than other hormones, and it also means that it behaves differently in the blood. While most estradiol, for example, is carried in the blood wrapped in the protein called sex hormone binding globulin (SHBG)—which renders it unavailable to cells—estriol doesn't bind with SHBG as easily, and thus more of it is available to the body. We know relatively little about how estriol is made in the body, but it seems to be converted directly from androstenedione and estrone in the ovaries and in the adrenal glands. During pregnancy, estriol is derived almost entirely from the androgens, completely circumventing production from estrone. Mother Nature obviously has a reason for avoiding estrone during pregnancy and producing estriol at levels ten times higher than the other estrogens, estradiol and estrone.

Why We Don't Know More about Estriol

What happened to estriol? Why don't women in the United States have unlimited access to this hormone, which seems to have most (if not all) of the benefits of conventional estrogen replacement therapy, but none or very few of its negative side effects? The answer lies in estriol's creator. Humans didn't create estriol; Mother Nature did. This raises the proverbial question of who would profit from marketing it—and the answer is that no one in the pharmaceutical industry would, because it can't be patent-protected. This is probably why you haven't heard more about it from your doctor. Most doctors' knowledge of hormones comes from the pharmaceutical industry, which develops and tests new drugs that can be patented. The pharmaceutical industry isn't going to tell you about the virtues of estriol because it could devastate their bottom line. So unless your doctor has been perusing the libraries for more effective ways of treating postmenopausal women with safe estrogens, don't expect him or her to bring the issue up when you ask about a body-compatible and safe form of ERT.

Estriol as an Alternative ERT

Estriol, as a form of ERT, has been around for a good 60 years in Western Europe. Way back in 1958, more than 40 years ago, an excellent review was written on the previous 20 years of estriol's clinical use. Such clinical use never became very popular here in the United States, other than among a few innovative scientists and clinicians, because no pharmaceutical company would touch it.

Perhaps the first notable clinical study (a study that uses humans) using estriol to treat menopausal symptoms was reported in 1961 by Christian Lauritzen, M.D., a gynecologist in Ulm, Germany. He has spent nearly five decades researching the effects of estriol on women. In his pioneering 1961 paper Dr. Lauritzen showed that an oral form of estriol is quite effective for relieving menopausal symptoms without causing the typical stimulation of the uterus seen with estradiol. A handful of clinical studies in the mid-1970s, primarily carried out in Western Europe, continued to show the benefits of estriol. But estriol was up against a tough rival, Premarin, a patented product derived from pregnant mares' urine that contains the human estrogen estrone, horse estrogen, and more than 100 other active ingredients. The patent on Premarin meant that its manufacturer put millions of dollars into its research, promotion, and marketing. It received FDA approval for use in hormone replacement therapy, and was backed by a well-trained sales force knocking on doctors' doors.

Because the pharmaceutical industry is not interested in a nonpatentable medicine like estriol, no matter how safe and effective it is, no serious multimillion-dollar clinical studies have been done on it, it has not been reviewed and approved by the FDA, no commercial brand-name product has been produced, no reader-friendly brochures are available to tell your doctor how to use it, and no sales representatives knock at your doctor's door to convince him or her that it's a safe and effective form of ERT.

Despite this great disadvantage, estriol did enjoy a flash of attention in 1980 when experts from around the world gathered to review its virtues relative to conventional estrogen replacement therapy, namely estradiol and conjugated horse estrogen (Premarin).

In his review of estriol, Dr. Robert Greenblatt, one of the foremost researchers in hormone therapy at the time, commented that "the ability of estriol to relieve vasomotor symptoms [hot flashes] and to improve vaginal maturation [prevent vaginal dryness] without inducing notable side effects, is sufficient reason for it to be included in the management of the postmenopausal syndrome." In other words, he felt that estriol should be considered an effective and safe form of ERT because it prevents menopausal symptoms such as hot flashes without causing side effects so common to conventional estrogen replacement therapy.

At the same conference Dr. Wulf Utian, now editor of the North American Menopause Society's journal *Menopause,* said, "Estriol, it would appear, has the potential for reduced risk but similar benefit to alternative estrogen or estrogen-progestin combinations." In his concluding statements Dr. Utian had the following to say about estriol: "The potential to minimize risks yet maximize most benefits places estriol in a unique category amongst the estrogens." The one drawback that prevented Dr.

Utian from giving estriol a sweeping endorsement is that it didn't appear to be as bone-protective as estradiol. This was the kiss of death for estriol, because at the time prevention of osteoporosis was "in" and clinical studies were showing that other forms of estrogens like Premarin were more effective in preventing bone loss. New research we will discuss below would suggest that estriol might be nearly as effective as estradiol for preventing bone loss if it's used in the correct dosage.

In 1987 Dr. Lauritzen presented the results of a five-year clinical trial of 2 mg oral estriol succinate in 940 postmenopausal women. As seen earlier in the smaller clinical studies, estriol was shown to be effective in relieving menopausal symptoms, while uterine bleeding occurred only rarely. More important, estriol was unequivocally shown to protect against cancers of the breast and uterus. During the five-year study period, only two breast cancers developed (three were expected), and no endometrial cancers were reported (three were expected). These results confirmed the benefits and safety of estriol as a form of estrogen replacement therapy.

Estriol Protects against
Breast and Uterine Cancers

That estriol is a very useful form of ERT wasn't news to Professor Henry Lemon. He and other clinical scientists had been saying this for more than 30 years. In fact, Dr. Lemon stated in a 1966 article published in the *Journal of the American Medical Association* that "Estriol offers a nontoxic, physiologic antagonist for ovarian estrogens, inducing little or no endometrial proliferation in postmenopausal women, which together with progesterone might simulate the protective effect of pregnancy upon subsequent breast cancer risk. In other words, estriol could be used as a form of ERT to protect the uterus and breast from cancer.

Dr. Lemon, a retired professor from the University of Nebraska, was best known for his extensive clinical and basic research on the protective actions of estriol, often referred to as the forgotten estrogen, in breast cancer. Dr. Lemon was an avid proponent of estriol as a form of estrogen replacement therapy and breast cancer preventive; he spent nearly his entire professional career researching the effects of estriol in preventing breast cancer.

In animal model studies of breast cancer, Dr. Lemon demonstrated that when rats were pretreated with estriol prior to exposure to cancer-causing radiation or chemicals, the development of mammary tumors was significantly reduced. The same protection was not seen with estradiol or estrone. This protective effect was attributed to estriol's ability to induce a more mature state of the breast glandular cells, rendering them less susceptible to damage by radiation and chemicals. This ability is the same mechanism by which early pregnancy results in as much as a 50 to 70 percent reduction in breast cancer later in life: pregnancy raises estriol levels dramatically.

Another mechanism by which estriol might be protective against reproductive cancers is that it appears to get preferential treatment on estrogen receptors. In other words, if estradiol, estrone, and estriol are all competing for the same estrogen receptor, it's likely that the estriol will get in, diminishing the cell-stimulating properties of the other estrogens.

Estriol for the Prevention of Breast Cancer?

In his animal studies Dr. Lemon demonstrated that estriol matures the breast cells, shielding them from damage by radiation, chemical carcinogens, and estrogens such as estradiol and estrone. This is precisely what estriol does to the breast ductal cells during pregnancy in humans: It's one of the factors that cause them to mature to a state less susceptible to development of cancer later in life.

High Levels of Estriol Mean Lower Risk of Breast Cancer

Over his 40-year research career, Dr. Lemon also published interesting work on the relationship between the production of estriol in a woman's body and her propensity for developing breast cancer. He discovered that women who produce very little estriol relative to estradiol and estrone are at increased risk of developing breast cancer. Asian women have a high estriol ratio, and they have a much lower incidence of breast cancer than Western women, which is one of the many reasons why we can't assume that their soy consumption is what protects them from breast cancer. Although we need more research to definitively prove this, we believe that when a woman has low estriol levels, it most likely means that her estrone and estradiol are being metabolized to the harmful catechol estrogens instead of to the harmless estriol.

Estriol as a Replacement Estrogen in Breast Cancer Survivors

Dr. Lemon also researched how effective estriol is in treating women who already have breast cancer. His rationale was that estriol, unlike estradiol or estrone, had not been shown in animal studies or human clinical trials to stimulate the uterus or breast cells, therefore making it an ideal candidate for ERT in very high-risk women whose breast tumors were estrogen-sensitive. A clinical trial of 2.5 to 5 mg per day of estriol therapy in 28 premenopausal and postmenopausal breast cancer patients demonstrated that estriol induced remission or arrest of metastatic tumors in six (37 percent) of the women.

In an article published in the journal *Cancer Research* in 1975, Dr. Lemon stated "2.5 to 5.0 mg/day of estriol might be a suitable minimum dose for prophylactic [breast cancer preventive] therapy in premenopausal women. Such a dosage is far less than the daily estriol production of pregnant women, who excrete upwards of 30 to 50 mg estriol per day."

This oral dosing of about 2 to 5 mg of estriol daily is similar to the oral dosing that has been shown in various clinical studies, performed primarily in Western Europe, to have beneficial effects on menopausal symptoms such as hot flashes and vaginal dryness, and yet not increase the risk of stimulating the growth of the breast or uterus.

Estriol Prevents Vaginal Atrophy and Urinary Tract Infections

A common problem at menopause is degeneration of the vaginal lining, which can make intercourse painful and renders the vagina more susceptible to invasion by bacteria, causing urinary tract infections. This is thought to be related to the rise in vaginal pH resulting from the loss of ovarian estrogen production and colonization of the vagina by unhealthy bacteria. Several studies clearly show that a vaginal estriol cream can prevent such urinary tract infections in postmenopausal women.

In an Israeli study published in 1993 in the *New England Journal of Medicine*, 50 women were treated with 0.5 mg of estriol in a cream every night for two weeks, and then twice weekly for the following eight months. Forty-three women were treated in a similar manner with a cream that did not contain estriol. The results of the study showed that estriol treatment resulted in a lowering of the vaginal pH, a marked rise in *healthy* lactobacilli bacterialflora, and a decrease in the *unhealthy E. coli* bacteria that are commonly associated with urinary tract infections. Vaginal pH decreased to a degree that was incompatible with survival of the bad bacteria. Out of 50 patients treated with estriol, there were 10 times fewer urinary tract infections than found among the 43 patients using an identical cream without estriol. Better yet, the side effects of the estriol treatment were rare. The only reason women discontinued treatment was irritating effects to the vagina caused by the carrier in the cream itself. It was concluded that 0.5 mg of estriol is safe and effective when delivered twice weekly after two to three weeks of daily dosing.

In a Swedish study published in 1994, 0.5 mg of estriol delivered vaginally was shown to be equally as effective as a low-dose vaginal estradiol ring in treatment of symptoms and signs of urogenital atrophy (degeneration of the vagina, vulva, and cervix) in postmenopausal women. Marked improvements were seen in vaginal dryness, painful intercourse, pain with urination (dysuria), and urinary urgency with both forms of estrogens.

Twelve women using the vaginal estradiol ring experienced vaginal itching, urinary tract infections, *Candida* (yeast) infections, and pressure in the vagina, while only one woman using estriol had any adverse side effects. Once again, vaginal pH decreased in both the estradiol- and the estriol-treated women. What this study tells us is that 0.5 mg estriol treatment twice weekly effectively eliminates problems of vaginal dryness and atrophy without the adverse side effects often seen with more potent estrogens like estradiol.

Estriol Helps Protect Your Bones

Let's now look at a few of the clinical studies published on estriol for treatment of menopausal symptoms and bone loss. As we mentioned, early studies seemed to indicate that estriol was inferior to estradiol and other forms of estrogens (conjugated estrogen such as Premarin) in preventing bone loss.

However, in mid-1996 three Japanese studies, one Taiwanese study, and one Italian study took a second look at the clinical effectiveness of estriol in preventing bone loss in postmenopausal women. All three Japanese studies reported essentially the same results, namely that 2 mg per day of oral estriol increased bone mass about 1 to 5 percent over a one-year period. This effect of estriol on bone is nearly equivalent to that reported historically for estradiol or estrone (as in Premarin). The Italian study reported that 0.5 mg per day of vaginal estriol was somewhat effective in preventing bone loss; the Taiwanese study found that estriol succinate was ineffective in preventing bone loss over a two-year study period.

Thus, estriol shows promise in preventing bone loss. One problem with it is bioavailability. When it's delivered through the skin, however—such as vaginally or topically—blood levels of estriol rise much higher than if it's taken orally (in a pill), and it may be this type of delivery system that will prove most effective for preventing bone loss. Clearly more research is needed to determine whether estriol in combination with natural progesterone, natural testosterone (if needed), resistance exercise, proper diet, and mineral and vitamin supplements is effective in preventing bone loss and subsequent fractures.

Estriol Relieves Hot Flashes and Night Sweats without Stimulating Uterine Growth

The five studies mentioned above demonstrated that estriol improved menopausal symptoms (relieved hot flashes and night sweats) in most of the women and did not stimulate abnormal growth of the uterine lining (endometrial hyperplasia), which is common when estradiol or Premarin alone is used for prevent-ing bone loss. These studies also demonstrated that less than 10 percent of the women experienced breakthrough menstrual bleeding, which can be a problem for postmenopausal women who take conventional estrogen replacement therapy. One of the studies using 2 mg estriol daily reported that it also im-proved blood lipids, resulting in lower total and LDL choles-terols, lower triglycerides, and increased HDL cholesterol. This is significant, because the other estrogens raise triglyceride lev-els, which is at least as important a risk factor for heart disease as is high LDL cholesterol. All five studies commented on the remarkable lack of side effects seen with estriol.

There have been a few studies that showed minor uterine stimulation and a slight increase in uterine cancer with high doses of unopposed oral estriol (no progesterone or progestin), but to our knowledge none of the studies using topical estriol in physiologic doses (with or without progesterone) showed such results. Since we always recommend that estriol, oral or topical, be used in physiologic doses and in conjunction with a proges-terone cream, uterine stimulation should not be a problem.

Estriol Doesn't Cause Blood Clots, but Other Estrogens Do

A very serious problem with using estradiol or estrone in a mi-nority of women (1 in 5,000) is that it increases the risk of death due to deep vein thromboembolism, which means the forma-tion of life-threatening blood clots in the veins. Estriol, on the other hand, has very little effect on the blood-clotting factors. Doses as high as 8 mg per day have not been found to increase the risk of blood clotting. Dr. Lemon also noted that estriol did not cause any problems related to thromboembolism in his clinical study exploring the use of estriol for treatment of menopausal symptoms in breast cancer patients. This was also the consensus of the review committee that met in the 1980s to review the clinical efficacy of estriol.

Estriol Protects the Skin from Aging

It's well recognized that the time around menopause is associated with more rapid aging of the skin. Estrogens are important for the structural proteins collagen and elastin, which give the skin elasticity and structure, as well as hyaluronic acid, a naturally occurring moisture retainer under the skin. Studies published in the mid- to late 1990s have shown that estriol, applied as a skin cream directly to the face, remarkably reversed wrinkling and other problems of skin aging associated with the onset of menopause.

In a study published in the *International Journal of Dermatology* in 1996, objective improvements (meaning that parameters were measured by precise objective testing rather than by patient report) in skin vascularization, skin elasticity and firmness, moisture content, wrinkle depth, and pore size were seen in 73 to 100 percent of 30 women using a 0.3 percent estriol cream for six months. Estradiol was equally effective, but it also increased the circulating concentration of the hormone prolactin, which is a risk factor for breast cancer. Small tissue sections were removed, and the skin was analyzed under the microscope for changes in collagen and elastin. The investigators found that there was a remarkable increase in type III collagen, which is widely distributed throughout the body but found predominantly in baby skin. The nearly thousandfold increase in the circulating concentrations of estriol found during pregnancy probably account for the softening of the skin known as the pregnancy glow.

Another interesting study worth mentioning was published in the *International Journal of Dermatology* in 1995. It showed that estriol skin creams are useful for the treatment of acne scars. Treatment of 18 men and women with 0.3 percent estriol cream resulted in 100 percent improvement in flattening of acne scars, 77 percent improvement in pore size, and a 47 percent improvement in skin moisture within seven to ten weeks of treatment. Neither prolactin nor estradiol levels increased during treatment with estriol, demonstrating that it had little if any systemic estrogenic effects.

The important point to be made in these studies is not so much that estriol will prevent aging of the skin associated with menopause, but rather that 0.3 percent (3 mg/g cream) estriol used on the skin does not have a significant enough systemic effect on the brain to cause increases in prolactin, which in combination with estradiol can stimulate the replication of breast cells and increase breast cancer risk. Topical estradiol, while it has the same benefits to the skin, has more pronounced systemic effects on the breast and uterus and would likely increase the development of cancers in these organs.

How to Take Estriol

According to Dr. Lemon, when the women in his studies took as much as 5 to 15 mg of oral estriol (a pill) daily, there was no increased proliferation of cells in the breast or uterus. The typical oral dose used in Western Europe is 2 to 5 mg daily, but because much of it is "dumped" by the liver immediately, this may only ultimately amount in 0.5 to 1 mg of estriol actually getting into the body.

Many clinicians use an estriol cream that delivers 2 to 5 mg. When made as a cream, the pharmacist should indicate on the container how much cream it takes to provide the 2 to 5 mg of estriol. When you deliver estriol to your body via a cream, it's delivered in a much steadier fashion than if taken orally, when it's subject to all the variables of how the digestive system and liver are working from hour to hour.

An estriol cream that delivers 0.5 mg, used every other day, has been shown very effective for treating vaginal atrophy and urinary tract infections. Published studies show that 0.5 mg estriol delivered every other day for two weeks is adequate for most women, and this is how estriol is used by most women in Western Europe. The reason estriol is used only every other day is that it doesn't clear from the body as fast as other estrogens; one dose lasts for two days. Using it every day could result in excessively high levels. Although estriol does not absorb through the skin as rapidly as estradiol or estrone, studies have shown that topical delivery of estriol is about 20 times more efficient than oral delivery.

The Best SERM Nature Has to Offer

Estriol has a place beside natural progesterone in hormone replacement therapy for women who have breast cancer but need some estrogen. Estriol fits the bill as a very useful "designer estrogen," or SERM, since it prevents or reduces bone loss, alleviates menopausal symptoms, improves skin texture, prevents vaginal atrophy and urinary tract infections, improves blood lipids, and helps prevent cancers of the breast and uterus.

Researchers spent nearly 40 years trying to construct a better progesterone for hormone replacement therapy, to no avail. No synthetic progestins have ever been shown to have all the benefits of progesterone—and all come with a host of unpleasant side effects. Unfortunately, the pharmaceutical industry that brought you synthetic progestins is now introducing all kinds of SERMs to the clinical marketplace and your doctor. We hope that the computer age's more effective dissemination of information will prevent us from making the same mistake in trying to develop a better SERM than estriol.

CHAPTER 9

THE NATURE
OF PROGESTERONE

The Great Protector

As you are already discovering, progesterone is an important factor in the prevention and treatment of breast cancer. The purpose of this chapter is to understand the nature of progesterone, the hormone so long neglected by conventional medicine.

Progesterone is one of the sex hormones, along with the estrogens and testosterone. The appellation *sex hormone* refers to the fact that most progesterone in humans is made by gonads, which are the ovaries in females and the testes in males. Smaller amounts of progesterone are produced by Schwann cells (for making myelin, the protective cover of nerves), brain cells (for making myelin in the peripheral nervous system), and adrenal glands (as a precursor for the synthesis of steroids such as cortisol). Prodigious amounts of progesterone are made by the placenta during pregnancy, being necessary both for the survival and development of the fetus and for preventing uterine contractions that otherwise might cause premature labor.

In nonpregnant ovulating women, progesterone production occurs from ovulation until a day or so before the menstrual period begins. Daily production ranges from 4 to 28 mg per day, the common range being 15 to 20 mg per day, usually from day 12 to day 26 of a 28-day menstrual month. It's a relatively weak hormone compared to estradiol, for instance, which is produced in amounts of only 0.3 mg per day, usually from day 8 to day 26 of the menstrual month. During pregnancy, placental production of progesterone rises to 300 to 350 mg per day in the last trimester.

Again in nonpregnant ovulating women, progesterone is produced by the corpus luteum (the remains of the follicle that produced the ovum or egg that month). Its function is to prepare and maintain the secretory endometrium (the blood-filled lining of the uterus) in anticipation of the arrival and implantation of a fertilized egg, and survival of the developing embryo. If fertilization doesn't occur within 12 days or so, progesterone production stops. The rapid decline of progesterone and estrogen levels is the signal for the shedding of the blood-rich endometrium (menstruation), leading to another monthly cycle. If fertilization does occur, the conceptus releases hCG (human chorionic gonadotropin), which signals the corpus luteum to increase its progesterone production to prevent shedding and uterine contractions, thereby helping ensure the survival of the pregnancy. It is this action of the hormone to protect and promote gestation that led to the name *progesterone*.

The role of progesterone isn't limited to its progestation effects. Progesterone, like other hormones, creates its effects by circulating through the bloodstream to bind to specific receptors in cells of programmed target tissues. Progesterone receptors are found in many tissues of the body, indicating that it has important effects throughout the body. It, like testosterone, is an anabolic steroid, meaning that it helps build tissue, creates energy, and is essential for the growth and repair of body tissues.

It should be remembered that hormones do not work in isolation: Each is part of a vast complex network of other hormones and metabolic mediators. This is especially true of progesterone and estrogen. They work essentially as a team despite the fact that a number of their respective roles appear to be opposing. The resulting effect of their respective roles is, in fact, due to the balance of the two hormones. This is not unlike the concept of yin and yang in the Taoist tradition. The following chart provides an indication of this teamwork between estrogen and progesterone.

PHYSIOLOGIC EFFECTS OF ESTROGEN AND PROGESTERONE

ESTROGEN EFFECTS	PROGESTERONE EFFECTS
Creates proliferative endometrium	Maintains secretory endometrium
Causes breast cell stimulation (fibrocystic breasts*)	Protects against breast fibrocysts
Increases body fat and weight gain*	Helps use fat for energy
Causes salt and fluid retention*	Acts as natural diuretic
Causes depression, anxiety, and headaches*	Acts as natural antidepressant and calms anxiety
Causes cyclical migraines*	Prevents cyclical migraines
Causes poor sleep patterns*	Promotes normal sleep patterns
Interferes with thyroid hormone function*	Facilitates thyroid hormone function
Impairs blood sugar control*	Helps normalize blood sugar levels
Increases risk of blood clots*	Normalizes blood clotting
Has little or no libido effect*	Helps restore normal libido
Causes loss of zinc and retention of copper*	Normalizes zinc and copper levels
Reduces oxygen levels in all cells*	Restores proper cell oxygen levels
Causes endometrial cancer*	Prevents endometrial cancer
Increases risk of breast cancer*	Helps prevent breast cancer
Increases risk of prostate cancer*	Decreases risk of prostate cancer
Restrains bone loss	Stimulates new bone formation
Reduces vascular tone (dilates blood vessels)	Improves vascular tone
Triggers autoimmune diseases*	Prevents autoimmune diseases
Creates progesterone receptors	Increases sensitivity of estrogen receptors
Relieves hot flashes	Necessary for survival of embryo
Prevents vaginal dryness and mucosal atrophy	Precursor of corticosteroid biosynthesis
Increases risk of gallbladder disease*	Prevents coronary artery spasm and atherosclerotic plaque
Improves memory	Causes sleepiness, depression**
Improves sleep disorders	Causes digestive problems**
Improves health of urinary tract	
Relieves night sweats	

* Indicates that these effects are caused by estrogen dominance, or an imbalance of estrogen caused by too much estrogen and/or too little progesterone.

** Indicates that these effects are caused by an excess of progesterone.

Note that many of estrogen's effects are, if not opposed by progesterone, undesirable. Note also that estrogen promotes the development of progesterone receptors, whereas progesterone helps restore normal sensitivity of estrogen receptors.

Estrogen stimulates the growth of endometrial cells, but unopposed estrogen leads to endometrial hyperplasia and, eventually, endometrial cancer. Progesterone is the protector. Bones are kept strong by two factors: restraint of bone resorption (an estradiol effect) and increase of new bone formation (a progesterone effect). The concept of maintaining a healthy estrogen-to-progesterone balance is evident throughout this list.

For progesterone to work optimally, it needs a little estrogen priming. Estrogens are needed to induce progesterone receptors to allow subsequent response to progesterone. This happens in each menstrual cycle: The first half of the cycle is dominated by estrogen, with very little progesterone being produced. During this time estrogen is priming the tissues to respond to progesterone by increasing the cellular levels of progesterone receptors. The second half of the cycle is dominated by progesterone through its own cellular receptors. Progesterone slows estrogen-regulated growth by down-regulating receptors for estrogen. By doing this, progesterone prevents estrogens from further stimulating cell division.

How Steroid Hormones Are Made in the Body

The biosynthesis of steroid hormones begins with cholesterol. In cells that make progesterone, cholesterol is converted first into pregnenolone, which is subsequently converted into progesterone. Within the ovaries are many thousands of follicles, which are tiny sacs each containing an immature ovum. With each menstrual cycle, approximately 120 follicles are stimulated to make an ovum ready for ovulation and conception. The first follicle to release its ovum immediately involutes, turns a yellowish color, and starts producing progesterone. The involuted empty follicle, now called a corpus luteum, is the "factory" for making progesterone in females. The rapid rise of progesterone concentration in the blood is a signal to both ovaries to stop further ovulation. This discovery of progesterone's effect of stopping ovulation was the concept underlying the development of the first birth control pills.

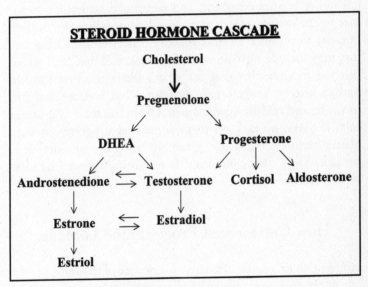

Progesterone is near the top of the steroid hormone cascade.

The body then uses progesterone for the biosynthesis of some of the other steroid hormones, including estrogens, testosterone, and the corticosteroids. This is what is meant when we say that progesterone is the *precursor* for other steroid hormones. Even without progesterone, however, the ovaries can produce estrogen and testosterone by other, more energy-expensive routes. But without healthy, fully functioning folli-cles, progesterone production fails.

By the age of 35, some 50 percent of women have dysfunc-tional follicles, leading to anovulatory cycles or luteal insuffi-ciency, along with lack of progesterone relative to estrogen. In previous books we have concluded that damage to follicle development due to environmental xenoestrogen exposure dur-ing embryo life is likely a major cause of this hormone imbal-ance. However, petrochemical pollutants can mimic other hormones besides estrogens, and continued xenobiotic expo-sure to the ovaries over a lifetime will also reduce the ovaries' capacity to produce a viable egg and progesterone. Other fac-tors may include nutritional deficiencies, bad diet, and stress. But the fact remains that for what's likely the first time in human history, progesterone deficiency has become rampant in young and middle-aged women. Given the many important roles it plays, it's rational to presume that progesterone sup-plementation should be given to progesterone-deficient women. Sadly, this conclusion is still being ignored by con-ventional medicine.

How Commercial Progesterone Is Made

Strangely to us, most physicians are unaware of the source of the hormones they prescribe. In brief, Russell E. Marker discovered, in 1939, a technique (called the Marker degradation process) for synthesizing progesterone identical to human progesterone from fats and oils in plants. By 1941 he found Mexican wild yams to be a good source of a special plant sapogenin called diosgenin, which could be used in the commercial synthesis of progester-one. Prior to this discovery, commercial progesterone cost $35,000 a pound. After pharmaceutical companies adopted the Marker degradation technique for producing progesterone, the cost fell to $7 per pound. Also, it was found that a similar technique was successful in synthesizing progesterone from fats of the soybean. The important fact is that the progesterone produced by commercial synthesis was identical to human progesterone.

The route of synthesis—wild yam or soybeans—is of no importance providing that the ultimate product, progesterone, is the same molecule.

Shortly after the discovery of commercial progesterone synthesis, the producers found that progesterone, being a natural substance, could not be patented. Pharmaceutical companies then devised chemical changes in the progesterone molecule to produce the synthetic, not-found-in-nature, and thus patentable progesterone-like compounds we now call progestins. These compounds may have some progesterone-like effects, but they don't convey the full range of progesterone benefits, and they all have undesirable side effects that don't occur with real progesterone, including increased risk of stroke and breast cancer. *Any* change in the molecular structure of a hormone molecule changes its actions.

The first commercially successful synthetic progestin was norethindrone, an oral birth control pill synthesized in 1951. There are now many different synthetic progestins. None of these synthetic versions should ever be used in treating patients with progesterone deficiency. There is no substitute for natural progesterone.

The great difference between progesterone and the various synthetic progestins is illustrated by the fact that progesterone is essential for successful implantation of the fertilized egg in the endometrium. (Ask any doctor who specializes in in vitro fertilization.) Progestins, on the other hand, can be used to abort a pregnancy during its early days, and they can cause birth defects. What further proof is needed?

How Progesterone Circulates in Blood

The progesterone molecule is smaller than a cholesterol molecule and, like cholesterol, is very fat-soluble and not water-soluble, meaning that it's repelled by water and attracted by fats. Cholesterol circulates in blood bound to proteins. The various forms are called lipoproteins (literally "fat-proteins"). Steroid hormones do the same. Estrogen is routinely bound to sex hormone binding globulin (SHBG). Progesterone, on the other hand, becomes bound to cortisol-binding globulin (CBG). Testosterone becomes bound to a mixture of several proteins, SHBG, and albumin. However, a portion of each hormone remains "free," or not bound to proteins. Only the free hormone is available to the body for use (bioavailable). Being lipophilic (fat-loving) and not water-soluble, the majority of free progesterone molecules are carried by red blood cells, whose membranes are made of fat, and not in the watery serum of the blood.

As we mentioned earlier, this situation is confusing to physicians who routinely measure hormones in serum. They don't realize that most of the free bioavailable hormone isn't found in serum. Thus, as Dr. S. R. Cummings and colleagues showed, serum testing (blood testing) of hormones is irrelevant—it doesn't reveal how much of the free hormone is present. Fortunately, the free hormone is soluble in saliva. When blood flows through the capillaries of saliva glands, the free hormone passively filters into the saliva. Saliva testing, therefore, provides an accurate measurement of free hormones that are actively filtering out of blood into tissues of the body.

A Semantic Problem for Physicians and Patients

As you may have noticed in the foregoing discussion of progesterone, we have consistently used the words *progesterone* and *testosterone* as singular hormones. *Estrogen,* on the other hand, is not the name of any particular hormone; it's a generic name for a family of hormones with estrogen-like activity. Each estrogen has its own name, such as *estrone, estradiol,* and *estriol.* Actually, humans make a number of estrogens, and different mammals make estrogens not found in humans.

However, progesterone is not the name of a class of hormones the way estrogen is. Many physicians mistakenly believe (thanks, in part, to misinformation from many drug company reps) that synthetic progestins are merely different forms of progesterone. None of them is progesterone. This error has led to many false conclusions. If a particular birth control pill results in facial hair growth, many physicians routinely claim that this is a progesterone side effect when, in truth, it's an androgenic side effect of the particular progestin used in the birth control pill. When the progestin medroxyprogesterone acetate (Provera) was found to cause an increased risk of breast cancer, some writers referred to this as a progesterone side effect when, in truth, real progesterone protects against breast cancer.

Progesterone Supplementation

Early on, researchers found that oral dosing of progesterone is unsatisfactory, since progesterone is rapidly metabolized in the digestive tract and liver before it ever reaches the bloodstream. In the process, 90 percent of it is changed into various metabolites; only 10 percent of the oral dose reaches the bloodstream. Injections were tried but, since the progesterone must be dissolved in some oil, they were often painful. Later it was found that progesterone is remarkably well absorbed through the skin when dissolved in an oil base, thus avoiding the loss of 70 to 90 percent of the hormone through the digestive tract and the liver when it's taken orally. Absorption through mucous membranes (mouth, rectum, vagina) is even more efficient. In a 1941 article the famous scientist Hans Selye, who recognized the calming properties of progesterone and its protection against stress-induced cardiovascular and immune system disease, wrote, "The fact that absorption of these water-insoluble, oil-soluble compounds may greatly be accelerated by administering them to surface membranes is perhaps of more than purely academic interest, especially since a similar improvement in absorption rate may perhaps be achieved in man by applying such compounds to mucous membranes." Selye was on the right track, but speed of absorption is not the most important factor. While rapidly absorbed via mucous membranes, the duration of effect is also shortened. When applied transdermally (on the skin), progesterone absorption into underlying fat is just as complete, but absorption into the bloodstream via capillaries in underlying fat is slower, leading to longer duration of effect. For this reason, transdermal application of progesterone is the superior delivery system.

Saliva testing confirms the excellent transdermal absorption of progesterone and most of the other steroid hormones. Estriol is the exception here: While it's well absorbed, it takes longer to absorb and isn't cleared from the body as fast. However, it is quickly absorbed through mucosa such as via mouth lozenges or troches, or by vaginal cream or gel.

It's difficult to understand why conventional physicians abstain from using transdermal progesterone. They routinely prescribe transdermal estradiol in the form of skin patches. In this form, the daily dose of estradiol is 0.05 or 0.1 mg. These transdermal doses are sufficient to match the estradiol effect of oral dosages of 1 or 2 mg per day. Is it not clear that transdermal dosing, in the case of estradiol, is 20 times more efficient than oral dosing? Why can't they see that progesterone dosing follows a similar pattern, particularly in light of the evidence that progesterone absorbs more efficiently through the skin than does estradiol?

Since the typical healthy ovulating woman makes 15 to 20 mg of progesterone per day from ovulation until a day or so before her period, there's little reason to exceed this dose of progesterone when supplementing progesterone-deficient women with transdermal progesterone. In the topical creams we prefer, each two-ounce jar or tube of cream contains 900 to 1,000 mg of progesterone. In typical menstruating women, progesterone needs to be applied only from day 12 to day 26 of the cycle. If the daily dose for these 14 to 15 days is 15 to 20 mg per day, the monthly dose is about 225 to 300 mg. This is about one-third of a two-ounce container. Thus, each two-ounce container will be sufficient for three menstrual cycles.

Women who have a shorter or longer cycle than 28 days should calculate their dosage as follows: Count backward two weeks from the expected first day of the period and begin the cream then. This is because the number of days in a woman's cycle from the first day of bleeding to the day of ovulation can vary tremendously, but the length of time from ovulation to the first day of bleeding is almost always two weeks.

In typical *post*menopausal women with less estrogen production, a transdermal progesterone dose of 12 to 15 mg is given for 24 to 25 days of the calendar month. Here again, the typical two-ounce jar will last for three months.

The two exceptions to this general plan are endometriosis and PMS. In treating endometriosis, the progesterone level should be raised to that of an early pregnancy, often 40 to 50 mg per day, from day 10 to day 26 of the cycle. In this case a monthly dose of 640 to 800 mg, or about two-thirds of a typical two-ounce container, will be required. For a fully detailed explanation of how and when to use progesterone according to our recommendations, please see chapter 13.

New research indicates that women with PMS may be unable to make enough allopregnanolone from progesterone. Allopregnanolone is the progesterone metabolite that binds to gamma-aminobutyric acid (GABA) receptors in the brain and has a calming effect. We have found that PMS is often relieved with higher doses of progesterone, which increases the level of metabolites and thus increases allopregnanolone. This can be accomplished by using transdermal doses of 40 mg per day from day 12 to day 25, often with a crescendo increase of 50 mg a day during the last three to four days before the period. Oral doses of 100 mg per day have also been successful in treating PMS, as reported by Dr. Joel Hargrove of Vanderbilt Medical School. We are hoping to soon discover a way for a woman to encourage the conversion of progesterone to allopregnanolone without having to use so much progesterone.

Progesterone's Protector Role

As can be seen from the list of estrogen and progesterone effects on page 155, progesterone protects against undesirable estrogen effects. Early in a menstrual cycle, estrogen causes a proliferation of the endometrial cells that line the uterus. At ovulation time, progesterone stops cell proliferation and converts them into a secretory endometrium with spiral capillaries full of blood for the nourishment of a possible implanted fertilized ovum (called a blastocyte at this stage). From this we can infer that progesterone protects against excessive endometrial cell proliferation (hyperplasia). In fact, 48 hours after ovulation and the surge of progesterone, all endometrial cell proliferation stops. This is the progesterone role that prevents endometrial cancer.

Emory University Medical School faculty conducted a meta-analysis of medical literature referring to hormone status and the risk of stroke. They found that unopposed estrogen was correlated with a 300 percent increase in stroke incidence compared to women with adequate progesterone. Progesterone protects against estrogen-induced strokes.

Estrogen dominance causes increased deposition of body fat and water retention. Women who are estrogen dominant are routinely overweight and troubled by edema of their feet. Farmers raising feedlot steers routinely give them supplemental estrogen: The steers get to market weight in less time and on less food. For the same reason, overweight estrogen-dominant women cannot easily lose weight by diet and exercise. Progesterone promotes utilizing fat for energy. When normal physiological levels of progesterone are restored, these same women can lose weight more readily.

Estrogen inhibits thyroid hormone action. Estrogen-dominant women frequently develop signs and symptoms of thyroid deficiency, yet their blood thyroid levels (T_3, T_4) are normal. Such women are routinely given thyroid supplementation despite their normal thyroid hormone levels. Progesterone, on the other hand, blocks the estrogen inhibition of thyroid hormone function. If such women are provided with proper progesterone supplements, their "thyroid" problem diminishes or totally disappears. Progesterone is protective against the thyroid inhibition caused by estrogen.

Cardiovascular disease is a case in point. Estrogen, though long touted as a protector against heart disease, is now discounted. Estrogen supplementation is found to have no effect on cardiovascular death rates and to offer no protection against atherosclerosis. Progesterone, on the other hand, has been neglected by conventional medicine despite excellent studies showing it to be cardioprotective. Hermsmeyer and colleagues at the Oregon Regional Primate Research Center convincingly demonstrated that, in rhesus monkeys that had their ovaries removed, medroxyprogesterone acetate (such as Provera) increased the risk of coronary artery spasm whereas progesterone protected against it. Additional research by Cheng, Lau, and Abumrad has found that, in cultured macrophages (special white blood cells), progesterone inhibits athero-genesis—the formation of cholesterol-containing plaque in the arteries, which eventually can lead to the blockages that cause a heart attack. Research by J. Koudy Williams at the Wake Forest University Bowman School of Medicine in Winston-Salem, North Carolina, reinforces these findings. Their research with monkeys also showed that medroxyprogesterone acetate likewise increased the risk of coronary atherosclerosis. At London's National Heart and Lung Institute, in a study by Peter Collins, women on HRT with progesterone could exercise significantly longer on a treadmill EKG test than those using HRT with Provera. There should be little doubt that progesterone protects against cardiovascular disease.

The immune system is also affected by hormone status. Autoimmune disorders are much more prevalent in women than in men, and more prevalent in women during the time of life when they are estrogen dominant than in women at other ages of life. Such disorders include rheumatoid arthritis, Sjögren's syndrome (dry eyes and dry mouth), Hashimoto's thyroiditis, Graves' disease, lupus erythematosus, and rosacea. It's not uncommon for women with these disorders to find that their symptoms gradually resolve when they balance their hormones with progesterone. Such cases strongly suggest that progesterone protects against autoimmune disorders caused by excessive estrogens.

Women who suffer from cyclical migraines that routinely occur only during the week or so before their menstrual period, or coinciding with its onset, often find relief by supplementing progesterone in the week or ten days before their period. Thus, progesterone protects against cyclical migraines.

Osteoporosis is rampant among U.S. women. Onset of the bone loss that characterizes osteoporosis commonly begins 10 or 15 years before menopause, at a time when women lose progesterone production but still produce plenty of estrogen. Estrogen treatment of osteoporosis may slow bone loss but cannot restore lost bone mass. Progesterone, on the other hand, stimulates new bone formation and can actually restore lost bone mass. This has been confirmed in both humans and test mammals. The mechanism for these hormone effects on bone has been found. Estrogen (particularly estradiol) inhibits the process by which old bone is removed to make room for new bone, called osteoclast-mediated bone resorption. In other words, it slows bone loss. Progesterone, on the other hand, stimulates new bone formation through special cells called osteoblasts. These are not opposing actions; both are needed for good bones. There's no doubt, however, that progesterone helps prevent and is needed to treat osteoporosis in women.

In both men and women, testosterone also builds bone. (For more on this topic, refer to *What Your Doctor May* Not *Tell You about Menopause*.) The clinicians we know who use a balanced and physiologic (what the body itself would make if it could) mix of estrogen, progesterone, and testosterone supplementation for women who have had a hysterectomy are having excellent results with building bone and maintaining bone density.

Hormones are important to brain function. Estrogen increases the excitability of brain cells, whereas progesterone decreases it. An excess or deficiency of either hormone results in less-than-optimal brain function. Excessive unopposed estrogen can cause anxiety, insomnia, and even panic reactions. Progesterone has been used successfully to control seizure disorders such as epilepsy. Excess estrogen causes edginess and an inability to concentrate. Progesterone and testosterone increase your ability to focus and concentrate calmly on the problem at hand. Grossly excessive progesterone can lead to mental lethargy. Grossly excessive testosterone causes aggressive outbursts, and lack of testosterone (as in men treated with castration and androgen blockade) can lead to depression and dementia. Each hormone has its role, and the right balance of hormones is the key.

Fibrocystic breasts are another good example of progesterone's benefits. This condition causes breast swelling each month, usually premenstrually, accompanied by considerable discomfort. The diagnosis can be validated by mammograms. Conventional treatments using synthetic androgens (male hormones) aren't very successful and promote androgenic side effects such as facial hair. In the late 1970s Dr. Regine Sitruk-Ware of France found that women with fibrocystic breasts were estrogen dominant: Their ratio of estrogen to progesterone was high compared to control women. He referred to the fibrocystic breast condition as benign breast disease. The BBD women were treated with transdermal progesterone, and Dr. Sitruk-Ware observed that the majority of them cleared and their breasts returned to normal within three to four months. This was published in *Obstetrics and Gynecology* in 1979. As the story goes, Dr. Sitruk-Ware was challenged to prove that the hormone ratio had been changed by the progesterone treatment, but blood (serum) tests did not reflect much change. The work of K. J. Chang, done in 1995 and described in chapter 6, proved through biopsy that not only was progesterone absorbed, but it also caused remarkable changes in breast cell replication, all without significant changes in serum progesterone levels. Because of the blood test results, Sitruk-Ware's critics discounted his good work, and his discovery of an effective treatment for fibrocystic breasts was lost for 16 years. Dr. Sitruk-Ware apparently did not realize that progesterone absorbed transdermally circulates in blood via red blood cells, not in the serum. However, Dr. Sitruk-Ware was correct: Estrogen dominance is the cause of fibrocystic breasts, and topical progesterone supplementation is the preferable treatment. Most physicians today are still unaware of this.

In breast tissue, estrogen stimulates breast duct cells to proliferate, whereas progesterone inhibits this proliferation and causes maturation and differentiation of the cells, making them more resistant to cancerous changes. Such effects have been demonstrated in both premenopausal and menopausal women. Breast duct cell proliferation is considered to be an early sign of the changes that lead to breast cancer. Therefore, it's reasonable to infer that progesterone protects against breast cancer. The evidence isn't hard to find. In 1981 L. D. Cowan and colleagues at Johns Hopkins published in the *American Journal of Epidemiology* their findings that women who were deficient in progesterone were 5.4 times more likely to acquire breast cancer, and 10 times more likely to develop cancer of any sort. In women with node-positive breast cancer, P. E. Mohr and coworkers found in 1996 that women with normal progesterone levels at the time of their breast cancer surgery had an 18-year survival rate—which was twice that of women with low progesterone levels at the time of their surgery. That is an extremely significant finding.

In March 1998 the National Cancer Institute convened a symposium on the role of estrogen as a cause of breast and prostate cancer. The various cancer research specialists who spoke reported finding the metabolic steps by which estradiol could indeed cause breast and prostate cancer. Two of the participants deserve special credit. Dr. Ercole Cavalieri of the University of Nebraska's cancer research center has discovered the metabolic steps that convert estradiol and estrone (but not estriol) into DNA-mutating catechol estrogen quinones leading to breast cancer. As we described in part I, Dr. Jose Russo of the Fox Chase Cancer Center in Philadelphia and professor of pathology at the University of Pennsylvania Medical School has demonstrated that human chorionic gonadotropin (hCG), a hormone released during pregnancy, prevents breast cancer by promoting maturation of breast lobules, making them less susceptible to estrogen-induced cancer. Also, in 1998 researchers B. Formby and T. S. Wiley of the Sansum Medical Research Foundation in Santa Barbara, California, showed in the *Annals of Clinical and Laboratory Science* that estrogen added to breast cancer cell cultures activated the oncogene (cancer-causing gene) Bcl-2, whereas progesterone activated the cancer-protective gene p53. In 1996 Dr. William Hrushesky of the Stratton VA Medical Center in Albany, New York, outlined in the *Journal of Women's Health* seven known metabolic mechanisms by which progesterone protects against breast cancer.

Studies such as these along with hundreds of supporting studies are the reason for this book. There can be little doubt that progesterone protects against estrogen-induced breast cancer. Further chapters in this book will detail the evidence that ignoring the factor of progesterone's protection against breast cancer has significantly fostered the present epidemic of breast cancer in women of industrialized countries. Success in preventing and treating breast cancer requires understanding the factors that cause and/or protect against breast cancer.

CHAPTER 10

THE NATURE OF THE ANDROGENS

The Part "Male" Hormones Play in a Woman's Hormonal Orchestra

Androgens are a class of hormones that include androstene-dione, testosterone, and dihydrotestosterone (DHT). Although dehydroepiandrosterone (DHEA) isn't, strictly speaking, an androgen, in a woman's body it can be quickly converted to androstenedione and testosterone, so we will include it as an androgen in this chapter. Androgens are commonly thought of as the male hormones, because they can have masculinizing effects, but they also play an important role in female health. Women make smaller amounts of androgens than men do, so they don't normally have the masculine traits of baldness, whiskers on the face, or a deep voice. The androgens bring many positive effects to a woman's body, and you'll find out more about those in this chapter.

Of the androgens made in a woman's body, about half are made in the adrenal glands, and the remaining half in the ovaries. When a woman has a total hysterectomy (both her uterus and ovaries are removed), her testosterone and DHEA levels usually drop to half of what's normal. Along with progesterone, the androgens are the most neglected hormone following total hysterectomy. Most women are given only unopposed estrogens despite estrogen-dominance symptoms and clear androgen-deficiency symptoms. The most common symptoms of low androgens following removal of the ovaries are low libido, depression, memory lapses, bone loss, vaginal dryness, and incontinence.

Androgens are also very important for the health of the skin. The cells of the skin (dermis), hair follicles, and sebaceous glands (glands that produce oils that lubricate the skin) contain high levels of androgen receptors. When androgens bind to them, this stimulates the skin cells to divide and thicken, the hair to thicken, and more oil to be produced. Because men produce more androgens, they have thicker skin, have more facial and body hair, and are more prone to acne. Women who suffer from polycystic ovary syndrome (PCOS) produce excessive amounts of androgens and have more facial and body hair, acne, and oily skin. These women generally tend to have greater muscle mass and are stronger.

There are many conjugates, or subcategories, of androgens that are intermediaries in the process of becoming one major steroid hormone or another, and although they don't have direct actions on cells, they circulate in the blood in higher amounts than testosterone does. These conjugates are one of the body's many systems designed to keep the steroid hormones in balance. Many of the androgens are conjugated in the liver, so impaired liver function (caused, for example, by taking multiple prescription drugs) can create an androgen imbalance.

Enzymes (referred to as aromatases) present in fat tissues can convert the androgens to estrogens. This is why women with more body fat have higher estrogen levels even after menopause, when the ovaries reduce their production of estrogens. This also is why many Western women have enough estrogen even after menopause; they have more than enough fat cells to make it. The conversion of androstenedione to estrogen in breast cells is an important piece of the breast cancer puzzle, and we'll explain why shortly.

Androgens are important in women as intermediates in the production of estrogen. In other words, the body makes cholesterol, which is converted to pregnenolone, which is converted to DHEA and progesterone, which are converted to androgens, which are then converted to estrogens. The estrogens are at the bottom of the steroid hormone cascade, and this makes the proper balance of androgens essential to the proper balance of estrogen.

If something biochemically interferes with the conversion of androstenedione to estrogen, it may cause symptoms of androgen excess, such as hair growth on the face, hair loss on the head, and acne. These symptoms, as we said, also appear as a symptom of polycystic ovary syndrome, which we discuss in more detail in chapter 4.

The effects of the androgens begin in the womb. All fetuses begin life morphologically as a female; if a Y chromosome sends out instructions to make androgens, the development of male physiology begins to take place. Later there are two phases of androgen production in boys: *adrenarche,* when the adrenals begin production of DHEA, and *puberty,* when the testes begin production of testosterone. Boys and girls begin adrenarche at about the same time. Boys produce only slightly more DHEA than girls. At puberty, a boy's testicles begin to produce more testosterone and DHT, while a girl's ovaries begin the cyclic production of estrogens and progesterone. The higher androgen levels produced by boys promote the characteristic male facial and body hair, thickening of whiskers, additional muscle, and deepening voice.

In girls estrogens suppress the expression of androgen receptors in the skin, hair follicles, and sebaceous glands, preventing the androgen expression so commonly seen in young boys as they transition through puberty. Progesterone produced by the ovaries also plays an important role in curbing excessive growth of facial hair and acne in young women by blocking the conversion of testosterone to DHT (dihydrotestosterone, the most potent form of natural androgen). Testosterone must be converted to DHT directly within the cells of the skin, hair follicle, or sebaceous gland before it can activate the androgen receptor in these cells. This conversion of testosterone to DHT is carried out by the enzyme 5-α reductase. Progesterone occupies the testosterone-binding site of 5-α reductase, preventing it from binding testosterone and converting it to the more potent DHT.

Young women who suffer from polycystic ovary syndrome ovulate less often than normal and experience irregular menstrual cycles, and instead of producing estrogen and progesterone, their ovaries manufacture testosterone at levels often equal to that of young males. They also experience the same androgenic effects as young males: male pattern facial and body hair growth, acne, oily skin, more muscle mass, thicker waist, and smaller hips. Women with PCOS also tend to have high insulin levels, which, as you read in chapter 4, can contribute to predisposing cells in breast tissue to become cancerous.

Androgens have what are known as anabolic effects, causing the growth of muscle, bone, and organs. The more muscle mass you have—whether you're a man or a woman—the more androgens your body will produce, and vice versa: The more androgens your body produces, the more muscle mass you'll have. This is why both male and female professional athletes dose themselves with androgenic hormones, because in many sports, more muscle mass means better performance.

Women who develop symptoms of androgen dominance such as thinning hair on the head, heavier hair growth above the lip, and a prominent belly may be lacking in the enzymes or enzyme cofactors (usually vitamins and minerals) necessary to convert androstenedione to estrogen. Androgen dominance can also be caused by eating too much sugar and refined carbohydrates, which chronically raises insulin levels. This is increasingly common in teenage girls.

DHEA

DHEA is a steroid hormone like estrogens and progesterone. It's made in the adrenal glands, which make more than 150 different hormones. Estrogens and testosterone are made primarily from DHEA, and to a lesser extent progesterone, throughout the body. The amount of DHEA made in our bodies is greater than that of any other steroid hormone. Ninety-five percent of the body's DHEA circulates in the blood joined to sulfur molecules (DHEAS), serving as a reserve that can easily be converted back into the active form. DHEAS is the primary source of androgen precursor for testosterone and DHT, but it apparently also has an important role in maintaining a healthy immune system independent of its role as an androgen precursor. We know that DHEA is important for the maintenance of health, but we don't yet have a complete understanding of its specific actions.

Between the ages of 20 and 25, DHEA production peaks. Men produce more than women, but both sexes make about 2 percent less every year after the age of 25. By the time a woman reaches her mid- to late forties, DHEA levels can be quite low, particularly in individuals whose adrenals have been exhausted from stress.

The onset of diseases such as cancer, heart disease, allergies, and diabetes, along with autoimmune diseases, correlates with this gradual drop in DHEA levels. We don't know yet if this means that lower DHEA levels play a causal role in these diseases, or if lower DHEA levels are a biomarker for aging in the same sense that gray hair and bifocals are. We do know that in elderly people, higher levels of DHEA mean better health and longer life span. When people with low levels of DHEA are given supplements, they tend to experience a significant boost in energy, immune function, digestion, ability to adapt to stress, feelings of well-being, and sex drive. Many feel that DHEA replacement actually takes years off their chronological ages.

There is also evidence that adequate DHEA levels help protect against osteoporosis, most likely because of its conversion to estrogens and androgens, both of which are important for healthy bones.

Before taking DHEA supplements, you should first check both DHEA (or DHEAS) and cortisol levels. If your cortisol is low, DHEA supplementation may not be as effective and may make an already low blood sugar (hypoglycemia, caused by low cortisol) worse. If this is the case, you need to consider lifestyle modifications (more sleep and laughter, less stress), better diet (more protein, less sugar), supplemental nutrients (particularly vitamins C and B$_5$, or pantothenic acid), and herbs (such as licorice), all of which help the adrenals produce more cortisol. You can also read the chapter on the adrenals in both *What Your Doctor May* Not *Tell You about Menopause* and *What Your Doctor May* Not *Tell You about Premenopause*.

If your cortisol is normal, you're over 40, and you are interested in possibly supplementing DHEA, ask your doctor to do a blood or saliva test to measure your DHEAS (the sulfur-bound form) levels. The normal blood range for women between the ages of 40 and 50 is 400 to 2,500 ng/ml; for women over 50, it falls to 200 to 1,500 ng/ml. These are pretty big ranges. If yours fall in or below the lower half of the range, and you are generally fatigued and have worked to balance your other hormones, diet, and stress levels, you might want to give DHEA a try. You can try using 5 to 10 mg of DHEA a day. Don't buy products advertising themselves as "DHEA precursors," including wild yam creams and pills, because your body cannot make the conversion, as much as these companies would like it to.

One word of caution: DHEA in excess can have masculinizing effects on women, and can also have the opposite effect of the low dosages—increasing your risk of diabetes and heart disease. This is much more true for women than men. If you start to see changes like acne, hair loss, or the growth of facial hair, cut back to 5 mg every other day or stop taking it. These side effects are entirely reversible with decreased dosage or discontinuation of DHEA. Have your DHEAS levels checked periodically as long as you're using it.

Testosterone

Women make about a tenth as much testosterone as their male counterparts. The adrenal glands and the ovaries are responsible for maintaining adequate testosterone levels in women. Testosterone gradually declines with age, with the steepest decline around the time of menopause. Testosterone levels of a perimenopausal woman tend to be about half those of a woman in her early twenties. After menopause, however, the ovaries continue to produce both testosterone and androstenedione.

Testosterone is one of the hormones responsible for maintaining libido, or sex drive, in a woman. Falling levels of testosterone around the time of menopause may result in a falling libido, although lack of sex drive is more commonly caused by estrogen dominance and associated thyroid deficiency. Studies of hormone replacement in women have shown that adding a low dose of natural testosterone can sometimes enhance the positive effects of other hormones and restore libido. The other side of this coin is that in many cases, as the ovaries wind down, women show signs of becoming more *androgen* (male hormone) dominant rather than estrogen dominant. Testosterone will only exaggerate this process.

Higher androgen production can occur in some menopausal women due to increased production by the ovarian stroma. The ovarian follicles no longer cyclically produce estrogens and progesterone, and the ovarian stroma begins to produce androgens in response to the increased levels of LH that occur at menopause. Facial hair and male-type pattern baldness are indicative of this shift. This can happen in premenopausal, estrogen-dominant women as well, because testosterone clearance from the body is partly controlled by the balance between estrogen and progesterone. Excess estrogen decreases testosterone clearance, and natural progesterone enhances it. (For those who are interested in biochemistry, this is because progesterone suppresses estrogen-induced SHBG, which would increase testosterone bioavailability, yet it also reverses androgenic changes because it blocks, via inhibition of 5-α reductase, testosterone conversion to the more potent DHT.)

If you've used progesterone cream for at least six months and still have a low libido, check your testosterone and DHEA levels to see if the problem could be due to low androgens. You should first check your androgen levels to make sure low libido is caused by low androgens, because this problem is often caused by other hormonal imbalances such as low levels of thyroid or high levels of stress hormones such as cortisol. In testing saliva, Dr. Zava has seen many cases in which women had perfectly normal or even high androgen levels and low libido. These women usually had other problems such as high stress and symptoms of low thyroid caused by estrogen dominance. Excessive estrogen or excessive natural progesterone replacement therapy can also suppress libido; if you're taking these hormones, check the levels of estradiol and progesterone to make sure you aren't using too much.

If you've balanced all of your other hormones and are still suffering from low libido (and you believe that it's a physical and not an emotional or psychological problem), then you might want to try a very small amount of some natural testosterone. It's easy to get it in a cream from a compounding pharmacist; some enterprising pharmacists are making testosterone lozenges, since it's well absorbed through the mucous membranes of the mouth. The optimal dose is usually in the range of 0.5 to 2 mg in the morning. If you find you're getting androgenic symptoms, reduce the dose, take it every other day, or stop taking it for a while.

Testosterone is available only by prescription. If you're interested, talk with your physician. Be sure to use only a natural form; synthetics such as methyltestosterone are powerful and can have unpleasant side effects.

Androstenedione

This steroid hormone is a precursor to testosterone and estrogens, and it can theoretically act as a DHEA precursor. Secreted from the adrenals and ovaries into the bloodstream, it has its own jobs to do before being converted into other hormones. In older women androstenedione travels from the ovaries to the fat cells, where it's converted to estrogen.

Androstenedione is a popular supplement for bodybuilders, who use it to boost their testosterone levels, increasing muscle mass and decreasing the length of time needed to recover from hard workouts. Many of the positive effects of supplemental testosterone—including enhanced energy, libido, and sense of well-being—have also been attributed to androstenedione, and this is due to its conversion to testosterone.

Androstenedione may also be involved in maintaining the strength of bones because it's converted to testosterone, which helps build muscles and bone, and to estradiol, which helps slow bone loss.

If you have testosterone-deficiency symptoms but aren't ready to try testosterone, androstenedione just might do the job. It's available in health food stores in oral and topical cream forms. Oral doses are usually in the range of 50 to 100 mg. Topical creams contain much less androstenedione (10 to 20 mg) but, according to Dr. Zava, they result in a much higher production of salivary testosterone than the oral products. How your body utilizes androstenedione is unique to your own metabolism. It will spill down the androgen and estrogen pathways, and how much of each is formed depends on your individual metabolism and, to some extent, your diet and body-fat content. The more body fat you have, the more likely androstenedione will get converted to estrogens by the aromatase enzymes present in fat tissue. The more you exercise and the more foods you eat or supplements you take containing natural aromatase inhibitors (such as soy isoflavones and chrysin) the more likely it is that androstenedione will spill down the androgen (testosterone) pathway. Some topical androstenedione products contain small amounts of natural progesterone, which is a natural aromatase inhibitor.

If you decide to try androstenedione, use very small oral doses, no more than 50 mg twice a week (or topical doses, no more than 10 mg daily), to see if your energy, libido, and mood are improved. Again, this can be a powerfully androgenic or male hormone, and it can increase estrogen levels, so it should be used with great care. Testing of saliva for testosterone and estradiol following androstenedione supplementation for several weeks will help you determine which direction the androstenedione is going.

Ovarian Androgens and Breast Cancer

Clinical studies have suggested that an excess of androgens made by the ovaries is connected to an increased breast cancer incidence. This stems from clinical research showing that breast cancer patients, and women at high risk for developing breast cancer, have higher urinary levels of testosterone and other androgens. High ovarian production of androgens is closely associated with chronic anovulatory syndrome (menstrual cycles in which a woman does not ovulate) and the consequent low production of progesterone. All of the studies that have found elevated levels of androgens in women with breast cancer have also reported a high incidence of anovulatory cycles, or a low ovarian production of progesterone. However, things are not always straightforward in biochemistry, and this association does not mean that androgens cause or promote breast cancer—quite the contrary. Scientists refer to this as an epiphenomenon, meaning that high androgens are coassociated with breast cancer but not related to its cause. In fact, the high androgens may be the body's attempt to correct the hormonal imbalance caused by estrogen dominance and a lack of progesterone.

Androgens inhibit the growth of normal breast tissue, and have been shown both in experimental studies of human breast cancer cells and in androgen replacement therapies in postmenopausal women to actually decrease the incidence of breast cancer.

In postmenopausal women whose high androgens are associated with increased breast cancer risk, follicle-stimulating hormone levels are usually elevated. FSH increases aromatase activity in some breast tissue, which converts ovarian androgens like androstenedione to estrogens. Thus, it is conceivable that *premenopausal* women who have polycystic ovaries, anovulatory cycles, and consequent high androgen levels may also be at higher risk of breast cancer as a result of local estrogen production in the breast tissue from androgens produced by the ovaries.

CHAPTER 11

THE PROBLEM OF ERT AND HRT

How Hormone Replacement Therapy Can Cause Cancer

Yes, you were right: HRT the way your doctor prescribes it *can* increase your risk of breast cancer. If you were one of the millions of women who refused to take HRT, or questioned your doctor about it, or felt queasy about taking it because you were afraid of getting breast cancer, you were right. To all the women who intuitively felt it was risky to take HRT but did anyway because their doctors insisted that the benefits outweighed the risks, you were right. And to all the women who took HRT against their own better judgment and then got breast cancer, this is a great opportunity to teach your female friends and relatives to trust their own judgment, to trust their intuition, to trust that sense of unease when you know something isn't right. HRT can increase your risk of breast cancer.

And furthermore, all those benefits your doctor told you were so important, such as avoiding heart disease and osteoporosis—those were highly exaggerated. In fact, the progestins in HRT could probably *give* you a heart attack, and you'll build at least as much bone lifting weights a few times a week at the YMCA as you will taking conventional HRT. The latest study on estrogen and Alzheimer's showed that the women taking estrogen actually did *worse* on cognitive tests. (There's no doubt that estrogen is good for the brain, but unopposed and/or in excess makes it difficult to concentrate and focus on much of anything. Most women know exactly what that feels like.)

As for those last few holdouts who are still trying to claim that conventional hormone replacement therapy might be okay for women who have had breast cancer, all we want to know is what happened to all their studies after the first two to four years? That's right. None of the studies done so far has gone on for more than four years; most have gone on for only two years. The silence from these researchers is deafening.

It's significant that HRT has a terrible rate of patient compliance, meaning that only about 15 percent of women who start taking it actually end up staying with it (we believe that for the past few years compliance with HRT has probably dropped to 5 to 10 percent). In contrast, compliance among women who use natural hormone replacement therapy (NHRT) is extremely high; most clinicians estimate that about 95 percent of their patients on NHRT stick with it.

Then there are those who claim that despite the increased risk of breast cancer in women who use HRT, women would be deprived if they didn't use HRT as they age; they should go ahead and ignore the risk and use it anyway. We encourage these physicians and scientists to at least consider natural hormone replacement!

In this book we distinguish among conventional ERT, HRT, and natural HRT (sometimes referred to as NHRT) because they are very different. ERT is estrogen replacement therapy, often prescribed by physicians for women who don't have a uterus due to a hysterectomy (surgical menopause). This is one of the deadliest and most costly errors in approach that conventional medicine makes. Estrogen should never be taken alone. Period.

Conventional HRT uses any number of types of estrogen— both natural and synthetic—usually in high doses, and it uses a synthetic progestin. In contrast, NHRT uses natural estrogen in the smallest possible dose when it's needed, and natural progesterone in small, physiologic doses that match what a woman's body makes when it's ovulating. Unfortunately, many alternative or holistic health care professionals resort to using high doses of progesterone when they don't get the results they're looking for with lower doses. This is not NHRT in any sense of the word—in the long term, high doses of hormones are not natural and are never a good idea. If NHRT isn't working, it could be due to adrenal dysfunction, low thyroid, chronic stress, or prescription drugs, for example.

The following is a composite that represents hundreds of pieces of mail (e-mail or otherwise) that Dr. Lee has received over the past few years from women with breast cancer, clearly defining the typical problems that can be caused by HRT:

> Dear Dr. Lee,
>
> I'm 47 years old and last year went to my doctor for my annual checkup. I felt fine but was having some irregular periods and trouble sleeping, so he put me on Prempro. In the next three or four months I gained 30 pounds, and became very depressed. My husband and I had no sex life, and my kids probably wished I would disappear because I was so cranky and tired all the time. I complained about this to my doctor and he insisted that it was not the hormones, that I was just depressed about "the change," and gave me a prescription for Zoloft. He said if I didn't keep taking the hormones I would have a heart attack and get osteoporosis and Alzheimer's. Then I still couldn't sleep so he gave me a prescription for Xanax. I was in a very mentally demanding job doing computer programming, and within six months I had to quit my job because I felt so awful and couldn't think anymore.
>
> As I write this it's clear that my problems started when I started taking the HRT, but it wasn't clear then because

my doctor was so insistent that it wasn't the hormones and I didn't even think to doubt him.

Then I found a lump in my breast. This was seven months after starting the HRT. It was big—about the size of a walnut. I'm pretty good about doing a breast exam in the shower at least once a month, so I can't figure out how it got there so fast. I had a biopsy done and it was malignant, and now my oncologist wants me to have a lumpectomy, and then radiation and chemotherapy. . . .

Here's the pattern in these letters:

1. A basically healthy middle-aged woman with some mild symptoms of estrogen dominance goes to see her doctor for a checkup and he or she puts her on conventional HRT (an estrogen and a progestin) without checking her hormone levels. In other words, he puts her on HRT whether she needs it or not, and regardless of symptoms. Much of the time the woman is given a dosage of estrogen higher than she needs.

2. The woman becomes estrogen dominant—and progressively sicker and sicker—but her physician won't admit (or doesn't realize, or doesn't want to realize) that it's the hormones that are creating her symptoms. These symptoms range from obesity and fatigue to gallbladder problems, dry mouth, and allergy. (See the list of estrogen dominance symptoms on pages 99–100.)

3. Within six months of being put on HRT, the woman finds a lump in her breast, and in some women it's malignant.

4. The woman has a lumpectomy or mastectomy, followed by radiation and chemotherapy. Her health is never really good again because of the radiation and chemotherapy.

5. After the surgery, the woman's body is no longer able to make hormones properly; her ovaries are damaged by the

chemotherapy or have been removed; her adrenals have also been damaged, resulting in lower DHEA and cortisol levels, and so she is hormone deficient. Because she's not producing hormones, she's at a higher risk for dementia, heart disease, immune system dysfunction, osteoporosis, and reproductive organ problems.

Giving conventional HRT with its high doses of estrogen and synthetic progestins to a woman who has been estrogen dominant on and off for years is, in our opinion, like throwing gasoline on a fire relative to breast cancer. What might have been a small breast cancer that her body was successfully keeping in check—and may have continued to keep in check for the rest of her life—suddenly blooms into a sizable lump. We hear repeatedly from women who found a good-sized lump in their breasts within six to nine months of starting conventional HRT. This is not scientific evidence, it's anecdotal, but when enough of the anecdotes pile up it's compelling evidence of a causal connection.

The History of Research of HRT and Breast Cancer

Researchers in the field of breast cancer and HRT started publishing articles in the late 1980s and early 1990s cautiously warning that long-term use of HRT could slightly or moderately increase the risk of breast cancer. The first studies found little risk in long-term use and a small risk in "current" use. The latest studies find the same small risk in current use, but also sharply increasing risk over time. These population studies are given added weight by dozens of studies showing that estrogen increases cell proliferation in the breast (see chapter 7 for details), and by a handful of studies showing that women with breast cancer had higher levels of circulating or urinary estrogens. Malcom Pike, M.D., even did a series of studies showing that in families with a genetic risk of breast cancer, the daughters of women with breast cancer had started menstruating earlier and had higher estrogen levels than normal. L. Bernstein, R. K. Ross, and M. C. Pike of the University of Southern California took two groups of women, one with breast cancer and one without, and found that those with breast cancer had 15 percent higher serum (blood) estradiol levels and 40 percent more urinary estradiol. The group also had 44 percent more urinary estriol. The fact that there was so much more estradiol in the urine may be an indication that the body is trying very hard to get rid of it. The excess levels of estriol may also be a protective mechanism: Estradiol that is converted to estriol would be safer, as estriol has not been shown to cause proliferation in breast cells.

Even in 1996 Dr. Lee was being castigated by his colleagues for insisting that HRT was causing breast cancer, but by early in 2000 the evidence was overwhelming. Noted Harvard epidemiologist Graham Colditz, M.D., who had in 1991 concluded that "current estrogen use increases risk of breast cancer to a modest degree," in January 2000 concluded, "Strategies for relief of menopausal symptoms and long-term prevention of osteoporosis and heart disease that do not cause breast cancer are urgently needed." His colleague Ronald Ross from the University of Southern California concluded in a similar study, "This study provides strong evidence that the addition of a progestin to HRT enhances markedly the risk of breast cancer relative to estrogen use alone. These findings have important implications for the risk-benefit equation in women using HRT." It's unfortunate that these brilliant researchers appear not to appreciate the value of NHRT.

The standard of care in conventional medicine is that when a woman has a uterus, she must add a progestin to her estrogen to protect her from uterine cancer. If she doesn't have a uterus (has had a hysterectomy), she's allowed to take estrogen alone. This is why the research showing that estrogen plus a progestin causes more breast cancer than estrogen alone is in some respects faulty: Virtually all of the women taking estrogen alone would have had a hysterectomy, which dramatically lowers all steroid hormone levels and thus lowers the risk of breast cancer. In other words, this research proves little about the risk of estrogen (ERT) and breast cancer, and everything about conventional HRT and breast cancer. British scientist Howard Jacobs, M.D., has called for using the lowest-possible dose of estrogen in HRT, which is at least a step in the right direction, but he's not quite there because he hasn't included the balancing role of natural progesterone.

In January 2000 the conservative *Journal of the American Medical Association (JAMA)* published a huge National Cancer Institute study (C. Schairer and colleagues) that examined more than 46,000 women, and showed that the conventional medical HRT regimen using estrogen and synthetic progestins (most often Premarin and Provera or Prempro) confers a higher risk of breast cancer than estrogen alone. The study received a lot of media attention, most of it shamefully misleading because the term *progesterone* was used to describe the progestins used in the study. Compared to no hormone use, the risk of breast cancer in women who use estrogen alone (ERT) is increased by 1 percent per year of use, whereas the risk in women using both estrogen and a progestin (HRT) is increased by 8 percent per year. This means that a woman who's on conventional HRT for five years has a 40 percent higher risk of breast cancer than a woman not using HRT. This is a *huge* increase, and yet there were still articles following the publication of this study suggesting that the benefits of HRT for heart disease and osteoporosis outweighed its risks. Not only have the benefits of HRT for heart disease and osteoporosis been exaggerated, both are almost entirely preventable with a healthy lifestyle.

This study was certainly not the first to show this strong a connection between HRT and breast cancer, but it was the first one so large and so statistically significant that it couldn't be ignored. In fact, Bergkvist (Sweden) reported similar findings in 1989; Willett, Colditz, and Stampfer found this in their Harvard Nurses Questionnaire study in 1995; and Oxford's Collaborative Group on Hormonal Factors in Breast Cancer study showed it in 1999.

Shortly after the publication of the *JAMA* study, the *Journal of the National Cancer Institute* published a study headed by Ronald K. Ross from the University of Southern California showing pretty much the same thing. This study was valuable because it did not include women who had undergone a hysterectomy—which automatically lowers breast cancer risk, with or without supplemental hormones, due to the fact that it lowers the entire hormonal milieu in the body. (This is not a good way to prevent breast cancer, however, because the lack of hormones increases the risk of heart disease, osteoporosis, allergies, and arthritis.) The study included 1,897 postmenopausal case subjects (women with breast cancer) and 1,637 postmenopausal control subjects (women without breast cancer) aged 55 to 72. The study showed that HRT was associated with a 10 percent higher breast cancer risk for each five years of use.

A Dutch study (C. J. Moerman and colleagues) that calculated the risks of women using HRT for 10 and 20 years starting at age 55 concluded that even for women with an increased risk of heart disease, the risk of breast cancer outweighs the benefits.

Perhaps with all of this evidence and the latest studies, this conclusion will finally sink into the minds of practicing physicians who prescribe HRT concoctions.

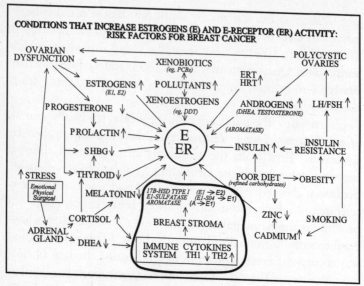

HRT occupies a small place on this chart but a large place in the causes of breast cancer.

Real versus Fake

The Schairer *JAMA* study was unique in that it finally directly targeted progestins as a cause of breast cancer. It bears repeating over and over: Progestins are not progesterone. Progesterone protects against breast cancer, progestins do not. Progestins are synthetic drugs that mimic some of progesterone's actions. They do protect the uterine lining from estrogen-caused cell overgrowth, but they don't protect the breast ductal cells from developing cancer. In fact, as we learned above, progestins can increase the risk of breast cancer.

As we've reported numerous times, there are many studies that show the difference between progesterone and the synthetic progestins, and, in particular, their differing effects on breast cells.

One of the most insidious reasons for the danger of conventional HRT is that many physicians have forgotten—thanks in part to constant lobbying by drug company reps and advertisements—that synthetic drugs are not the same as natural or bio-identical drugs. We hear over and over again from women whose physicians contemptuously informed them that the synthetic progestins are the same as progesterone. For these women, we have a suggestion.

The differences between progesterone and progestins have been clearly outlined in chapter 9, but sometimes the Socratic method of questioning works better to illuminate an issue, especially when speaking to a physician. Those who still insist that progestins and progesterone are the same, or that *progesterone* is a generic term that also covers progestins, can ponder the following questions.

If progesterone and progestins are the same:

- Why do fertility doctors always use progesterone and not progestins?
- Why do progestins cause birth defects, while progesterone is essential for a viable and healthy pregnancy?
- Why don't synthetic progestins show up in blood and saliva tests for progesterone levels? In other words, why doesn't taking a progestin raise progesterone levels in the body?
- Pregnant women are making 300 mg of progesterone daily in the last trimester. Why don't they have higher rates of breast cancer, as women do who use progestins?
- Why doesn't natural progesterone cause the side effects listed for medroxyprogesterone acetate (Provera), the most commonly used synthetic progestin for HRT?

For those who want an even deeper explanation of how hormones work, please refer to the appendix on page 427, where Dr. Lee has written a basic explanation of how molecules are put together (complete with diagrams) and how steroid hormones function in relationship to their structure and to each other.

Some doctors commenting on the Schairer *JAMA* study have suggested that women and their doctors should interpret this data to mean that they should use unopposed estrogen for a few years at menopause. Since it is widely known that unopposed estrogen causes endometrial cancer, blood clots in the veins, strokes, gallbladder disease, and weight gain, these doctors must be confused or uninformed. Furthermore, estrogen alone has also been proven to increase the risk of breast cancer—just not as much as estrogen-progestin combinations. This study should be interpreted as a clarion call to doctors to stop using progestins and start using progesterone.

It would also be prudent to give serious thought to how safe it is to take the progestins found in birth control pills. Depo-Provera, a long-term injectable form of birth control, is medroxy-progesterone acetate, the same progestin used in HRT. We already know Depo-Provera causes devastating side effects in many women, and there are no long-term studies of its effect on breast cancer risk that we're aware of. This *JAMA* study is a very good reason to stay away from Depo-Provera and reconsider oral contraceptives in general.

> An aside: About 6,000 women were excluded from consideration in this study because they were using "shots, patches, or creams." This probably means women who weren't using Premarin or Provera were excluded, but we also suspect there were many women in this group using transdermal and oral natural progesterone. We have not received a reply to our requests for more information on this matter.

Finally, it's appropriate to remember that menopause is not a disease, and specifically not a disease of estrogen deficiency. As S. R. Cummings and colleagues reported, two-thirds of women aged 60 to 85 continue to make plenty of estrogen. The problem, they found, is that many women produce enough sex hormone binding globulin to inhibit the activity of the estrogen they make. Progesterone researcher and clinician Helene Leonetti, M.D., found that in women around the age of menopause, hot flashes (classically considered a true sign of estrogen deficiency in early menopausal women) respond nicely to low-dose transdermal progesterone supplementation. Older women who have less estrogen, and who still have hot flashes, don't respond as well. It's inappropriate to treat all postmenopausal women with estrogen. A rational approach to hormone treatment would include tests of free hormone levels so that hormone supplements are used only for women truly hormone deficient, and in doses that restore normal physiologic levels, rather than the "one-dose-fits-all" approach. Conventional medicine projects a dilemma: how to supplement estrogen without increasing estrogen-induced risk. The dilemma may be a mirage created by overdosing. With proper endogenous hormone balance during premenopausal years, women remain healthy. Why wouldn't the same be true if proper hormone balance is achieved during postmenopausal years?

Since the benefits and safety of progesterone, and the disadvantages of synthetic progestins, are so clear, why are physicians so reluctant to use it in HRT? One reason often put forth is that physicians are waiting for a double blind, placebo-controlled study to prove to them that topical progesterone does indeed prevent estrogen-induced endometrial proliferation as, for example, medroxyprogesterone acetate (MPA) does. They need to wait no longer. Dr. Helene Leonetti and colleagues have published just such a study, finding that both vaginal and transdermal progesterone, in low physiologic doses, effectively blocks endometrial cell proliferation in postmenopausal women receiving Premarin.

The Politics of HRT

It's clear that the scientific research has been telling us for about a decade that HRT increases the risk of breast cancer, but few conventional doctors have listened. More recently, large-scale studies published in top medical journals have provided strong evidence that can no longer be ignored. This is a good example of how biased drug company research can influence medical thinking and treatment for years before independent, non-drug-company studies catch up with the truth. In the meantime, people become convinced that these drugs are safe.

It took the medical community a generation to realize that the unopposed estrogen given to women from the mid-1960s to the mid-1970s was causing an epidemic of endometrial (uterine) cancer that killed thousands of women. It's taken another generation and thousands more deaths for the medical community to *begin* to admit that unopposed estrogen also causes breast cancer, and that even the HRT combination of estrogen and a progestin increases the risk of breast cancer.

We've already explained how most scientific research about hormones is controlled by drug companies, and how medical treatment for breast cancer is controlled by what one physician we know calls the "cancer industrial complex." Thus, physicians have had little to no evidence to turn to when they don't want to recommend Premarin and Provera to a menopausal woman. Prescribing Prempro (for example) to a menopausal woman is the standard of care in conventional medicine.

An aside: In case you have any doubts as to the extent to which drug companies are controlling physicians, did you know that pharmacies sell prescribing information to drug companies? That's right. A drug company rep can purchase a list of all the doctors who are filling prescriptions at a particular pharmacy, and find out exactly what they're prescribing. How's that for an invasion of privacy?

Most physicians don't even want to hear about natural hormones, mostly because they're afraid of the negativity from other conventional doctors and drug company reps that will accompany their decision to use them. The irony is that all the physicians we know who've switched to natural hormones have become the busiest doctors in town, with women waiting for months to see them. This is because women talk to each other about health issues, and once they find a doctor who's willing to listen to them and prescribe natural hormones according to their individual needs, they rapidly spread the word to other women. (Women also tell each other about how awful they feel using HRT.)

CHAPTER 12

TAMOXIFEN AND RALOXIFENE

Why Synthetic Drugs Create New Problems

The drug tamoxifen (Nolvadex), now widely used in conventional medicine in attempts to both prevent and treat breast cancer, is a perfect illustration of how economic forces can exert control on breast cancer research and treatments. Thanks to tireless promotion by its manufacturers, and an embarrassing lack of approved and effective breast cancer treatments, tamoxifen is the newly installed fourth tier of conventional medical treatment for breast cancer, after surgery, radiation, and chemotherapy.

What Is Tamoxifen?

Tamoxifen is a synthetic, nonsteroid, synthetic drug that competes with estrogens for binding to the estrogen receptors in some parts of the body, including the breast. When estrogens bind the estrogen receptors in cells of the breast or uterus, for example, this activates cell growth and division. When tamoxifen occupies the estrogen receptor in place of an estrogen, it paralyzes the receptor, preventing it from triggering the events that result in cell division. In this sense, tamoxifen is an estrogen antagonist or anti-estrogen.

It might help us understand how tamoxifen has become a part of breast cancer treatment if we examine its history. Much of the rationale for using tamoxifen to treat breast cancer came from research involving the effects of tamoxifen on human breast cancer cells in tissue culture flasks in the laboratory. During the past 30 to 40 years great efforts have been made to find accurate, reproducible ways to study human breast cancer in tissue culture. Several human breast cancer cell lines were cultured from the breast tumors of women, and these have been widely used for decades in research on human breast cancer. Some of the breast cancer cell lines contain receptors for estrogens and progesterone, giving us a wealth of information about the interactions of these hormones with their receptors.

Early on, researchers discovered that tamoxifen very effectively inhibited the growth of the cancer cells in the flasks that contained tissue with estrogen receptors, but had little effect on the growth of the cancer cells that did not contain estrogen receptors. Eventually the researchers discovered that tamoxifen did not kill the cancer cells, but put them into a deep sleep or quiescence. Scientists call this a cytostatic drug. The negative side of this type of drug is that when estrogen is added back, the cells begin to divide again.

Since 70 to 80 percent of all breast cancers contain estrogen receptors, this provided a strong impetus to test tamoxifen's anti-cancer effects in women with breast cancer, and clinical trials with tamoxifen began in the early 1970s. After the first studies it was clear that following five years of use, the cancer-protective benefit waned. It was also clear that tamoxifen didn't work for breast cancer tumors that weren't estrogen-driven, or when the cancer had spread to the lymph nodes. Further, numerous serious side effects of the drug emerged. It has been clearly established in both animal and human studies that tamoxifen quickly causes thickening of the uterus (considered a precursor to cancer) in virtually all test subjects, and in the first studies a significant number of women died of endometrial (uterine) cancer. In response, the World Health Organization has listed tamoxifen as a cancer-causing drug.

In other words, tamoxifen is not a really an anti-estrogen; rather, it has selective anti-estrogen properties in parts of the body for a limited period of time, and potent estrogenic effects on other parts of the body. Thus it became known, along with raloxifene, as a Selective Estrogen Receptor Modulator (SERM).

Other side effects of tamoxifen include a tripling of the risk of potentially fatal blood clots in the lung, and an increased risk of stroke, blindness, and liver dysfunction. And in fact, it has never been shown that tamoxifen reduced the mortality rate of women using it long term, regardless of its protection against breast cancer. In other words, if you use tamoxifen, it may reduce your risk of breast cancer for a while, but there's an approximately equal chance that it will cause you to get something equally serious or to die of something else. As far as we can tell, the so-called mortality benefit of tamoxifen was created by statistically lumping together DCIS patients with patients having a palpable cancer tumor. As we explained in chapter 3, DCIS isn't really even a true cancer and has a 99 percent ten-year survival rate regardless of treatment. It's probable that if you take the DCIS out of the tamoxifen mortality statistics there would be no mortality benefit. Furthermore, except in 10 to 15 percent of women under the age of 60 with node-negative cancer who've had a hysterectomy, tamoxifen doesn't prevent a recurrence of breast cancer, it only delays it—and at the high price of a nearly 2 percent risk of potentially fatal blood clots and endometrial cancer.

In a large study funded by the National Cancer Institute known as the Breast Cancer Prevention Trial, 13,000 women *without breast cancer* were given either tamoxifen or a placebo for six years or less (the average was three years). Reportedly, 154 of the women receiving the placebo developed invasive breast cancer, while only 85 women on tamoxifen did. The study had been planned to extend longer but was cut short, it's claimed, so those women on the placebo could switch to tamoxifen.

Among the women taking tamoxifen, 33 developed uterine cancer compared to only 14 in the placebo group, and those women over the age of 50 were at the highest risk. Women taking tamoxifen in this trial also had three times the chance of developing a pulmonary embolism (blood clot in the lung) as women who took the placebo (18 women taking tamoxifen versus 6 on placebo); three women taking tamoxifen died from these embolisms. Women in the tamoxifen group were also more likely to have a deep vein thrombosis (a blood clot in a major vein) than women on placebo (35 women on tamoxifen versus 22 on placebo). Women taking tamoxifen also appeared to have an increased chance of stroke (38 women on tamoxifen versus 24 on placebo). All of these side effects are well-known effects of excess estrogen. And remember, all of the above women were *healthy* when they entered the trial!

Other less life-threatening but very unpleasant side effects of tamoxifen include phlebitis (inflammation of the blood vessels), depression, nausea and vomiting, hot flashes, severe vaginal dryness, and vaginal discharge. Hot flashes and depression are very common side effects.

Spokesmen for the multicenter NCI study admit that tamoxifen for preventive use is indicated only in women with increased risk of breast cancer, determined primarily by family history. They estimate that only about 0.3 percent of women 39 years of age or younger would be candidates for tamoxifen treatment. Further, because of the increased risk of side effects with years of use, most doctors wisely don't prescribe it for longer than five years. And yet it's estimated that 60 percent of women in the United States with breast cancer have been put on tamoxifen.

We can draw two new conclusions from this study: first, that the effectiveness of a selectively anti-estrogen drug like tamoxifen further underscores the powerful role estrogen plays in causing breast cancer; and second, that because of the risks it carries, tamoxifen isn't the real answer to the problem of opposing estrogen's cancer-causing effects.

The European Tamoxifen Studies: Why Are Their Results So Different?

Two European placebo-controlled clinical trials, smaller but of longer duration than the earlier U.S. Breast Cancer Prevention Trial, failed to confirm that the incidence of breast cancer is reduced with the preventive use of tamoxifen. This difference may be due to a younger population in these two trials, to patient compliance rates, or to differences in the populations studied, especially in risk levels and in family history. Nevertheless, the results of these two longer trials, combined with the serious side effects of tamoxifen, cast doubt on the wisdom of taking tamoxifen for breast cancer prevention.

In the study by U. Veronesi and colleagues, while there was no significant difference in breast cancer frequency between the group that took the placebo (22 cases) and those who took tamoxifen (19) after 46 months of the study, there was a statistically significant reduction of breast cancer among women receiving tamoxifen who also used hormone replacement therapy. Among 390 women on HRT and allocated to placebo, eight cases of breast cancer developed compared to one case among 362 women allocated to tamoxifen. However, compared to the placebo group, there was a significantly increased risk of vascular events (such as blood clots and strokes) and hypertriglyceridemia (high triglyceride levels) among women on tamoxifen. Since all participants had previously been hysterectomized, tamoxifen's risk of endometrial cancer wasn't a factor in this study.

In the study by T. Powles and coworkers, 2,471 women aged 30 to 70 with a family history of breast cancer were given either tamoxifen or placebo, and followed for 70 months. The overall frequency of breast cancer during the trial was the same for women on tamoxifen and placebo (tamoxifen 34, placebo 36). Participants who were already on HRT when they entered the study had an increased risk of breast cancer compared to non-users, whereas those who started HRT after entering the trial had a significantly reduced risk.

The higher overall frequency of breast cancer in women in this trial compared to the Veronesi trial may reflect the difference in eligibility. Eligibility for the Powles trial was based predominantly on a strong family history of breast cancer. Of interest in the latter study is the fact that four cases of endometrial cancer occurred in the tamoxifen group compared to one in the placebo group.

In an editorial in the British medical journal *The Lancet,* Kathleen Pritchard of the University of Toronto suggests that the difference in the U.S. and European results may be due to the fact that tamoxifen only temporarily suppresses the growth of tumors, and that if the American women were followed for longer periods of time, the results might be more similar.

The Window of Benefit Narrows Even More

A year or so after the Breast Cancer Prevention Trial was halted early, the NCI published a report concluding that most women over the age of 60 have a better chance of being harmed than helped with tamoxifen, and even women younger than 60 who still have a uterus are in danger. Although the conclusions in the report are somewhat convoluted, it's clear that while women under age 50 are less likely to be harmed by the drug, the early glowing reports of a 49 percent lower risk of breast cancer recurrence aren't being borne out, and in the vast majority of women more harm than good is done by this drug.

This study was followed a few months later by one in *The Lancet* by van Leeuwen and colleagues showing that when tamoxifen was taken long term, not only did it increase the risk of uterine cancer by 6.9 fold in women who took it for at least five years, but these cancers were significantly more likely to be deadly. The authors of the study "seriously question widespread use of tamoxifen as a preventive agent against breast cancer in healthy women."

Despite this study, just a few months later the FDA approved the use of tamoxifen in the treatment of ductal carcinoma in situ (DCIS), which as you'll remember was already "99 percent curable" with the standard treatments of surgery, radiation, and chemotherapy (or more likely despite radiation and chemo). To illustrate the confusion that runs rampant in the breast cancer industry, the company that manufactures tamoxifen released a statement to the press announcing the FDA's approval of its use to treat DCIS. The release stated that DCIS accounts for nearly 20 percent of all newly diagnosed breast cancer cases, and that "the approval of tamoxifen to reduce the risk of *invasive breast cancer* in women with DCIS is an important advance" (italics ours). One paragraph later, the press release said that "DCIS is a *non-invasive* breast cancer" (which is true). And so far we have no evidence that women with DCIS are more likely to progress to invasive cancers than women in the normal population—in fact, one study showed just the opposite. Thus, we have a highly toxic treatment being given to women with a cancer that's already 99 percent curable, to prevent an invasive breast cancer, even though no studies show an increased likelihood of invasive breast cancer in these women. Obviously the cure is worse than the disease. This would be somewhat akin to giving a woman chemotherapy because she had a Class II mildly abnormal pap smear (an indication of a few abnormal cells that calls only for a repeat pap smear in six months), or cutting off your finger because of a hangnail.

One of the scenarios that we frequently get mail about: A

woman around the age of 55 with a malignant breast cancer that hasn't spread to her lymph nodes has had a lumpectomy, followed by radiation and chemotherapy. Her uterus and ovaries have been permanently damaged by radiation and chemotherapy, and she's having terrible symptoms of hot flashes, night sweats, mood swings, and depression. Then she's put on tamoxifen, and the symptoms become unbearable. However, her doctor, who *insisted* that she take HRT a few years earlier, now won't put her on any type of HRT to relieve her symptoms because he's afraid of a cancer recurrence (not to mention liability should there be a recurrence). If the side effects of the radiation, chemotherapy, and tamoxifen don't kill her, she has the potential to live another 30 years or so, but without her ovaries and without hormone replacement her risk factors for many chronic diseases increase dramatically.

It's tragic for these women that their doctors don't understand that progestins and natural progesterone are not the same, and that progesterone not only is likely to prevent a recurrence of breast cancer, but will often relieve most of the above symptoms as well. Women whose ovaries are completely nonfunctional often also need some supplemental estriol and maybe even some testosterone; recommendations on supplementing hormones in general are given in part III.

Misleading Tamoxifen Advertising

In a letter to the FDA, Cindy Pearson, executive director of the National Women's Health Network (NWHN), elegantly laid out the truth about an ad for tamoxifen that appeared in *Newsweek,* which no doubt inspired many women at risk for breast cancer to run to their doctors and beg for tamoxifen. The ad is also an excellent example of how statistics are deceptively used both in advertising and in writing abstracts of published studies:

The ad is misleading because of the shifting use of absolute and relative risk numbers. By juxtaposing text reading "women who took Nolvadex [tamoxifen] had 44% fewer breast cancers than women taking sugar pills," with text asserting that health threatening side effects "occurred in less than 1% of women," Zeneca is deliberately creating an inaccurate impression of the risk/benefit ratio of this drug. The average consumer reading this text would understand that she has a 44 percent chance of benefiting from taking tamoxifen and less than a 1 percent chance of experiencing the associated risks.

If the ad used relative risk consistently, it would say that women who took tamoxifen had 44 percent fewer breast cancers and 253 percent more endometrial cancers. Or alternatively, if Zeneca wants to use the absolute numbers to assert that women have a less than 1 percent chance of being harmed by tamoxifen, the ad should also explain that in absolute terms the women have only a 1–2 percent chance of benefiting from the drug depending on their underlying risk of getting breast cancer in the first place.

. . . We hope that the FDA will act quickly and strongly. We are especially concerned because we believe that Zeneca has demonstrated a pattern of misrepresentation in its promotion of Nolvadex. This is not the first misleading advertisement of this promotional campaign. Though the FDA has issued warning letters to the company regarding previous advertisements, the company is continuing to promote tamoxifen to consumers in ways that mislead women and put their health at risk.

Tamoxifen is not a risk-free drug. Healthy women have already died as a result of taking tamoxifen.*. . .

*Reprinted with permission of the National Women's Health Network.

The Public Citizen Health Research Group petitioned the FDA to revise the labeling on tamoxifen in regard to using it to prevent breast cancer in women at high risk of the disease because ". . . in the clinical trial testing the effect of tamoxifen in lowering the incidence of breast cancer, the number of potentially fatal reactions caused by its use was approximately equal to the reduction in the number of breast cancer cases that occurred in women." Another way they explained this was, ". . . Nolvadex produced a reduction of 2.9 cases of breast cancer per 1,000 women per year (the benefit) but also increased by 2.8 the number of life-threatening adverse events such as uterine cancer, blood clots, and stroke. . . . There was no difference in survival and no difference in the number of women dying of breast cancer (6 on placebo and 7 on tamoxifen). These numbers apply to the women who participated in this trial, 75 percent of whom had a risk of 2.0 or greater. Women with a lower risk would expect to have less benefit."

We know from research that tamoxifen halts some of the growth factors that are stimulated by estrogen, and this is a good piece of the puzzle to have. However, with its long list of serious and even potentially deadly side effects, we believe that the only reason tamoxifen is used at all is because conventional medicine has so little else to offer women with breast cancer. Within a generation, we believe it will be seen as a national scandal that this dangerous drug was prescribed to healthy women deemed at risk for breast cancer.

Just in case you're wondering about the profitability of a drug like tamoxifen, it's estimated that at least 60 percent of women with breast cancer are taking tamoxifen, and at a cost of about $1,000 per year each, that's $1,000,000,000 or a *billion* dollars a year into the pockets of the drug company that manufactures it. In this perspective, the few hundred million dollars a year that the drug company is putting into advertising and PR, and supplying tamoxifen for research trials and studies, seem like a drop in the bucket next to the profits that are being raked in.

The tamoxifen freight train is rolling, and despite the harm it does and its very debatable benefits, it will take years, if not a decade, to slow it down again. Many doctors prescribe it as a matter of course to virtually all women with breast cancer, regardless of age or whether they have a uterus, and apparently without regard to the NCI study warning against such indiscriminate use.

Tamoxifen and Progesterone?

Many women write to tell us that they're taking tamoxifen, and wonder whether they can also use progesterone. There's no contraindication that we know of, and it would probably help offset some of the estrogenic side effects, but the truth is that we just don't know for sure and have no way of knowing for sure without lots of clinical experience and/or studies of women using both tamoxifen and progesterone. We would much rather see studies of women with breast cancer using just progesterone, in which we believe women would get all the estrogen-opposing effects and none of the harmful side effects!

Raloxifene: The Other SERM

Raloxifene (brand name Evista) is a Selective Estrogen Receptor Modulator similar to tamoxifen. Although raloxifene doesn't appear to cause uterine cancer the way tamoxifen does, and doesn't increase breast density on mammograms, its side effects are still considerable. Its use is associated with a slightly statistically significant higher incidence of influenza syndrome (the flu), hot flashes, leg cramps, peripheral edema (swelling in the legs and arms), and endometrial cavity fluid. Of greater significance, however, is the finding that women receiving raloxifene were over three times more likely than the placebo users to experience venous blood clots: Raloxifene apparently shares with natural estrogens their well-known proclivity to cause venous thromboemboli (blood clots in the veins). This side effect of un-opposed estrogen shouldn't be taken lightly: Pulmonary emboli (blood clots in the lungs) can be life-threatening.

Raloxifene also appears not to have estrogen's beneficial effects on the brain, or its anti-inflammatory effects on blood vessels. Its overall effects on bone are more neutral than beneficial.

Although raloxifene isn't FDA approved for treating breast cancer as of this printing, this hasn't stopped a well-orchestrated public relations campaign designed to convince the public and doctors that it will work as well as or better than tamoxifen. A New York judge finally ordered the makers of raloxifene to stop advertising that their product prevents breast cancer, but the cat was already well out of the bag; women began clamoring for it and doctors began prescribing it.

A huge breast cancer prevention trial known as STAR is recruiting healthy women at high risk for breast cancer to compare the efficacy and safety of tamoxifen and raloxifene. The implication that women entering the trial will be "stars" would be entertaining if the potential for unnecessary tragedy wasn't also present.

We don't recommend that you become a drug company guinea pig by taking a not-found-in-nature synthetic hormone. It doesn't help prevent bone loss as well as real estrogen does, it can *cause* hot flashes, it raises the risk of blood clots, and we just don't know how good it is at preventing or stopping breast cancer. (Thanks to a study on the effects of raloxifene on bone that also looked at breast cancer incidence, chances are good it will be found to have a similar profile to tamoxifen's effects on breast cancer, with less risk of uterine cancer.) Being a synthetic drug, it's also hard on the liver, and *The Lancet* has reported a case of hepatitis in a woman who took it.

PART III

PRACTICAL ADVICE
FOR PREVENTING
AND HEALING
BREAST CANCER

CHAPTER 13

HOW AND WHEN TO USE NATURAL PROGESTERONE

The Guardian Angel of Breast Cancer

In parts I and II we've given you detailed information on the politics of breast cancer, risk factors, and how hormones work for and against you when it comes to breast cancer. In part III we're going to get down to some practical, hands-on recommendations for how to find out if your hormones are out of balance and if so, which ones, how to use natural hormones, how to eat and exercise for optimal health, and how to clean up the environment immediately around you to minimize your risk of not just breast cancer, but cancer in general, as well as chronic degenerative diseases such as heart disease, diabetes, and arthritis.

This chapter will give you detailed guidelines for how to use natural progesterone, if you need to. We'll address the specific needs of women who have their ovaries, women who have had total or partial hysterectomies, women who have endometriosis, fibroids, menstrual migraines, or PMS, and women using estrogen for irregular periods.

Our recommendations for progesterone aren't going to change if you've had breast cancer: It's always optimal to strive for balance to prevent a recurrence of cancer. Whether you want to reduce your risk of breast cancer or prevent a recurrence, balancing your hormones with natural progesterone could be your single biggest ally.

If you've had breast cancer, that's a good indication that something has been out of balance in your body. The imbalance may have been caused by your mother's exposure to pesticides when you were a fetus; it may have been too many chest X rays as a child; it may have been birth control pills used when you were a teenager or inappropriately prescribed HRT. It could be genetics, chronic stress, poor diet, or exposure to toxins in the workplace. It may be a combination of the above and more. Some of these factors you can do something about, some you can't. For example, you can manage stress better, exercise more, choose an optimal diet, and create hormone balance. For a perimenopausal woman, balancing hormones may seem more like a juggling act than a balancing act (read the book *What Your Doctor May Not Tell You about Premenopause* for details), because hormones are constantly fluctuating, but every small increment of positive change can make a major difference in your health. Finding the dose and timing of natural progesterone that's right for your body is important to hormone balance, and this chapter will help you do just that.

How and When to Use Natural Progesterone

Women differ in almost every aspect of their physiologies. Although genetically all humans are 99 percent the same, that 1 percent difference can account for an astounding variation in how the details work. It's not rational for a doctor to order the same dose of any given medicine for every patient, and the same is true of natural progesterone.

While medical professionals can give you guidelines to work within, it's up to you to find the best dose for your body. Ideally, you should be able to find the minimum amount you can use to gain and sustain relief from your symptoms. Because natural progesterone is so safe, it won't hurt you to use a little more than your optimal dose. That gives you plenty of room for experimentation.

On the other hand, as with most substances, too much progesterone can cause problems. As the use of progesterone has increased in popularity, health care professionals have developed many different schools of thought about how to use it, and many of them prescribe very high doses of progesterone. This practice is counterproductive and leads to further hormone imbalance, not to mention a handful of interesting theories about why the progesterone isn't working the way Dr. Lee says it does. Here's the answer, folks: It's the overdose!

Chronically high doses of progesterone over many months eventually cause progesterone receptors to turn off, reducing its effectiveness. Using excessive doses of progesterone can also cause the side effects listed below. But keep in mind, not all women suffer from these side effects when they use excessive doses of progesterone.

POSSIBLE SIDE EFFECTS OF EXCESSIVE PROGESTERONE

- **Lethargy or sleepiness.** This is probably an effect of allopregnanolone, a by-product of progesterone, on the brain.
- **Edema (water retention).** This is probably caused by excess conversion to deoxycortisone, a mineralocorticoid made in the adrenal glands that causes water retention.
- *Candida.* This is the bacterium present in a yeast infection; excess progesterone can inhibit anti-*Candida* neutrophils (white blood cells).
- **Bloating.** Excess progesterone slows gastrointestinal (GI) transport, and with the wrong kind of gastrointestinal flora, such as *Candida,* this can lead to bloating and gas. (During pregnancy the high levels of progesterone slow food transport through the GI tract to enhance absorption of nutrients.)
- **Lowered libido.** Excess progesterone blocks an enzyme

called 5-α reductase that allows conversion of testosterone to DHT, and thus overinhibits the conversion. This happens primarily to men who are using too much progesterone.

• **Mild depression.** Excess progesterone down-regulates estrogen receptors, and brain response to estrogens is needed for serotonin production.

• **Exacerbated symptoms of estrogen deficiency.** Excess progesterone down-regulates estrogen receptors and desensitizes tissue to estrogen. Because progesterone receptors are dependent on estrogen priming through the estrogen receptor, excess progesterone in the absence of estrogen can cause a lot of problems. Dr. Zava especially sees this in women who have very low estradiol and are taking large doses of progesterone.

Progesterone deficiency reduces the sensitivity of estrogen receptors. Many perimenopausal women with symptoms of estrogen deficiency (such as hot flashes) find relief by adding progesterone cream in physiologic doses, which are doses that match what the body of a healthy, premenopausal woman would be making.

Then there's the question of progesterone metabolites (some mentioned in the list above), the by-products created by excessive progesterone. In addition to the above-listed side effects, they certainly put an extra and unnecessary burden on the liver as it works overtime to excrete them. This happens most frequently when women use oral progesterone (pill form). As much as 90 percent of an oral dose is destroyed in the gastrointestinal tract within 15 minutes or so of taking it. The progesterone that's destroyed becomes by-products or metabolites that enter the liver, where they and the real progesterone are transported into the bloodstream. Several research groups, including one in France (Nahoul) and another in the United States (Levin), using highly sophisticated methods of analysis, came to the conclusion that about 80 percent of what's measured as progesterone by conventional blood tests is really inactive metabolites of progesterone. Therefore, if you're taking 100 mg of oral progesterone and your blood test comes back as 10 ng/ml, the real progesterone level is more likely only to be about 2 ng/ml and the rest of it inactive metabolites, or metabolites that are causing side effects rather than benefits. These metabolites aren't as likely to get into saliva, and therefore a measurement of bioavailable progesterone (through a saliva test) will give a disproportionately lower—but more accurate—level than blood progesterone tests.

We hear the most from women who are taking too much progesterone, but there are creams out there with virtually no progesterone in them (5 to 10 mg per jar of cream), and women who use these creams are underdosed. We know that 10 mg of progesterone per jar of cream isn't enough to oppose the effects of estrogen, or to build bone. These creams are *not* recommended.

Before we begin on the next section of this chapter, we'd like to emphasize that we *always* prefer that women work in partnership with a skilled and competent health care professional when balancing their hormones. It's notoriously difficult to be objective in diagnosing and treating yourself and tracking whatever changes might be taking place. This is particularly important if you have breast cancer. With or without a health care professional to work with, it's a great idea, at least for the first few months of a hormone balance regimen, to keep a daily journal that records what you ate, what you took in the way of supplements, and how you felt.

Dosage Recommendations for Progesterone

All the dosage recommendations in this chapter are based on using a two-ounce container of progesterone cream that contains a total of 900 to 1,000 mg of progesterone (a 1.6 to 2 percent progesterone cream). This amounts to about 40 mg per ½ teaspoon, 20 mg per ¼ teaspoon, and 10 mg per ⅛ teaspoon.

Most women only need 15 to 20 mg of progesterone daily—about what the body would make if it were making its own progesterone. Some women do better with closer to 30 mg, and others do fine with closer to 10 mg. People and their metabolic needs differ.

Another way of looking at it is this: If a premenopausal woman uses 20 mg of progesterone per day for 14 days each month, the monthly dose is 280 mg, approximately one-third of the two-ounce container. When using the creams with the concentration Dr. Lee recommends, this 20 mg dose is found in ¼ teaspoon of cream. This is commonly a very acceptable dose. Dr. Lee doesn't recommend the super-high-dosage creams that contain 3,000 mg, which are typically listed as 10 percent creams and contain about 100 mg of progesterone per ¼ teaspoon. It's way too easy to get too much progesterone with these doses, and we're striving for balance.

If you're taking a physiologic dose (an amount approximating what your body would make itself under normal circumstances) and your symptoms don't go away after four to six months, or if they return, it's best to work in partnership with a competent health care professional to find out why. In many cases other hormone imbalances need to be corrected, most commonly estrogen deficiency, androgen deficiency (particularly problematic in women who've had a complete hysterectomy), poor adrenal function causing low or high cortisol levels, or thyroid deficiency. (See *What Your Doctor May* Not *Tell You about Menopause* and *What Your Doctor May* Not *Tell You about Premenopause* for details on supporting adrenal function.) There's never a reason to give an estrogen supplement to a woman still having monthly periods; the very fact that she is menstruating is evidence that she's making plenty of estrogen.

After menopause, the ovaries continue to make small amounts of estrogen and testosterone. In addition, estrogen continues to be made by body fat. In two-thirds of women after menopause, estradiol levels are sufficient.

A progesterone-deficient woman who starts using natural progesterone cream in the recommended doses will find that, in three to four months, her body's progesterone level will reach physiologic equilibrium. Most women will be able to judge for themselves, based on symptoms, whether the previous hormone imbalance is now corrected.

In a menopausal woman (who isn't preparing her uterus for pregnancy), about one-half of a two-ounce container used up in 24 to 25 days of the calendar month, about ¼ teaspoon per day, will usually restore good physiologic levels of progesterone in one to two months. After that, one-third of a container (closer to ⅛ teaspoon per day) will maintain these levels. Women who are closer to actual menopause may need higher doses to counter the excessive amounts of estrogen that can be sporadically produced by the ovaries at this time.

Ultimately, how you achieve your monthly dosing goal will probably come down to personal preference, and perhaps the personal preference of your health care professional. How you're feeling will be a good indicator of whether it's working for you. In a very few women, the first few weeks of starting a hormone balance regimen can involve some worsening of symptoms and even new ones, but this phase generally passes quickly.

The cream can be applied once or twice a day. Dr. Lee advises a divided dose, with a larger dose at bedtime and a smaller dose in the morning. Getting each dab of cream to be exactly the right size isn't that important here, because there's a buffering effect as the progesterone is absorbed into subcutaneous (under-the-skin) fat. The release of the hormone from body fat serves to make the progesterone effect relatively steady even if daily doses vary a little.

How to Get the Most Out
of Your Progesterone Cream

Here are some general guidelines on how to get the most out of your progesterone cream dose:

- The larger the area of skin the dose is spread on, the greater the absorption.
- Apply the cream to thinner skin with high capillary density—such as places where you blush. Through testing at his lab, Dr. Zava has found that the best spots are the palms (if they aren't callused), chest, inner arms, neck, and face. The soles of the feet are also good if they're not thickened from walking barefoot.
- Progesterone cream should always be applied after, not before, a warm bath or shower.
- If you use the cream at bedtime, it can be calming and help you sleep. If you want to apply it twice a day, use a larger dab at night and a smaller one in the morning.
- Since other ingredients of the cream are generally not absorbed, continual use of any single skin area will eventually saturate that area, which might reduce progesterone absorption. Rotate among three or four different skin sites on different days.

When During the Month
to Use Progesterone Cream

In this section we're going to first give you general information on when to use progesterone cream, and then we'll get into different ways of using it for specific problems. These guidelines will apply whether you have breast cancer or want to regain hormone balance to help prevent breast cancer. All the information we have right now tells us that, in relationship to breast cancer, it won't be helpful, and may be harmful, to use too much progesterone.

Guidelines for Postmenopausal Women

Postmenopausal women can use progesterone cream for 24 to 26 days of the calendar month. Women who experience a recurrence of hot flashes or other symptoms during the break can try reducing the dose gradually over a two- to three-day period before taking the break; if that doesn't work, reduce the break time to just three days completely off. The monthly break is important, since postmenopausal women still make estrogen; the addition of progesterone may cause the recurrence of menstrual periods. It's wise to allow complete shedding, which usually occurs when you allow the progesterone to fall for several days. If regular periods resume, then return to the premenopausal schedule of using progesterone two weeks each menstrual month, stopping a day or two before the expected period. When the periods stop for three to four months, then you can resume the 24 to 26 day schedule again. If spotting continues, it's wise to consult with your doctor.

Guidelines for Premenopausal Women

If you have signs of estrogen dominance and progesterone deficiency, you can use progesterone during the two weeks prior to your period, stopping a day or two before the expected period. When a woman is progesterone deficient, estrogen receptors become less sensitive. When progesterone deficiency is corrected, these estrogen receptors regain normal sensitivity. In some women this can cause breast swelling and tenderness for two to three months. This breast swelling is due to the estrogen effect in breasts that causes fluid retention in breast cells, and again, it usually resolves in two to three months. Dr. Lee often advises women with this problem to use smaller doses of the progesterone cream.

If you have an average 26- to 30-day menstrual cycle, you can begin your first month of progesterone cream use between day 10 to 12 of your menstrual cycle, counting the first day of your period as day 1. Continue until a day or two before your expected period, which for most women is between 26 and 30 days. (If you don't know how long your cycle is because you've had irregular bleeding, or if your cycles have been very short or very long, use your intuition and pick a day.) If your period starts before your chosen last day, stop using the cream and begin counting again to day 10, 11, or 12. It may take two to three cycles to find the synchrony your body desires.

It can be perfectly normal to have a menstrual cycle as short as 18 days and as long as 32 days. If your cycle is shorter or longer than average, use the following method to determine when to take the cream: Use the calendar to figure out when the first day of your period is expected, and then count backward two weeks. This is when you should start taking the cream. The reason for this is that the number of days from day 1 of your period to the day you ovulate can vary greatly, but for nearly all women the number of days between ovulation and the start of the next period is 14 days. The closer you can get to taking the progesterone when you ovulate or just after, the more in tune with your own cycle you'll be.

Even if you can tell that you've ovulated, it doesn't mean you don't need progesterone supplementation. Ovulation does not guarantee continued progesterone production throughout the luteal phase. In many women progesterone production falls shortly after ovulation and they become estrogen dominant again in the week before their period. This is called luteal phase failure and is very common in U.S. women after age 35. It's a frequent cause of irregular cycles and infertility.

It may take up to three months of progesterone use to restore normal menstrual cycles. As women approach menopause, estrogen production often becomes more variable. Under such circumstances, it may be unrealistic to expect regular cycles, even with progesterone cream.

It's best to synchronize your natural progesterone supplementation with your body's own hormonal cycles as much as possible. Menstrual dysfunction is usually the result of more than just progesterone deficiency. Factors such as stress, diet, and cortisol or thyroid hormone play important roles in this matter. The cooperation between the hypothalamus (the part of the brain that controls the endocrine system), the pituitary gland (the "master gland" that sends out instructions to other glands throughout the body), and the ovaries may be out of sync because the body is out of balance. Adding progesterone at the right times in the right amounts helps this complex system regain its equilibrium.

Ovulation often begins to be irregular eight to ten years before actual menopause. Each anovulatory cycle sends a woman deeper into estrogen dominance as body-fat progesterone stores are depleted. Very thin women with little body fat go into estrogen dominance much more quickly. In women with long-standing progesterone deficiency, the body fat is devoid of progesterone. In such women the first one or two months of transdermal progesterone are used to replenish body-fat stores, so it makes sense to use higher doses during this time. After two to three months of progesterone use, the dose can usually be reduced with good effect. Women who use ¼ teaspoon of cream twice a day (40 mg per day) for the two weeks prior to their period usually find that they can cut the dose in half (20 mg per day) for these same two weeks each month and continue to have good results.

We can't emphasize enough that the bottom line in progesterone dosing is always observed physiologic effects. Are your PMS symptoms improved? Are you gaining less weight before your periods? Are your breast or uterine fibrocysts getting smaller? Are your moods steadier? Are you less anxious? It's all about working to find the dose that corrects the problem, then reducing that dose to the minimum needed to maintain the desired effect.

Guidelines for Menopausal Women

Menopausal women can simply use 10 to 15 mg of progesterone daily for 24 to 26 days in a row of the calendar month. Many women find it easiest to start using the cream on the first of the month and stop from day 24 to 26 until the next month. Other women prefer to take their hormone break the first five to six days of the calendar month and then use the cream until the end of the month. It's best to use the cream in divided doses: half before bed and half in the morning. If that doesn't work well for you, however, don't be concerned; just pick one time of the day when it's most convenient to use it and use the whole dose.

Guidelines for Premenopausal Women Who Are Menstruating but Not Ovulating

Salivary assays done during the luteal or midcycle when progesterone levels would normally be at their highest can determine whether you're having anovulatory cycles. If your progesterone levels are low, this indicates either that you haven't ovulated or that the follicle is unable to produce the proper amount of progesterone. Dr. Zava finds with saliva testing that anovulation is usually associated with both low estradiol and low progesterone, and occurs frequently in women who have been on birth control, particularly Depo-Provera. These women often suffer from symptoms characteristic of both estrogen and progesterone deficiency.

In contrast, ovulation with luteal insufficiency is associated with normal to high estrogen and low progesterone, along with a host of estrogen-dominance symptoms. If you have estrogen-dominance symptoms, that's a pretty good indicator that your progesterone production is inadequate. Your health care professional can help you determine where you are.

In one study on a group of 18 regularly cycling women with an average age of 29, seven of them (39 percent) were found to be anovulatory, and weren't producing progesterone during the luteal phase. A lot of women who appear normal for their age group are actually not ovulating and have very low progesterone levels.

If this is you, try using one-third of a two-ounce container of cream that contains approximately 900 to 1,000 mg per container during the time from presumed ovulation to a day or so before your expected period (⅛ teaspoon twice daily). This will provide you with about 300 mg of progesterone per month. Since the daily progesterone produced by women with well-functioning ovaries ranges from 12 to 24 mg per day, your goal is to restore progesterone to these normal levels.

Women's sensitivity to hormones differs tremendously, so your dose will depend upon your individual sensitivity. Since progesterone is such a safe hormone, don't be afraid to experiment a bit to find the dose that serves you best. What's normal for one women is not necessarily normal for another.

As mentioned above, in premenopausal women who've been progesterone deficient for years, it's common for the initial application of progesterone to cause water retention, headaches, and swollen breasts—symptoms of estrogen dominance. This happens because the estrogen receptors shut down by progesterone deficiency are "waking up." It's important to remember that these symptoms will usually disappear in two weeks to two or three months.

Guidelines for Women with Endometriosis

Endometriosis involves small islets of endometrial tissue scattered here and there about the uterus, other pelvic organs, the wall of the colon, and even in the lungs. While the cause isn't clear, these islets of endometrial tissue respond to estrogen just as the endometrial cells in the uterus do—they fill with blood each month, causing severe pain that recurs monthly. During pregnancy, endometriosis recedes, only to recur after the pregnancy when normal periods return. This suggests that the higher levels of progesterone during pregnancy inhibit estrogen-stimulated endometriosis.

During regular menstrual cycles, estrogen production rises around day 7 to 8 of the cycle and falls a day or so before your period begins. Progesterone production, on the other hand, starts after ovulation (around day 12), reaching levels several hundred times greater than estrogen, and falls abruptly a day or so before your period. Using this concept as a model for treating endometriosis, progesterone can be given in doses similar to that of early pregnancy, starting at day 8 and continuing until day 26 of a usual 28-day cycle. Experience shows that this treatment is often effective in relieving the symptoms of endometriosis. Your goal is to find the lowest dose of progesterone necessary to control endometrial stimulation.

During the early weeks of pregnancy, progesterone production doubles or triples, from the normal 12 to 24 mg per day to 40 to 60 mg per day. These levels are easily reached using ¼ teaspoon of progesterone cream twice or three times a day during these 18 days of the cycle. Many women find success using a two-ounce jar or tube of the recommended cream each monthly cycle. Improvement is usually noted after several months of using progesterone cream in this manner. If improvement isn't found in two months, the dose can be raised to one ounce per week. It can take up to six months for symptoms to be controlled, and even then they may not dissipate entirely. If the symptoms eventually disappear, the progesterone dose can be decreased gradually to find the lowest effective dose. (Otherwise use the dose that's most effective to control symptoms.) This must be continued until menopause is passed, since recurrences are common if the progesterone protection is lowered too much. If a flare-up occurs, increase the dose to the previous effective level. If high doses of progesterone cream make you sleepy, that's an indication that you're taking too much. Reduce the dose until the sleepiness goes away.

Guidelines for Women with Uterine Fibroids

Fibroids (benign tumors that grow in the uterus) are the most common reason that women visit a gynecologist in the ten or so years before menopause. Fibroids tend to grow during the years before menopause and then atrophy after menopause. This suggests that estrogen stimulates fibroid growth, but we also know that once they get larger, progesterone too can contribute to their growth. Many doctors prescribe Lupron injections to block all sex hormone production. This causes the fibroids to shrink, but they regrow when the injections are stopped. The anti-progesterone drug RU-486 is also used to reduce the size of larger fibroids.

Women with fibroids are often estrogen dominant and have low progesterone levels. In women with smaller fibroids (the size of a tangerine or smaller), when progesterone is restored to normal levels the fibroids often stop growing and shrink a bit, which is likely due to progesterone's ability to help speed up the clearance of estrogens from tissue. If this treatment can be continued through menopause, hysterectomy can be avoided.

However, some fibroids, when they reach a certain "critical mass," are accompanied by degeneration or cell death in the interior part of the fibroid, and will have an interaction with white blood cells that ends up with the creation of more estrogen within the fibroid itself. It also contains growth factors that are stimulated by progesterone. Under these circumstances, surgical removal of the fibroid (myomectomy) or the uterus (hysterectomy) may become necessary. When you think of treating smaller fibroids, you should be thinking in terms of keeping your estrogen milieu as low as possible; when treating large fibroids, all hormones should be kept as low as possible.

The last thing you want to do if you have fibroids is take estrogen, which will stimulate them to grow. If you're estrogen dominant, then it's important to use a supplemental progesterone, usually in doses of 20 mg per day during the luteal phase of the cycle. Sometimes this approach works to slow or stop fibroid growth, and sometimes it doesn't. It is worth a try. Reducing stress, increasing exercise, and reducing calories are also good strategies for slowing fibroid growth.

There are a number of techniques for removing fibroids without removing the uterus. If your doctor doesn't know about these, find another one who does! The difference in recovery time alone between laparoscopic removal of fibroids (for example) and hysterectomy is three weeks versus three months.

Ultrasound tests can be obtained initially and after three months to check results. A good result would show that the fibroid size hadn't increased, or had decreased by 10 to 15 percent. With postmenopausal hormone levels, fibroids usually atrophy.

Guidelines for Women with Breast Fibrocysts

Breast fibrocysts are an overgrowth of normal breast tissue and are primarily due to excessive exposure to estrogens over a prolonged period of time. This is a sign that your ovaries aren't producing enough progesterone. Breast fibrocysts respond remarkably well to topical progesterone, a fact that the French first recognized some 30 years ago.

Progesterone cream at 15 to 20 mg per day from ovulation until the day or two before your period starts will usually result in a return to normal breast tissue in three to four months. You can apply the progesterone cream to your breasts every few days if you find that this helps. You can also take 400 IU of vitamin E at bedtime every night, as well as 300 mg of magnesium and 50 mg of vitamin B_6 a day. For many women it helps to cut out caffeine (coffee and certain soft drinks) and reduce sugar and refined starches in the diet. Once the fibrocysts are under control, taper down the natural progesterone to the minimum dose needed to prevent recurrence.

Guidelines for Women Using Estrogen Supplements

Some women who have irregular bleeding are prescribed estrogen by their doctors. This is a misguided approach. Irregular periods are due most often to progesterone deficiency. Without the normal rise and fall of progesterone each cycle, the uterus just doesn't know when to shed its lining. There's really no good reason to give estrogen to women who are still menstruating. Unless you're close to actual menopause and experiencing blatant estrogen deficiency symptoms such as hot flashes, night sweats, and vaginal dryness, the very fact that you're menstruating indicates that you're not deficient in estrogen.

You can try reducing your estrogen dose by half when you add progesterone, then gradually taper off the estrogen completely, if possible. If you're using estrogen tablets, simply cut them in half or take one every other day.

Estrogen patches deliver a low steady state of estrogen and in this sense more closely mimic production by the ovaries. However, many women find that even this small amount of estrogen creates estrogen-dominance symptoms. Other than side effects of estrogen overdosing, the most common reason for women to discontinue the patch is skin irritation caused by the adhesive in the patch.

Some women have found that removing the cover and allowing the adhesive to air overnight reduces this problem. Others have found that overdosing can be dealt with by using patches that can be cut to reduce dose delivery by cutting out a dime-sized, circular piece of tape that will cover half of the patch. Place the tape over the skin and put the patch over it. Some women who try this complain of skin irritation from the tape; if this happens, ask your doctor to switch you to oral estrogen while you decrease your dosage over time.

Guidelines for Specific Premenopause Problems

For Women with PMS

PMS usually involves stress and higher levels of the hormone cortisol. Excessive cortisol not only reduces progesterone production but also competes with progesterone for common receptors, so you may need a higher progesterone dose than usual. For the first month or two, use up to a full two ounces a month, taking progesterone from day 10 to 12 to day 26 to 30. Dr. Lee advises women treating PMS to use the cream in a crescendo pattern, with small dabs at night starting on day 10 to 12 and gradually increasing to two dabs per day morning and night. Finish off the last three or four days with bigger dabs, or applying the cream three times a day. When symptoms subside, the dose may be reduced to find the lowest effective dose. Since PMS is a syndrome with multiple causative factors, it's wise to seek guidance in matters of stress management, diet, and other nutritional advice.

For Women with Menstrual Migraine

Use natural progesterone during the ten days before your period (day 16 to 26). When you feel the characteristic "aura" that usually precedes migraines, apply ¼ teaspoon of cream every three to four hours until your symptoms cease (usually this happens in only one or two applications). You can also apply the cream directly to your neck or your temples.

Guidelines for Women Who've Had a Hysterectomy or Ovariectomy

Complete hysterectomy, a term some doctors use inappropriately to refer to removal of both the uterus and the ovaries, is also known as surgical menopause, and its abruptness is hard on the body. If you've had your ovaries surgically removed, all the ovarian hormones are lost. Hormone replacement in these circumstances should include low-dose estrogen if needed and natural progesterone cream in normal physiologic doses for 24 to 26 days of the calendar month. Many women, after removal of their ovaries, also have testosterone deficiency, causing low energy levels, depression, and lack of libido. The best way to confirm the diagnosis is by measuring free testosterone levels (as in a saliva hormone assay), and not by regular blood tests. If it's present, testosterone deficiency can be effectively treated by transdermal testosterone in doses as low as 0.15 mg per day. (See chapter 14 for details on supplemental testosterone.)

Restoring hormone balance in castrated (ovaries removed) women requires attention to all three of the sex hormones. If only the uterus was removed (hysterectomy), progesterone levels fall in one to two months, and estrogen levels fall in one or two years, as in normal menopause. Since hysterectomy seriously reduces the blood supply to the ovaries, hormone balancing is a bit more complex than with ordinary menopause. Attention must be paid to estrogen, progesterone, and testosterone, as in the hormone loss from ovary removal (oophorectomy). As stated before, under no circumstances should estrogen be given without progesterone.

Can I Use Natural Progesterone if I'm Taking Birth Control Pills?

The honest answer to the above question is that we just don't know for sure. We suspect that the more potent progestins in the birth control pills will block progesterone from its receptors, but progesterone has many effects in different parts of the body, so it could have some benefit anyway. On the other hand, we really don't know whether progesterone will interfere with the action of oral contraceptives. We suspect it won't, but we don't know for sure. We hope that somebody studies this question sometime soon.

Where to Find Natural Progesterone

At this time, natural progesterone cream is available over the counter and by prescription at compounding pharmacies. You can usually find it in health food stores, and it's easy to find on the Internet. Be sure that you're getting the real thing. If the label says "wild yam extract," don't buy the product without calling or e-mailing the company and confirming that it contains progesterone and not diosgenin or dioscorea, which are precursors of progesterone in the laboratory but do *not* convert to progesterone in the body. Pregnenlone also *cannot* be used as a substitute for progesterone.

Your doctor can order a progesterone cream from a compounding pharmacist, but be careful of the 10 percent creams that contain very high amounts of progesterone. Taking a higher-than-recommended dose doesn't contribute to hormone balance. Dr. Lee recommends a 1.6 percent cream by weight, with about 450 to 500 mg of progesterone per ounce. In ¼ teaspoon of cream this amounts to about 15 to 20 mg of progesterone.

Many natural progesterone creams contain ingredients other than progesterone that may be active, including wild yam extract—which is usually diosgenin—as well as a variety of herbs and aromatic oils. We don't know which are active and which aren't, or what biochemical effects these ingredients may or may not have, nor do we know what effect they may have when used by women who are pregnant or nursing. In an extensive screening of hundreds of herbs traditionally used for hormonal imbalances, Dr. Zava has yet to identify one whose activity is similar to natural progesterone. For this reason, we feel that progesterone creams containing herbs should be avoided by women who are trying to get pregnant, who are pregnant, or who are nursing. These women are advised to use one of the creams that contain only progesterone as the active ingredient. (This is not to say that the other ingredients aren't helpful for women with hormone imbalances—we suspect they probably *are*.)

Some herbs have traditionally been used to stop pregnancy (abortifacients), induce menstrual periods (emmenagogues), or induce labor. In his research Dr. Zava has found that these herbs interact with progesterone receptors but don't activate the receptor in the same manner as natural progesterone. In fact, many behave more like an anti-progesterone, which is consistent with their use.

If a progesterone cream feels grainy or sandy, it probably means the progesterone has precipitated out. We recommend that you return or exchange it. We don't recommend creams that contain DHEA or any other hormone besides progesterone, unless you're under the supervision of an experienced health care professional.

In the Resources section at the back of this book you'll find a list of progesterone creams that contain our recommended dose of progesterone and no other hormones. It doesn't cost anything to be on this list; most of the companies listed are those we've known for years, and we offer the list as a service to our readers. There are plenty of perfectly good progesterone creams that aren't on this list, many of them private-label versions of these creams. Due to space limitations we can't list them all. None of the authors of this book sells progesterone cream or makes any money from the sale of any progesterone cream.

A Final Reminder

In this chapter we've covered a lot of ground concerning the use of natural progesterone. We have explained why transdermal progesterone is the preferred delivery system. Oral dosing is inefficient and results in excessive progesterone waste products. With creams there is the advantage of slower absorption and avoiding the first pass loss through the liver. Sublingual drops and vaginal suppositories of progesterone are absorbed very quickly and also excreted more quickly than transdermal cream application. Keep in mind that individuals differ; we aren't all stamped out of the same cookie cutter. Individualization in hormone balancing is a necessity. Knowing how things work is a great advantage in getting them right. We trust your wisdom to help you make the right decisions in your health care.

CHAPTER 14

HOW AND WHEN TO USE OTHER HORMONES

Estrogen, DHEA, Pregnenolone, the Corticosteroids, Testosterone, and Androstenedione

If you've had breast cancer or are at a high risk for it, supplementing with any hormone except progesterone can be risky. There's so much we don't know about the hormonal details of how cancer is initiated and promoted that great caution and a conservative approach are essential. More than ever it's important that you use small physiologic doses of natural hormones that approximate what the body makes, rather than large pharmacologic doses of synthetic hormones. A general rule to follow is that if you are truly deficient in a steroid hormone, it's probably a good idea to supplement it, but never to the point that you create an excess. Always remember when supplementing steroid hormones: Optimal balance means minimal risk. This means having a saliva hormone level test when you begin supplementing. If your symptoms resolve, then your hormone levels are probably fine; if not, you may want to have another test six months after supplementing to see what's still out of balance.

In general our recommendation is that if you're at risk for breast cancer or a recurrence of the disease, don't use supplemental hormones (except for progesterone) unless your hormone levels are well below normal. Even then, if you know you're not going to carefully track your hormone levels for as long as you're taking supplemental hormones, then *don't* do it.

If you've had a complete hysterectomy, are plagued by hot flashes and night sweats, have no libido at all, or are losing bone mass, even when using progesterone cream, then supplemental estrogen and/or testosterone is a consideration. It's important to have a saliva hormone level test first to make sure that the symptoms you're experiencing are truly a hormone deficiency and/or imbalance. For example, if you've had breast cancer, your low libido might have as much to do with emotional trauma as with low testosterone, and you don't want to add testosterone to your body unless you truly need it.

Estrogen

About a third, or 35 percent, of postmenopausal women (usually those with less body fat) may benefit from low-dose estrogen supplementation. HRT doses of estrogen are typically greater than a postmenopausal woman needs. Overdoses of estrogen prescribed to postmenopausal women are a large factor in causing many of the illnesses they experience.

After a total hysterectomy (ovaries also removed), the problem is a bit different. With the ovaries removed, all the ovarian hormones are removed. Commonly, physicians prescribe only estrogen. This is an error; these women certainly need progesterone, not only for its own benefits but also to balance supplemental estrogen. No one should be taking unopposed estrogen without progesterone.

As you've probably noticed, throughout this book our message is that estrogen is the smoking gun when it comes to breast cancer. Granted, it's not estrogen per se but rather unbalanced estrogens, synthetic forms of estrogen, and estrogens forced down harmful biochemical pathways that do the damage, but there's no doubt that it's the primary culprit in this disease. Thus, our advice is that if you've had breast cancer or are at high risk for it, don't use any type of estrogen except estriol, and even that should be used sparingly. We'll give recommendations for use below.

There are always exceptions, and the exception to the "no-estrogen" advice is that if you're very deficient in estradiol and/or estrone, and you have serious estrogen-deficiency symptoms, you might need to use *small* doses of estrogen. As Dr. S. R. Cummings and colleagues found in 1998 in an article published in the *New England Journal of Medicine,* when measuring estradiol levels in postmenopausal women aged 65 to 80, only one-third were actually deficient in estrogen. It was also found that conventional ERT or HRT estrogen doses were eight to ten times higher than needed. In a recent report from *The Lancet,* for example, the dose of estradiol for optimal bone effect in women with osteoporosis was 0.25 mg per day rather than the 1 to 2 mg usually given. Keep in mind the fact that progesterone won't work without at least a little bit of estrogen to prime its receptors!

Although the concept of an estrogen patch is great, the usual estrogen patch is far too highly dosed. Apparently those who make them don't realize that transdermal absorption is 10 to 20 times more efficient than oral doses. Until recently, the patch doses could not be reduced by cutting the patch in half, since all the estrogen ran out of the cut portion during the first day. Some of the newer patches with honeycomb construction can be cut into smaller portions for smaller doses, and they will work adequately.

If you are so inclined, you can try using some of the gentler phytoestrogens first, such as eating some soy (see chapter 16 for details) or red clover extract, and see if these help relieve your symptoms.

If you aren't at risk for breast cancer, then it's fine to use appropriate amounts of estrogen *if you need it.* You'll find even more detailed recommendations on how to tell if you need estrogen in *What Your Doctor May* Not *Tell You about Pre-menopause*. (Yes, menopausal and postmenopausal women can also benefit from this book.)

Natural estrogens (for humans) are estrone, estradiol, and estriol. All of the available evidence we have so far indicates that estriol is safe to use to control menopausal symptoms, and that it may even be protective against breast cancer. The research is divided on whether estriol builds bone, but indications are that it does have at least some bone-building properties. If you're experiencing vaginal dryness, night sweats, or hot flashes and you want to try some supplemental estriol, please read chapter 8, which is about estriol and includes recommendations on how to use it.

We can't emphasize strongly enough that no woman, with or without a uterus or ovaries, should ever take estrogen alone. It should *always* be combined with natural progesterone.

DHEA

DHEA, or dehydroepiandrosterone, is a steroid hormone like the estrogens and progesterone are. It's made in the adrenal glands, which make more than 150 different hormones. Estrogens and testosterone are made from DHEA (or progesterone) throughout the body. The amount of DHEA is greater than that of any other steroid hormone. All but 5 percent of it is bound to sulfur molecules (DHEAS), making it more soluble in blood plasma and providing us with ample reserves to draw from. We know that DHEA is important for the maintenance of health, but a complete understanding of its specific actions has so far eluded researchers.

Between the ages of 20 and 25, DHEA production peaks. Men produce more than women, but both sexes make about 2 percent less every year after the age of 25. By the time a woman reaches her mid- to late forties, DHEA levels can be quite low.

When people with low levels of DHEA are given supplements, they tend to experience a boost in energy, immune function, ability to adapt to stress, feelings of well-being, and sex drive. DHEA in excess can have masculinizing effects on women, and in excess it can have the opposite effect of the low dosages—increasing your risk of diabetes and heart disease. This is much more true for women than men. If you start to see changes like acne, hair loss, or the growth of facial hair, stop taking it. These side effects are entirely reversible with discontinuation of DHEA.

The downside of DHEA for women at risk for breast cancer is that it can convert to estrogen and theoretically could increase estrogen levels more than you want. Recent research even shows that DHEA itself has a stimulatory effect on breast cells, particularly when estrogen is low. However, other studies have shown an association between low DHEAS levels and metastatic breast cancer, and epidemiological studies haven't found an association between DHEA levels and breast cancer.

Thus, if your DHEA levels are *low* (the normal range for middle-aged women is quite broad), taking enough to restore midnormal levels may be beneficial, but keep in mind that an excess of DHEA could be harmful. If you decide to use it, keep a close watch on your overall hormone balance levels, testing every six months or so.

The recommended dose of DHEA for women is 5 to 10 mg a day. If you have your DHEA levels checked with a blood test, remember that DHEAS is the relatively inactive form. Saliva DHEA testing is a more accurate measurement of the active DHEA in the blood.

Pregnenolone

Pregnenolone is made from cholesterol by mitochondria and is the compound within cells from which DHEA, progesterone, estrogens, cortisol, and testosterone are created. It would seem that taking large doses of pregnenolone would be a good way to reach hormone balance, giving the body what it needs to make its other steroid hormones. Unfortunately, it doesn't necessarily work that way. Pregnenolone is an intermediary in the biosynthesis of other steroid hormones. If the ovaries or testes have lost the ability to create these other steroid hormones, the presence of pregnenolone will not change that situation. In other words, if your ovaries are functioning properly, then supplemental pregnenolone may be turned into other steroid hormones. If your ovaries are malfunctioning, however, they may not be able to use pregnenolone to make other hormones—pregnenolone is not a reliable way to supplement hormones.

Pregnenolone does appear to have some benefit for rheumatoid arthritis symptoms. Those who have this autoimmune disease can try 10 to 50 mg three times daily. Give it at least a month to work. Some clinicians use doses of 100 to 200 mg daily, but please use these amounts only under the supervision of a health care professional who will monitor your health.

Researchers have recently discovered that pregnenolone blocks receptors for the neurotransmitter gamma-aminobutyric acid. High GABA levels can have the effect of blocking memory, and pregnenolone seems to offset this effect. It also increases brain cell activity. Those who have problems learning or remembering may benefit from 50 to 100 mg of pregnenolone between meals, but again, at these doses please work in partnership with a health care professional and monitor your hormone levels.

The Corticosteroids

Corticosteroids are made by the adrenal cortex in response to long-term stress. They include cortisol, which is a glucocorticoid that regulates immune response, opposes insulin, and stimulates conversion of proteins to glucose in the liver (gluconeogenesis). Other corticosteroids such as corticosterone help regulate mineral balance. Aldosterone is the most potent of these, acting on the renal tubule (kidney) to promote retention of sodium and the increased excretion of potassium. You might also see these hormones referred to as cortisones, which has become a generic term for adrenal cortex hormones.

These hormones respond to any stressors that increase energy requirements. Fasting, infection, intense exercise, pain, or emotional stress stimulates the secretion of a releasing hormone from the hypothalamus in the brain, which tells the adrenals to secrete extra cortisol. There's also a regular daily cycle of cortisol release into the bloodstream, with peaks in the morning and late afternoon and lows in midafternoon and during deep sleep.

Cortisol is extremely important to survival when stress of any sort is present. If an animal can be made stress-free, the lack of cortisol is not life-threatening. But without the corticosteroids, we couldn't survive even the slightest stress. People who have had their adrenal glands removed or whose adrenals don't make enough cortisol are in danger of death from even mild illness. These people must use cortisol replacement for the rest of their lives, increasing their dose at any sign of extra stress or infection.

Excessive cortisol, on the other hand, creates a broad range of undesirable side effects including truncal obesity, elevated blood glucose, hypertension, "moon" face, a fatty accumulation called a buffalo hump behind the neck and upper thorax, osteoporosis, easy bruising, a susceptibility to fungal infections, and disorders of the immune system. If produced by excessive stimulation by pituitary hormones, the resulting disease is called Cushing's disease. If resulting from excessive adrenal production independent of pituitary control, the disease is called Cushing's syndrome.

Chronic stress leads to chronic high levels of cortisol in the bloodstream, which leads to a greater need for both DHEA and progesterone to maintain balance. In addition to the symptoms of Cushing's disease and syndrome, chronic excessive cortisol is toxic to brain cells in high concentrations and can cause short-term memory loss. A lifetime of high cortisol levels may be a primary cause of Alzheimer's disease and senile dementia. High cortisol is also a primary cause of osteoporosis, because it blocks the bone-building effects of progesterone.

As with the other steroid hormones, an excess of cortisol is associated with a poorer survival outcome in breast cancer patients, while cortisol deficiency is associated with breast cancer risk. Optimal balance means minimal risk.

The way this hormone is used in conventional medicine is another good example of the dramatic difference between physiologic and pharmacologic dosing with hormones. People who take powerful synthetic cortisone drugs such as prednisone, prednisolone, and dexamethasone for their anti-inflammatory effects suffer side effects like swelling of the face, acne, unwanted hair growth on the face and body, lowered resistance to infection, weight gain around the midriff, menstrual irregularities, and psychological problems ranging from depression to anxiety to outright psychosis. With long-term use, these medications cause adrenal cortisol production to shut down completely, so that stopping the drug can cause fatal complications.

In contrast, natural hydrocortisone, or cortisone acetate, used in small doses several times a day has very little incidence of side effects, and has been used successfully to treat symptoms of adrenal insufficiency. For more details on adrenal insufficiency and how to treat it, please read *What Your Doctor May* Not *Tell You about Menopause* or *What Your Doctor May* Not *Tell You about Premenopause*.

Supplementing natural hydrocortisone or cortisone acetate in doses of 2.5 to 5 mg two to four times daily can be a safe and effective way to replenish depleted adrenals. (Too much taken later in the day can cause insomnia, so adjust your dosage accordingly, or don't take it later in the day.) Proper use of natural cortisols can correct problems as diverse as asthma, rheumatoid arthritis, and chronic fatigue. However, it's very important to combine the cortisone supplementation with lots of rest, good nutrition, and hormone balance, with the goal of healing the adrenal glands and not having to use it every day. Once you've brought your body back into balance you can use it occasionally as needed, which you'll know by your symptoms.

We suggest that you use natural cortisone supplementation under the guidance of a health professional, because even natural cortisone isn't safe if you take too much, and it's a delicate balance to maintain. If you take it when you don't really need it, it can cause problems. If your doctor doesn't know about William McK. Jefferies's groundbreaking book, *Safe Uses of Cortisol*, inform him or her that it contains all the necessary information on how and when to prescribe physiologic amounts of natural cortisone.

If you don't have the symptoms of cortisol deficiency but are living an extremely hectic life, working and playing too hard and not taking time to get enough sleep and to relax, you're probably making too much cortisol. Even if your adrenals can sustain this kind of energy without ever running down, you're still at risk from chronically high cortisol levels. Optimal health is achieved with a balance of activity and rest.

Testosterone

Women make about a tenth as much testosterone as their male counterparts. The adrenal glands are responsible for maintaining adequate testosterone levels in women.

As is the case with most other hormones and aging, female production of testosterone decreases with age. Studies of hormone replacement in women have shown that adding a low dose of natural testosterone can sometimes have a positive effect. The other side of this coin is that in many cases, as the ovaries wind down, women show signs of becoming more *androgen* (male hormone) dominant rather than estrogen dominant. Testosterone will only exaggerate this process.

Facial hair and male-type pattern baldness are indicative of this shift. This can happen in premenopausal, estrogen-dominant women as well, because testosterone clearance from the body is partly controlled by the balance between estrogen and progesterone. Excess estrogen decreases testosterone clearance, and natural progesterone enhances it. In estrogen-dominant women testosterone hangs around in the body for a longer time, and the end result is as though more testosterone were being made. This is why progesterone cream tends to reverse the androgenic changes mentioned above.

Testosterone can be converted to estrogen in the body, and like estrogen it's a hormone that encourages cell growth, so it should be used with great caution if you're at risk for breast cancer. Research on testosterone and breast cancer is inconclusive: Some studies correlate high testosterone levels with breast cancer. Again, this is more evidence that it's hormones *in excess* that cause problems.

Dr. Zava has found through saliva testing that the majority of women who have had total hysterectomies suffer from low androgens (testosterone, DHEAS, and androstenedione). Testosterone deficiency can cause loss of energy, depression, memory lapses, vaginal dryness, incontinence, and loss of libido. Similar symptoms to those listed above for testosterone deficiency can also be caused by adrenal exhaustion or thyroid deficiency. These too should be sorted out by a physician.

The only two conceivable reasons to use testosterone in the face of breast cancer risk would be if you've had no libido at all for more than a year (and you would like some), or if you've experienced steady bone loss that hasn't been helped by any of the many approaches suggested by Dr. Lee. As a precautionary measure you should have your estrogen and testosterone levels checked at least every six months if you are supplementing; if you get any androgenic symptoms, you should cut back on your dose by half or stop using it.

These days testosterone is available as a transdermal patch, which is the preferred delivery system. A recent study found that after complete hysterectomy (ovaries removed) women often suffer low energy, depression, and lack of libido. Testing free testosterone (but not the usual serum testing) showed that these women were testosterone deficient. Transdermal testosterone, in doses of 0.15 mg per day, raised their free testosterone levels fivefold and effectively relieved their symptoms. Clinicians report to us that they successfully use doses of 0.15 to 1 mg per day.

A compounding pharmacist can make up testosterone creams of similar dosage. In questioning practicing clinicians who use supplemental testosterone, we've found that combining testosterone and progesterone into one cream isn't recommended. It's so easy for women to get too much testosterone that they need to be able to adjust their dosage if they notice symptoms of excess.

Testosterone is available only by prescription. If you're interested, talk with your physician. Be sure to use only a natural form, as synthetics like methyltestosterone are powerful and can have unpleasant side effects.

Androstenedione

This steroid hormone is a precursor to testosterone and estrogens, and it can theoretically act as a DHEA precursor. Secreted from the adrenals and ovaries into the bloodstream, it has its own jobs to do before being converted into other hormones in the liver. In older women it travels from the ovaries to the fat cells, where it's converted to estrogen.

Androstenedione is a popular supplement for bodybuilders, who use it to boost their testosterone levels, increasing muscle mass and decreasing the length of time needed to recover from hard workouts. Many of the positive effects of supplemental testosterone—including enhanced energy, libido, and sense of well-being—have also been attributed to androstenedione.

Androstenedione may also be involved in maintaining the strength of bones. It's converted to estradiol in the bones themselves, and estradiol helps slow bone loss.

We recommend that you not use androstenedione if you're at risk for breast cancer, as it can so easily be converted to estrogen in women.

CHAPTER 15

TESTING AND SYMPTOMS

How to Determine Your Hormone Balance

Before you can correct a hormonal imbalance, you need to know which hormones are out of balance, and the best way to do this is through a combination of testing and recognizing symptoms. In this chapter we'll explain the best way to test your hormone levels and give you a Hormone Balance Test to help you notice what your symptoms are and determine what they may mean.

Testing for Hormone Levels

Here's a very typical scenario of a woman who begins using progesterone cream and then goes to see her doctor: She reports to her doctor that her lumpy and painful breasts have cleared up, her insomnia has disappeared, and her premenstrual bloating and irritability are almost entirely gone. The doctor does a blood test that measures her serum levels of progesterone, and when her progesterone levels turn out to be low, concludes that: (1) the progesterone does not absorb; (2) it's just coincidental or due to the placebo effect; (3) they should increase the progesterone dose so some change in serum progesterone can be measured to validate the clinical response.

Had the doctor measured salivary progesterone, there would

have been no question that it absorbed through the skin. Instead of thinking about increasing the dose, the doctor would be thinking about scaling it down. Many women are overdosed with progesterone because of misunderstandings over how remarkably effective and efficient transdermal hormone delivery can be.

\The best way to test your hormone levels is with a saliva test. You don't need a prescription for a saliva test; you can order it yourself. You can find out how to order a saliva test at the end of the book under Resources. However, if the results of the test are confusing to you, it's probably best to discuss them with a qualified health care professional and work in partnership with him or her to create a program for restoring hormonal balance.

Saliva tests are more useful than blood tests because they measure the bioavailable (free) hormone in the blood. After steroid hormones (progesterone, cortisols, estrogens, DHEA, testosterone) are manufactured by the ovaries, adrenal glands, or testes, they're released into the bloodstream, where they attach or bind to very specific hormone carrier proteins and, to a lesser extent, to red blood cells. Progesterone and cortisol bind to cortisol binding globulin (CBG). The estrogens (estradiol, estrone, estriol) and testosterone bind to sex hormone binding globulin (SHBG). All of the steroids also bind to albumin, which is a protein present in very high concentrations in the blood. For every 100 steroid molecules bound to these carrier proteins, only about 1 to 5 percent escape the binding proteins and make it into the cells during circulation through the blood. The small 1 to 5 percent of steroids that escape the binding proteins are considered the free or bioavailable hormones, and these are what you want to measure, because they represent the amount of hormone that the tissue actually receives and responds to.

Some of the steroids also bind to red blood cells. The more fat-loving a steroid hormone is, the more likely it is to hitch a ride on a red blood cell. Steroids hang on less tightly to red blood cells than they do to carrier proteins. This means that steroids bound to red blood cells will dissociate more easily and therefore are more bioavailable for use by your cells. Studies have shown that when red blood cells pass through the capillaries of tissues, the steroids bound to them can dissociate and enter tissues within milliseconds.

When steroid hormones are delivered through the skin with topical creams or gels, most of the steroid, as it enters the bloodstream, is picked up by red blood cells and transported rapidly to tissues. Remember, it takes only about 20 seconds for blood to circulate completely throughout the body. Those who have experienced almost an instantaneous response from sublingual hormone therapy will appreciate just how fast hormones can circulate in the body when they enter directly into the bloodstream. We've heard from many women who were estrogen dominant for years and applied progesterone cream. They report, "It was as if my body immediately breathed a huge sigh of relief." This is because the progesterone cream is entering the bloodstream almost immediately and having a calming effect on the brain.

Now that you understand what happens in your body when you apply progesterone cream, you'll be able to understand why blood tests don't work to measure topically (skin) applied hormones—particularly the ones that are highly fat soluble like progesterone. When hormones are delivered topically, they enter the bloodstream, bind to red blood cells, and are rapidly transported to tissues of the body, one of which is the salivary duct—which in turn delivers them to the saliva. This makes saliva testing an accurate measure of your free hormones. In contrast, when blood is measured for hormones, what do you think is first removed to create the serum used for testing? You guessed it, red blood cells. Thus, blood tests completely miss the free hormones bound to your red blood cells.

A group of French-Taiwanese researchers illustrated this testing discrepancy beautifully in one of their published studies. They were interested in determining if progesterone (25 mg) delivered topically in a gel to the breasts of women would result in progesterone uptake into the breast tissue and change how fast the breast ductal cells were replicating, or dividing. (A high replication rate increases cancer risk.) What they found after only 10 to13 days was that 25 mg of topical progesterone (the dose recommended by Dr. Lee) resulted in a 100-fold increase in progesterone in the breast tissue and a significant reduction in cell division. What the researchers simultaneously discovered is that when they did blood tests of these women's hormone levels, progesterone in serum did not increase. Had they known to measure progesterone levels in saliva before and after applying the progesterone gel, they would have found a dramatic rise in salivary progesterone levels. A number of subsequent studies have shown that topical application of progesterone increases saliva levels dramatically, whereas the serum levels show little or no change. Thus, by measuring hormones in saliva it's possible to determine not only how much hormone is bioavailable but also how much is entering tissues throughout the body.

When to Take a Saliva Test

Testing your saliva simply requires spitting into a plastic tube at a time when you haven't recently been eating or drinking, and sending it off to the lab. However, it's important to time your saliva test correctly if you're having menstrual cycles and/or if you're already using progesterone cream. If you're taking hormones you intend to test, such as topical progesterone, you should have been actively taking the hormone for at least two weeks.

• *Premenopausal women.* You want to test your saliva hormone levels during the luteal phase of your menstrual cycle, when progesterone production should be at its peak. For most women this is between day 19 and day 21 of the cycle, counting the first day of menstruating as day 1.

• *Perimenopausal women.* If you're having irregular cycles, then you'll need to use your intuition and make your best guess as to when you are in the luteal phase. It should be about seven to ten days before you expect to start your next period.

• *Menopausal women.* You can take a saliva test at any time.

If you already know that you're progesterone deficient, then it doesn't make sense to test your saliva hormone levels when you aren't using progesterone; this will tell you only what you already know—you need progesterone. What you want to know is what your hormone levels are when you're using the cream.

The test will be most helpful if you time it according to when you last used progesterone cream. Saliva testing has given us an accurate picture of what happens to your hormone levels after you apply progesterone cream. When scientists measure the absorption of transdermal progesterone hour by hour after application of the cream, they find that saliva levels rise within two or three hours, achieving their peak about three hours after application. These peak levels last about three hours and then begin to drop, indicating that the liver is processing the progesterone for excretion. This is a normal function of the liver. After 12 to 15 hours about 90 percent of the absorbed progesterone from a single application has been processed by the liver for excretion.

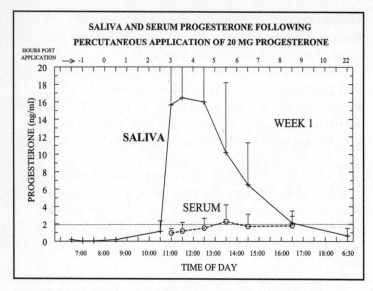

Topical progesterone barely shows up on a blood (serum) test but saliva testing gives an accurate portrayal of its presence in the body.

This teaches us several important lessons. The fall in progesterone 12 to 15 hours after application suggests that progesterone cream doses should be given in two small doses daily rather than a single bigger dose each day.

If the saliva sample is obtained two to three hours after application, the progesterone level will be at its peak. If the saliva sample is obtained 15 hours after application, over 90 percent of the absorbed progesterone will have passed through the body and the saliva level will be lower. For this reason, it's ideal to standardize saliva collection time at 8 to 10 hours after application to measure progesterone at the halfway point of the curve. Subsequent testing results will be meaningful only if the same collection time (relative to application time) is used at each testing.

In reality, many women use progesterone cream only in the morning, and if other hormones besides progesterone are being tested, they should be collected first thing in the morning. Thus,

Dr. Zava's lab tells women to collect their saliva sample at 8 to 24 hours following their last dose, in the morning, before applying the cream. Based on testing, his lab has established a range (500 to 3,000 pg/ml) that 80 percent of women should fall within if they use 10 to 30 mg of progesterone and take the test within 8 to 24 hours.

What's most important is that the saliva testing laboratory establishes ranges based on topical hormone delivery, because these ranges will be higher than normal. When levels fall below this range, then it's possible that the progesterone just isn't absorbing well or is cleared more rapidly than in the average individual. If symptoms of estrogen dominance persist in concert with low progesterone, despite dosing of 10 to 30 mg, then it will be important to consider the following:

- Check to make sure the product contains adequate amounts of progesterone.
- Apply the progesterone to parts of the body that blush (where capillaries are more numerous and closer to the surface) and apply it when your body is warm (as in after a warm bath or shower.
- Increase the dose or apply progesterone more than once during the day.

If progesterone testing shows the level to be above the expected range, then a reduction in the dose is called for, especially if you're having problems such as bloating or excessive sleepiness. Both saliva levels and symptoms should be used in concert to help you and your health care professional make educated decisions about whether to increase or decrease your progesterone dosing, or leave it the way it is.

Finally, the graph also recorded the progesterone serum levels during the hours when saliva progesterone was high. As you can see, the serum levels didn't reflect the obvious rise of saliva progesterone. This is a clear example of why blood tests are irrelevant in this scenario.

Interpreting the Results of a Saliva Test

As we mentioned earlier, it's ideal if you can interpret and analyze the results of your saliva hormone level test with a health care professional. However, as we know from the mail we receive from women around the world, many of you don't have access to a health care professional who is willing or qualified to help. We'll give suggestions on finding a doctor in your area at the end of the book under Resources. Here are some general guidelines to use.

The normal physiological luteal range of saliva progesterone in a woman who has ovulated is 0.1 to 0.5 ng/ml, which is equal to 100 to 500 pg/ml. Since topical progesterone creams create higher saliva levels, the expected range in women using 10 to 30 mg topical progesterone 8 to 24 hours after using it is 0.5 to 3 ng/ml, which is equal to 500 to 3,000 pg/ml. At the 3-hour peak saliva levels in those using topical progesterone can range as high as 5 to 30 ng/ml, which is equal to 5,000 to 30,000 pg/ml.

For this reason, we can't make it a goal to reach "normal" luteal levels of progesterone when using progesterone cream, because topically applied progesterone has its own unique graph, which is different from the graph produced when endogenous (made-in-the-body) levels of progesterone are tested. The goal is to use physiologic levels of progesterone, and use the saliva test and symptoms to help adjust dosing if necessary.

Since saliva estradiol is usually measured in picograms per milliliter (pg/ml), it's helpful if the lab also records progesterone levels in pg/ml. The normal saliva estradiol range is 1 to 5 pg/ml (average 2.5). In progesterone-supplemented women where the expected range for salivary progesterone is 500 to

3,000 pg/ml, the average ratio of progesterone to estradiol should therefore be in the range of about 200 to 1,000. This ratio should be used only as a guidepost in combination with symptoms to determine if thought should be given to increasing or decreasing the progesterone or estrogen dose.

To determine what your hormone levels are, you simply look at the "normal" expected ranges on your results to find out whether your hormone levels fall within these parameters. If you're only marginally excessive or deficient and you feel fine, then don't be concerned. If you have an excess or deficiency of a hormone and you're also having symptoms of that imbalance (see the Hormone Balance Test on page 256), then it may be time to consider supplementation.

Other Factors in Hormone Balancing

Stress can make hormone balancing problematic. Chronic stress is usually accompanied by higher levels of adrenaline and/or cortisol. Cortisol inhibits progesterone production by the ovaries. If you're progesterone deficient, excess cortisol will do more damage than it will if you have adequate progesterone. Adequate progesterone levels protect against excess cortisol because the progesterone sits on the cortisol receptor and thus protects against the negative side effects of excess cortisol. Supplemental progesterone can be of great benefit in situations where excess cortisol is causing bone loss and affecting the hippocampus, causing symptoms such as memory loss and mood swings.

Stress comes from many sources, including situational problems, trauma, and inflammation. Inflammatory bowel disease, for example, can induce high levels of cortisol that can significantly reduce progesterone production and cause estrogen dominance.

Thyroid hormone is another problematic factor. Thyroid

hormone regulates cellular metabolism. Many women with estrogen-dominance symptoms (normal to high estrogen and low progesterone) have symptoms of low thyroid levels, and recent research is showing us that excess estrogen, or estrogen not properly balanced with progesterone, inhibits thyroid function. Correcting the estrogen dominance with progesterone frequently corrects the thyroid hormone inhibition problem.

If your estrogen level is higher than normal, effort should be taken to reduce it. By far the most common cause of excess estrogen is an overdose of supplemented hormones, usually Premarin or estradiol. The solution to this is simple—reduce the dose to the lowest level that resolves symptoms. Excess estrogen not caused by HRT can be lowered by preventing excess calorie intake (remember, fat cells make estrogen), avoiding sugars and refined carbohydrates, and maintaining a high-fiber diet, including supplementing with high-fiber products such as psyllium or rice bran if necessary.

Excess estrogen can also be caused by a liver that's not efficiently excreting estrogens. It's important, therefore, to find a nutritionally oriented health care professional to prescribe the nutrients that support the liver in this process. (You can also read more about supporting your liver function in chapter 18 on xenohormones.)

Why Your Doctor Isn't Using Saliva Hormone Testing

Many people ask us why their doctor doesn't use saliva hormone testing. When the subject comes up with doctors, they say that it's not what they're used to, or the test results are confusing to them; many still think blood tests are the gold standard. When questioned further, it often becomes clear that they're unaware that blood (serum) testing does not distinguish between the non-bioavailable protein-bound hormone and the free or bioavailable hormone present in blood. Neither does it measure the free hormone carried by red blood cells. The typical physician has not yet learned of the curve pictured on page 250 showing the rise and fall of progesterone when absorbed transdermally. As a result, they don't know the importance of standardizing the saliva collection time relative to the time the cream is applied. It's no wonder that doctors are confused about the test results.

Another problem doctors have with saliva tests is that topical progesterone levels are generally higher than endogenous (made in the body) levels and they don't know how to interpret the results. At the same time, and somewhat ironically, the topical progesterone doesn't show up at all in blood tests! And yet millions of women can attest to the fact that a physiologic dose of progesterone, 10 to 30 mg, applied topically to the skin, can help correct many hormonal imbalances.

Any woman asking her doctor to check her hormone levels must expect that she might have to educate him or her about the advantages of saliva testing.

Determining Hormone Imbalance with Symptoms

Assessing and tracking your symptoms can be as important as testing your hormone levels. Many laboratories that test hormones in blood or saliva provide you only with numbers and no explanation as to what they mean. For most laypeople as well as some health care professionals unfamiliar with hormone profiles, this can be confusing, frustrating, and quite frankly a waste of money. Hormone levels can provide a road map to your hormonal health but should always be combined with knowledge about your symptoms, age, and menopausal status, along with what hormones you're taking. Without this information, hormone testing is much less likely to be helpful.

Hormone profiles should also, for the most part, parallel symptoms. For example, estrogen dominance should in most cases be associated with an imbalance in progesterone to estradiol (too much estradiol relative to progesterone). Estrogen-deficiency symptoms should be associated with low estrogens, particularly estradiol. Likewise, androgen deficiency or excess should be reflected in hormone levels for testosterone, androstenedione, and DHEA. In short, hormone profiles and symptoms should show similar patterns.

Ideally, symptoms should be documented at the time of saliva collection and reported in concert with and correlated to the hormones tested. This will allow the health care provider to examine what you feel are your most significant problems and how this relates to the hormones tested. Imbalances can then be corrected with conservatively and thoughtfully applied natural hormones.

The vast majority of women with breast cancer have been estrogen dominant for one reason or another, often for many years. They only have to read the list of symptoms that are common with estrogen dominance on pages 99–100 to find themselves.

The Hormone Balance Test

While a saliva hormone test can give a very accurate picture of which hormones are out of balance, it's always best to compare this to symptoms. For this reason, we have devised a Hormone Balance Test that can give you a good sense of which hormones are out of balance, based on your symptoms alone. Ideally you would be working with a health care professional both on determining which hormones are out of balance and on using natural hormones to bring your body back into balance.

Read carefully through the list of symptoms in each group, and put a check mark next to each symptom that you have. (If you check off the same symptom in more than one group, that's fine.)

Go back and count the check marks in each group. In any group where you have two or more symptoms checked off, there's a good chance that you have the hormone imbalance represented by that group.

The more symptoms you check off, the higher the likelihood that you have the hormone imbalance represented by that group. (Some people may have more than one type of hormonal imbalance.)

SYMPTOM GROUP 1

☐ PMS
☐ Insomnia
☐ Early miscarriage
☐ Painful and/or lumpy breasts
☐ Unexplained weight gain
☐ Cyclical headaches
☐ Anxiety
☐ Infertility

___ TOTAL BOXES CHECKED

SYMPTOM GROUP 2

☐ Vaginal dryness
☐ Night sweats
☐ Painful intercourse
☐ Memory problems
☐ Bladder infections

☐ Lethargic depression
☐ Hot flashes

___TOTAL BOXES CHECKED

SYMPTOM GROUP 3

☐ Puffiness and bloating
☐ Cervical dysplasia (abnormal pap smear)
☐ Rapid weight gain
☐ Breast tenderness
☐ Mood swings
☐ Heavy bleeding
☐ Anxious depression
☐ Migraine headaches
☐ Insomnia
☐ Foggy thinking
☐ Red flush on face
☐ Gallbladder problems
☐ Weepiness

___TOTAL BOXES CHECKED

SYMPTOM GROUP 4

A combination of the symptoms in groups 1 and 3. (If you've checked two or more boxes in each of these two groups, you may belong to symptom group 4.)

___TOTAL BOXES CHECKED

SYMPTOM GROUP 5

☐ Acne
☐ Polycystic ovary syndrome (PCOS)
☐ Excessive hair on the face and arms
☐ Hypoglycemia and/or unstable blood sugar
☐ Thinning hair on the head
☐ Infertility
☐ Ovarian cysts
☐ Midcycle pain

___TOTAL BOXES CHECKED

SYMPTOM GROUP 6

☐ Debilitating fatigue
☐ Unstable blood sugar
☐ Foggy thinking
☐ Low blood pressure
☐ Thin and/or dry skin
☐ Intolerance to exercise
☐ Brown spots on face

___TOTAL BOXES CHECKED

If you've checked two or more boxes in one or more symptom groups, read the following to find out what type of hormonal imbalance(s) you may have.

ANSWERS

SYMPTOM GROUP 1

Progesterone deficiency. This is the most common hormone imbalance among women of all ages. You may need to change your diet, eliminate synthetic hormones (including birth control pills), and begin to use some progesterone cream.

SYMPTOM GROUP 2

Estrogen deficiency. This hormone imbalance is most common in menopausal women, especially if you're petite and/or slim. You may need to make some special changes to your diet and take some women's herbs (see *What Your Doctor May* Not *Tell You about Premenopause*); some women may even need a bit of natural estrogen (about one-tenth the dose usually prescribed by doctors).

SYMPTOM GROUP 3

Excess estrogen. In women this problem is most often solved by getting off the conventional synthetic hormones most often prescribed by doctors for menopausal women. Adding progesterone often helps relieve symptoms and balance hormones.

SYMPTOM GROUP 4

Estrogen dominance. This is caused when you don't have enough progesterone to balance the effects of estrogen. Thus, you may have low estrogen—but if you have even lower progesterone, you can have symptoms of estrogen dominance. Many women between the ages of 40 and 50 suffer from estrogen dominance. You may want to try using some natural progesterone cream.

SYMPTOM GROUP 5

Excess androgens (male hormones). This is most often caused by too much sugar and simple carbohydrates in the diet, and can often be dealt with through simple dietary changes.

SYMPTOM GROUP 6

Cortisol deficiency. This is caused by tired adrenals, which are usually caused by chronic stress. If you're trying to juggle a job and a family, chances are good you have tired adrenals. Please read either *What Your Doctor May* Not *Tell You about Menopause* or *What Your Doctor May* Not *Tell You about Premenopause* book for detailed recommendations on restoring tired adrenals.

Now that you have a better idea of which of your hormones may be out of balance, you can read up on our recommendations for balancing these hormones in the rest of part 3.

CHAPTER 16

THE LIGHT AND DARK SIDES OF SOY

How to Eat Soy So That It Helps

Today it's all but impossible to find a health-related magazine or TV show that doesn't shout out the benefits of soy foods for the prevention of menopause symptoms, breast and other cancers, heart disease, and osteoporosis. In the past decade the soy industry has poured hundreds of millions of dollars into the research, marketing, and advertising of soy foods, and it has been well rewarded for its efforts. However, while we agree that certain soy foods, eaten in moderation, can be a healthy addition to the diet, we believe that women who are eating soy with every meal, or even every day, may be damaging their health. Soy has its good side, but it also has its bad side, which has been largely ignored by those rushing to cash in on this nutritional fad.

Traditional Asian soy foods such as tofu, tempeh, and miso have been a dietary staple in that part of the world for centuries, and they're increasingly found in Western diets. Western food manufacturers have also developed a slew of new soy foods, using these little beige beans as an ingredient in protein powders, hot dogs, burgers, cheese, cereals, sports bars, and other convenience foods. Soy milk, texturized soy protein, and soy cheese have been touted as nutritious alternatives to cows' milk products and meat. Supplement companies create pills from soy phytochemicals and advertise them as natural medicines for relief of menopause symptoms, or as protection against cancer, heart disease, or osteoporosis. Soy powders are sold as supposedly healthy meal alternatives. Some of these products are good for you, and some are best avoided. In this chapter you'll find out how to eat soy foods so they enhance your health.

Soy Foods and Breast Cancer Risk

One of the first studies that showed a clear link between soy food consumption and reduced breast cancer risk was carried out in Singapore by nutritional epidemiologist and professor H. P. Lee. Lee and his coworkers compared the diets of 200 women with breast cancer to the diets of 420 healthy women. They found that *premenopausal* women who ate the most soy had only about one-third the risk of developing breast cancer compared to other women of Singapore who were in the same age range.

Lee and coworkers took detailed dietary surveys to get an idea of the foods the women were consuming regularly. The most important findings of this study were that the women who ate the most red meat had a risk of breast cancer almost three times higher than those who ate the least, and that soy didn't seem to help prevent *postmenopausal* breast cancer—by far the most common kind—at least not among Asian women living in Singapore.

In a study carried out in the Shanghai and Tianjin provinces of China, no connection between soy consumption and breast cancer risk was found. A Japanese study found that women who ate more miso soup had lower risk; tofu also seemed to help reduce risk, but not as much as miso did. A more recent study carried out by the University of California in San Diego found that Chinese women living in the United States who ate more soy foods (primarily as tofu) had a 30 percent lower breast cancer risk. These researchers cautioned that other elements of diet and lifestyle could easily account for the differences in breast cancer rates they found. In other words, the women who ate more tofu might also have eaten more vegetables, or they might have included more green tea and herbs in their everyday fare.

The most abundant phytoestrogens in soy, genistein and daidzein, are also known as isoflavones (EYE-soh-FLAH-vones). Soy isoflavones have been shown to slow the growth of breast cancer cells in test tube studies, and they're more abundant in soy than in any other food. While some of these test tube studies have had positive results, others have shown no effect, and still others show a possible *increase* in the growth of breast cancer cells with genistein. Another test tube study showed that breast cancer apoptosis (cell death) increased with the addition of genistein, which is a favorable result. Other research suggests that the estrogenic phytochemicals in soy could in fact *stimulate* the growth of estrogen-sensitive breast tumors. Confused? You should be. The research on this subject is very conflicting. However, these and other studies on the soy–breast cancer relationship just don't show any strong evidence in favor of soy as a breast cancer preventive. Any effect it does have appears to be small and difficult to separate from other dietary, lifestyle, and genetic factors.

Problems with Interpretation of Dietary Studies

All of the important studies that have found a link between eating soy foods and lower breast cancer risk involved Asian subjects, who eat a lot of soy foods but who also seem to have a lower overall genetic propensity for developing breast cancer. One of the most common claims made by the soy industry is that Asian women have less breast cancer than Western women, and since they eat more soy than Western women, this is evidence that soy protects against breast cancer. This argument raises some important questions about research into diet–disease connections.

The typical Asian diet, soy or no soy, is rich in other foods known to help protect against cancer (which we'll discuss in detail in chapter 17). Anti-cancer foods such as garlic, green and herbal teas, sea vegetables, and herbs are frequent additions to the Asian diet. Asian women also tend to be much slimmer than Western women, and they tend to get more exercise and consume fewer calories. It's simply not possible to factor out how these food and lifestyle factors contribute to cancer risk. There aren't any long-term data on the benefits of soy foods in the context of the typical Western diet, or in women who are of non-Asian ethnic backgrounds.

Lifestyle, genetics, and other differences in diet probably play a more important role in decreased breast cancer risk than soy foods. Today, as Asians Westernize their diets by abandoning traditional foods and adding more hydrogenated oils, refined flours, and sugar, the number of breast cancer cases in this population is on the rise.

Soy and Menopausal Symptoms

With all that we know about the pitfalls of conventional medicine's treatment of women in menopause, it makes sense that women are turning to natural approaches to relieve menopausal discomforts. The beneficial effects of estrogen on these discomforts are indisputable, but as women become more informed they see that the risks—especially of breast cancer—may be too great to justify its use. Others stop using conventional HRT because of side effects, then look to natural remedies to help them control their menopause symptoms.

This growing interest in natural solutions for treating menopausal symptoms has prompted the food and supplement industries to develop alternatives to conventional pharmaceutical estrogens such as Premarin. The soy foods industry has been poised to benefit most from this search for natural remedies for menopause because of soy's high phytoestrogen content.

The lay press and the soy industry have widely promoted the message that soy phytoestrogens act, in effect, as surrogate estrogens. Such a message gives women the impression that they can use soy to naturally relieve symptoms of falling estrogen levels at menopause. While the research does show that isoflavones behave like estrogens in the body, the conclusion that they're all the medicine a woman needs to help her through menopause is not borne out by recent clinical studies on soy and menopausal symptoms.

Soy phytoestrogens have very little effect on vasomotor symptoms such as hot flashes, night sweats, and vaginal dryness. In one comprehensive study from the Bowman Gray School of Medicine in North Carolina, researchers looked at the effects of soy phytoestrogens on women aged 45 to 55 with menopausal symptoms. This study was big news because the women who took a phytoestrogen-rich soy supplement reported a 50 percent decrease in the severity of their hot flashes. What most news stories didn't mention, however, is that the placebo group reported a 35 percent reduction. Furthermore, this study showed small reductions in the *severity* of hot flashes, but none in their *frequency*. In other words, these women were having just as many hot flashes as they did before they added soy foods or supplements, but the intensity of these hot flashes was diminished. While decreased intensity is certainly a good thing when it comes to hot flashes, soy estrogens are clearly not as potent as many forms of conventional estrogen replacement, which often eliminate hot flashes quickly and completely.

A recent study of women with vasomotor symptoms at the Mayo Clinic showed no benefits from soy protein isolates, which have high levels of phytoestrogens. This has also been Dr. Zava's experience in analyzing saliva hormone level results accompanied by detailed questionnaires: Soy phytoestrogens simply don't work well to control vasomotor symptoms. The isoflavones in soy *are* aromatase inhibitors that lower the levels of estrogens made by the body, which is counterproductive to controlling vasomotor symptoms.

Soy phytoestrogens *do* have the estrogenic effect of stimulating the growth of breast cancer cells in tissue cultures. Several studies presented at a recent soy symposium showed that soy protein isolates stimulate the growth of normal breast cells much the way that natural estrogens do, and of course this would add to breast cancer risk if progesterone isn't present.

The Estrogen "Set Point"

Asian women are much less likely to have a troublesome menopause. This may be due in part to the fact that Asian women experience less of a drop in estrogen levels when they reach menopause because they have naturally lower estrogen levels throughout life than Western women do. When a woman has a hot flash, it's because her ovaries have slowed the production of estrogens and her brain is adjusting to a new level of estrogen in the bloodstream. Over two to five years the brain readjusts to the lower estrogen levels, and symptoms begin to drop off in their frequency and severity. Western women tend to have higher estrogen levels throughout their reproductive lives than Asian women do, and their brains become conditioned to those levels—a sort of estrogen "set point." At menopause the drop from this set point is more dramatic in Westerners because they started at a higher level. On the other hand, Asian women have less estrogen to begin with, a lower set point, so the decrease at menopause isn't as great.

A good example of another biochemical set point is coffee. If you drink two or three cups of coffee every morning, your brain develops a set point for caffeine. If you withdraw this daily dose of caffeine, your brain will definitely notice the difference. On the other hand, if you drink only one cup a day, the adjustment if you stop drinking it altogether will be smaller. The same goes for estrogens: If your body has consistently high estrogen levels throughout your reproductive years, as do many Western women, your brain will notice the difference at menopause more than if your levels are low, as they are in Asian women.

During perimenopause, the few years around the time that menopause is occurring, women often experience steep highs and lows in their estrogen production as the brain and ovaries attempt to regulate hormone levels. Chronically low progesterone contributes to the erratic production of estrogen. These changes in hormone production can be confusing to treat, because they create symptoms of both estrogen dominance and estrogen deficiency. Although supplemental progesterone cream doesn't always completely eradicate symptoms, it can substantially reduce the extremes of estrogen fluctuations and reduce symptoms considerably.

Soy's Effect on Cholesterol Levels

The FDA now allows soy manufacturers to make medical claims that soy lowers cholesterol levels. For people with normal cholesterol levels, however, soy has little or no effect.

In 1995 James Anderson, M.D., and his colleagues at the University of Kentucky did a metanalysis, combining the data from 29 of the 38 studies that had been published on soy and cardiovascular disease. Their results, published in the *New England Journal of Medicine,* revealed that textured soy protein and soy protein isolates significantly reduced blood levels of total cholesterol, LDL (bad) cholesterol, and triglycerides. They also found that soy foods slightly raised levels of HDL (good) cholesterol.

Cholesterol fell more in subjects who had very high cholesterol to begin with. In fact, almost no change was seen in women or men with cholesterol counts of 127 to 200. The researchers concluded that 30 grams of soy protein a day would lower cholesterol in those who began with high cholesterol. Eight ounces of tofu contains 30 grams of soy protein.

A more recent study from the University of Guelph in Canada showed that the consumption of 60 grams of soy protein isolate a day for a month had virtually *no effect* on the cholesterol or triglyceride levels of 20 healthy men. The soy supplement also didn't reduce the stickiness of red blood cells. (When red blood cells stick together to form clots, they can block blood flow through vessels and cause heart attacks or strokes.) Genistein (one of the isoflavones found in soy) levels in the blood of the subjects rose almost 100-fold during the soy supplementation, to nearly three times normal levels found in Japanese people eating a traditional soy-based diet. Later in this chapter you'll see why such high genistein levels could cause problems in the body.

In a 1997 study Dr. Kenneth Carroll and colleagues at the University of Western Ontario reported that soy foods lowered the LDL-to-HDL cholesterol ratio by 14 percent and increased HDL by an average of 9 percent. Again, the benefits were seen only in men and women with very high LDL levels.

From these studies, we can conclude that soy will improve unhealthy cholesterol counts but won't lower numbers already in the healthy range. Considering the possible hazards of very low cholesterol—remember that steroid hormones, including estrogen and progesterone, are made from cholesterol—this is good news.

Protection against Blood Sugar Imbalances

A potential cardiovascular benefit of soy foods is the effect of soy protein on insulin and glucose levels. Chronically high blood sugar and insulin levels are increasingly common in aging people who eat less-than-ideal diets, are overweight, and don't exercise.

In these people insulin stops doing its job of moving glucose into the cells, dramatically increasing the risk of type II diabetes and cardiovascular disease.

A study published in 1997 in the journal *Metabolism* investigated the effects of dietary soy protein, in combination with the estrogen estradiol, on heart disease risk factors in monkeys. They discovered that soy protein in combination with conjugated estrogens significantly improved the monkeys' cholesterol levels and their ability to move blood sugars into the cells. This combination also reduced cholesterol oxidation in the animals' arteries. All of these changes are associated with decreased risk of cardiovascular disease in both monkeys and humans. In monkeys treated with estradiol only, fatty deposits in the aorta (the major artery leading away from the heart) decreased, along with total body weight, abdominal body fat, and LDL cholesterol. The smallest fatty deposits were found in the aortas of monkeys that got both soy and estradiol, suggesting that the best protection against buildup of deposits in the arteries is a combination of soy and estradiol.

These results provide some evidence that soy foods and estrogen replacement therapy can help protect against cardiovascular disease. The evidence in favor of soy's protective effects on blood vessels provides the strongest scientific support for adding it to your diet.

Soy and Bone Health

Osteoporosis is another disease that strikes Westerners more than it does Asians. Could this be due to differences in the amount of soy foods eaten? This is what the soy industry claims. The fact is, there's very little evidence that soy foods protect the bones of Asian women against osteoporosis and the fractures it causes. Contrary to popular belief, epidemiological studies show that the bones of Asian women are no denser than those of their

Western counterparts. While Asian women do get osteoporosis, their fracture rate is not as high as that of women in the industrialized West. Some experts attribute the lower fracture rate to the Asian plant-based diet; others point to the fact that Asian women get more weight-bearing exercise. It's also been said that Asian women squat more in their daily activities, and so the muscles and connective tissues in their hips are stronger and more resilient than in Western women who sit in chairs and cars most of the day.

One way in which soy could improve bone health is as a replacement for animal protein in the diet. The high sulfur content of meats creates an acidic environment in the body, and calcium is drawn from the bones to neutralize this acidity if there isn't enough calcium in the diet. Soy supplies high-quality dietary protein but doesn't increase the body's acidity.

We also know that the isoflavone daidzein found in soy appears to have a positive effect on bone mass in humans. Isoflavones may act similarly to estrogens in slowing bone loss. Ipriflavone, a commercial synthetic derivative of daidzein, has been shown to increase bone mass in the forearm and prevent bone loss in the spine in postmenopausal women. However, overall soy studies show only minimal effects in preventing bone loss. Isolated isoflavones might offer more bone benefits. If you've been diagnosed with osteopenia or osteoporosis, adding soy foods to your diet could help, but we don't recommend relying on soy alone to build bone mass.

The Dark Side of Soy

As you can see, the research simply isn't compelling enough to justify the great press soy foods have been getting. This doesn't mean soy foods aren't good foods, but stocking your larder with soy and soy supplements isn't going to offer you top-notch protection against breast cancer, menopause symptoms, cardiovascular disease, or osteoporosis.

A substantial number of nutritionists don't agree with all of the soy-industry-fueled, unconditionally positive press soy has been getting. This small coalition of scientists believes not only that soy's benefits have been overstated but also that some soy foods can be quite *unhealthy* for some people. Just as you don't read a lot of negative press in your doctor's office about synthetic progestins, you won't read a lot about the possible adverse effects of soybeans in the popular press.

Why the Chinese Didn't Eat Soybeans for 2,000 Years

Some of the earliest writings about the soybean date back to 3000 B.C. The Chinese emperor Shen-nong, the so-called King of Farming, wrote about the great virtues of the soybean plant, listing it as one of the five sacred crops. Apparently, the soybean plant was recognized as sacred because it regenerated the soil for future crops. Drawings in the text showed that it was the root, not the bean, that was considered beneficial. These ancient texts suggest that the Chinese recognized that soybeans were not fit for human consumption in their natural form.

Two thousand years later it was discovered that with proper preparation, soy could be a rich source of nutrients. Processes that removed toxins—which today are known as anti-nutrients—were developed to make soybeans into nutritious staples. Some astute scientist or hungry commoner figured out that a mold, when allowed to grow on the beans, destroyed the toxins and made the nutrients in the beans available to the body. This process became known as fermentation and led to the creation of tempeh, bean paste, and natto.

Later a simpler process was developed to prepare soybeans for human consumption. After lengthy soaking and cooking, the beans were treated with nigari, a substance found in seawater. The end product was what we now know as tofu. By about 1400 A.D., during the Ming dynasty, soy appeared in the Chinese Materia Medica as a nutritionally important food and an effective remedy for many common ailments.

Anti-nutrients in Soybeans

Soybeans, in their natural form, contain phytochemicals that have toxic effects on the human body. Phytates, goitrogens, and enzyme inhibitors are the major anti-nutrients found in soy. They are thought to have some positive effects, but can also act as toxins.

Anti-nutrients are produced by the soybean plant to protect it from the sun's radiation; from bacterial, viral, or fungal invasion; and from being eaten by animals. In essence, these anti-nutrients act as the plant's immune system and protect it from overforaging by animals. All plants contain some anti-nutrients, but some contain far more than others. Soy is especially rich in these toxic phytochemicals, and if they aren't removed by careful preparation (long soaking and cooking or fermentation), soybeans aren't really fit for regular human consumption.

Phytic Acid or Phytates

Soybeans are one of nature's richest sources of phytic acid. (Most legumes contain it.) In the gastrointestinal tract this phytochemical binds tightly to essential minerals such as zinc, copper, iron, magnesium, and calcium. It's especially fond of zinc, a mineral that supports wound healing, protein synthesis, reproductive health, nerve function, and brain development. In fact, it has been said that people living in third-world countries are shorter than those in more developed nations because of zinc deficiency caused by too much phytic acid from legumes. Some scientists believe that mental development could be stunted by a high-phytate diet.

Enzymes in the fungus used for fermentation break down the phytates in soybeans. Soaking also reduces phytate content, although not as much. Fermented soy foods such as miso and tempeh have the least phytic acid of all the soy foods. Tofu, whole soybeans, soy milk, soy chips, soy protein isolates, and soy flour contain much higher levels of phytates. This doesn't mean miso and tempeh are the only worthwhile soy foods; thousands of years ago the Asians figured out that eating tofu with mineral-rich sea vegetables and some animal protein could make up for its mineral-depleting effects.

Anytime you consume soy foods with higher phytic acid content, accompany them with kelp or seaweed and some low-fat protein, such as from fish.

Enzyme Inhibitors

Whole soybeans and unfermented soy products are rich in enzyme inhibitors that can diminish your body's ability to digest carbohydrates and protein. Digestive enzymes from saliva and the pancreas are secreted into the gastrointestinal tract to help break down the foods you eat. These enzymes—amylase, trypsin, and chymotrypsin—are inhibited by phytochemicals in soy. If foods can't be broken down by these enzymes, they can't be absorbed into the body and used for energy and tissue repair. When foods are incompletely digested because of enzyme inhibitors, bacteria in the large intestine try to do the job, and this can cause painful and potentially embarrassing bouts of gas.

The content of enzyme inhibitors in soy varies widely, depending on where the soybeans were grown and how they've been processed. In a single soy food source, such as the soy protein isolates commonly used in infant formula, levels of enzyme inhibitors can vary by as much as twentyfold. There's no method for measuring or standardizing foods for enzyme inhibitor content. Fermentation partly destroys them, and heating does so to a lesser extent. Individuals with low levels of digestive enzymes, such as the elderly, would be likely to suffer the most from soy's enzyme-inhibiting actions.

Goitrogens

Low thyroid activity—also known as hypothyroidism—is quite common in American women, especially those who are approaching menopause. Thyroid hormones drive the energy-generating systems in every cell of the body. Without them, the cellular furnaces called mitochondria are unable to burn fats, carbohydrates, and proteins for fuel. Low thyroid activity shows up as an inability to generate heat; the skin is cold and body temperature is low. Some substances found in foods can inhibit the ability of the thyroid gland to make its hormones. These goitrogens (so named because they can cause goiter formation) are abundant in unprocessed soybeans. In the early twentieth century the goitrogenic effects of soybeans on animals were well known.

The isoflavone genistein found in soy can block thyroid production. This is likely to be the reason that people who consume soy are more likely to have the autoimmune disease Hashimoto's thyroiditis. Phytic acid can add to these effects by binding zinc and copper, both of which are needed to make thyroid hormones.

Soy Can Slow Your Brain

Glucose, the simplest form of sugar, is the fuel your cells need to function. The brain is especially dependent on a steady supply of glucose and has several very complex fail-safe mechanisms to ensure that it always has enough—even if it means diverting it away from other parts of the body.

A transport protein, GLUT1, sits on the outside of cells, waiting for glucose to float by in the bloodstream. As soon as GLUT1 senses glucose, it snatches it up and sends it into the body of the cell, where it's used to generate energy. New studies show that the activity of this transport protein is shut down by the phytoestrogen genistein. (Daidzein does not have this effect.)

These studies were done in test tubes with soy products that contained quite a lot of genistein—more than the average person would get from eating moderate amounts of traditionally prepared soy foods. Soy protein isolates and other unfermented soy foods have much higher genistein content than Asian soy foods.

A recent study from Hawaii by White and coworkers of 8,000 Asian men over a 35-year period showed that those consuming the highest amount of tofu had smaller brain size and nearly three times the rate of senile dementia (mostly Alzheimer's). If soy isoflavones are responsible for this brain effect, which is supported by the biochemistry outlined above, we have to ask ourselves whether we are accelerating the aging of our brains by consuming high doses of soy isoflavones in pills and soy protein isolates.

Genistein's Cancer-Fighting Properties Affect Normal Cell Function

In the 1980s a group of Japanese scientists discovered that genistein, an isoflavone found in soy, is a potent inhibitor of tyrosine kinases, enzymes involved in the transfer of energy from one molecule to another. They play important roles in virtually all energy-generating processes in normal cells, driving cell division, memory consolidation, general tissue repair and growth, and blood vessel growth. The activity of tyrosine kinases is very tightly regulated. When cells begin to grow in an uncontrolled way and stop differentiating—when they become cancerous— this regulation has gone wrong. Among other things, cancer cells overexpress tyrosine kinases, and the result can be that they multiply out of control. When the role of tyrosine kinases in cancer was recognized, researchers began to look at ways in which cancer growth might be slowed by inhibiting the activity of these enzymes in cancer cells. Genistein, with its tyrosine-kinase-inhibiting effects, came along about the same time.

As research on genistein's possible anti-cancer effects began to accumulate, the soy industry began to develop products that would appeal to the Western palate and also provide a rich supply of genistein. In the midst of all of this excitement little attention has been paid to the potential adverse effects of genistein on tyrosine kinase activity in normal, noncancerous cells.

Genistein, Tyrosine Kinase, and Normal Brain Function

Tyrosine kinase activity is important for communication pathways in the brain through specific binding sites called GABA A receptors. These receptors are abundant in parts of the brain involved in memory processing, such as the hippocampus. We are now learning from test tube studies that genistein is capable of inhibiting tyrosine-kinase-related functions of GABA A in brain cells. This inhibition could mean that, if genistein levels rose high enough in the bloodstream, the activity of brain cells important for memory would be impaired.

Obviously, genistein-rich foods such as tempeh and miso haven't induced brain stupor in Asians. But Asians have never pushed the genistein content of their soy foods to the limits we've pushed it to in the West. Some Westernized soy foods contain 20 to 60 mg of genistein per serving, while Asians are estimated to eat only 4 to 10 mg of genistein a day. We just don't know the long-term effects of consuming genistein-enriched commercial products on the brain or elsewhere in the body.

Women are being encouraged to use such products through and beyond their menopausal years to thwart menopause symptoms, heart disease, and breast cancer. It's possible that this course of action could end up advancing age-related memory loss. Only time will tell, but you don't have to be one of the guinea pigs in this experiment. Stick with soy foods prepared in the traditional Asian ways and avoid soy supplements or Westernized soy foods with high levels of genistein.

An aside: Too much genistein in your diet may have dire consequences for both the inside and the outside of your cranium. Many normal cell processes require unfettered tyrosine kinase activity, one of which is hair growth. One study examined the effects of various chemicals on the growth of human hair follicles and found that genistein decreased hair growth by 60 to 80 percent!

Genistein and Blood Vessel Growth

Genistein also appears to suppress blood vessel growth, an action probably related to tyrosine kinase inhibition. Several test tube and animal studies have shown that genistein suppresses the growth of blood vessels toward tumors, which is a positive effect if you have cancer. You'll recall from chapter 3 that some types of tumors need to set up their own blood supply to grow beyond their early stages. By preventing this, you could effectively starve a tumor that needs its own blood vessels to grow, invade other tissues, and metastasize.

While this action of genistein is an advantage when it comes to tumor growth, it could be a disadvantage in normal cells. Genistein doesn't discriminate. It blocks the growth of normal blood vessels too. A genetically inherited abnormality called hereditary hemorrhagic telangiectasia (HHT) involves the growth of abnormal blood vessels in the gastrointestinal tract and nasal passages. These areas become engorged with blood, causing frequent, excessive bleeding. Migraines, caused by the same overabundance of blood vessels, are also common in HHT sufferers. When people with HHT were treated with about 60 g of isolated soy protein a day, they all found significant—in some cases, complete—relief from nosebleeds, gastrointestinal bleeding, and migraines. This is an excellent illustration of genistein's profound effect on blood vessel growth throughout the body. This isn't an effect that you necessarily want to have every day!

The point here is that it isn't difficult to consume enough soy protein isolate to affect blood vessel growth in healthy tissues. An advantage for someone with HHT or a tumor could be a liability for the average person. Another study found that genistein reduced blood vessel formation in the eyes. Before we load up on genistein, we need to ask more questions: Will this phytochemical, in excess, have an adverse effect on vision? Could it affect the microvascular systems in other organs?

You Say Genistein, I Say Genistin

Many soy product labels boast that they contain more isoflavones than others, but as it turns out, most of the isoflavones in nonfermented soy foods are unavailable to the body.

Most Western soy enthusiasts don't realize that when they eat foods such as whole cooked soybeans, soy flour, textured vegetable protein (TVP), soy milk, and tofu, most of the isoflavones are not bioavailable. Most of the isoflavones in soy are bound to carbohydrate molecules called glucosides. In this form genistein is actually called genistin. Think of genistin as genistein locked in a sugar coating that must be digested to make it available to the body. Sugar-bound isoflavones can enter the bloodstream, but they can't enter the tissues in this form.

Fermentation is what transforms genistin into genistein. It also reduces antinutrients such as phytic acid and trypsin inhibitors. The isoflavones in fermented soy foods such as miso, tempeh, and soy natto are low in antinutrients, and 40 to 90 percent of the genistein in these foods is unbound with sugars and freely available to the tissues. The content of unbound genistein in whole soybeans, soy flour, and roasted soybeans is only about 2 to 6 percent of the total genistein content.

Many soy products sold in the United States don't distinguish between genistein and genistin on their labels. Most of the isoflavone content is sugar-bound and unavailable to the tissues unless it's first broken down by enzymes in the body. Although some genistin is converted to genistein by bacteria in the body, fermentation in the gastrointestinal tract is much less efficient than the traditional methods of fermentation used to make miso and tempeh. Some people's bodies are more efficient at this than others. A healthy gastrointestinal tract, however, is more likely to transform genistein into genistin by attaching sugar molecules, rather than working the other way around. It's unlikely that much unbound genistein will make it into your system if you eat unfermented soy or take pills that contain genistin improperly labeled as genistein.

GENISTEIN FACTS: THE BEST AND WORST

Here's a quick summary of what we know about genistein:

- Genistein has some estrogenic effects. This may help relieve menopausal symptoms, but may—like estradiol—stimulate the growth of estrogen-sensitive breast tumors.
- Genistein inhibits thyroid peroxidase, the enzyme that places iodine on tyrosine, and thus blocks thyroid production.
- Genistein inhibits the formation of blood vessels in tumors (angiogenesis). This will prevent tumor growth but may also have some negative impact on normal processes of vascularization required for vision and hair growth.
- Genistein is a potent antioxidant, and its free-radical-scavenging activity could be expected to help prevent diseases of aging such as heart disease and cancer.
- Genistein inhibits tyrosine kinase activity. While they're important for tumor growth, tyrosine kinases are also needed for the proper functioning of neurotransmitters and memory. High doses of genistein could impair brain development or memory.
- Genistein inhibits glucose uptake, possibly slowing tumor growth. Tumors thrive on glucose, but so do brain cells. This, too, could slow mental function.

How to Get the Nutritional Benefits of Soy

Americans tend to believe that if a little of something is good, then a whole lot more is better. The evidence is strong that this isn't the case with soy foods, just as it isn't the case with hormone balance or certain vitamins. A little natural progesterone and estrogen in the right amounts caɪ bring many women through menopause with a minimum of symptoms, but not enough or too much of either will diminish the benefits. Vitamins A and D are vital for good health, but if taken in excess they can be toxic. Genistein is beneficial in the moderate amounts found in the typical Asian diet, but has the potential to do harm in higher doses.

In China, Indonesia, Korea, Japan, and Taiwan, about 3.4 to 13 kilograms of soy is consumed per person per year. If we generalize to 10 kg per person, we can estimate that each person eats 30 grams (3,000 mg)—about an ounce—of soy a day. An ounce of tempeh contains about 10 mg of free (unbound) isoflavones, including 4 mg of genistein. For miso or fermented bean curd (soy natto), an ounce a day would contain about 20 to 30 mg of free isoflavones and 8 to 12 mg of genistein.

Based on what we know about Asian diets and the potential hazards of overdosing on genistein, we recommend that women consume natural soy foods (miso, tempeh, tofu, natto). This will be enough to take advantage of genistein's cancer-protective effects, but not enough to cause the potential problems discussed in this chapter. Avoid genistein or soy isoflavone pills and soy protein isolates unless you have specific reasons to take them. See the table on page 284 for more specific recommendations and isoflavone content of soy foods.

The overblown positive press on soy has led to the creation of soy hot dogs, soy cheeses, soy yogurt, and soy snack bars, all of which may be high in anti-nutrients—there's really no way of knowing. These foods may be more nutritious than other foods with regard to their fat and protein content, but they won't do much to prevent breast cancer.

Avoid soybean oil, which has essentially no isoflavones and is usually hydrogenated. Soy sauce is also virtually devoid of iso-flavones.

Tofu is a good food, rich in protein and low in fat. Eat it with a small amount of animal protein, preferably fish, and some sea-weed or kelp to supply minerals that can be bound by phytates.

Soy allergy is not uncommon. It's estimated that up to 30 percent of the Western population may be allergic to soy. If you find that soy foods don't agree with your digestive system, or if you have headaches or other symptoms when you eat soy, you may want to avoid them.

For those of you who aren't allergic to soy, here are some guidelines to help you choose soy foods that are low in anti-nutrients and good for disease prevention.

GENISTEIN CONTENT IN VARIOUS SOY FOODS

Values represent milligrams of the sugar-free, unbound form of genistein per 3 ounces (about 100 grams) of soy product. The sugar-bound form of genistein, correctly termed genistin, can comprise more than 90 percent of the total isoflavones in unfermented soy products.

SOYBEAN FOOD TYPES	GENISTEIN CONTENT milligrams/3 oz	ANTI-NUTRIENT CONTENT	FAVORABLE SOY FOOD
COOKED SOYBEANS	1–2	HIGH	NO
ROASTED SOYBEANS	5–6	HIGH	NO
SOY OIL	TRACE	HIGH	NO
SOY FLOUR	1–2	HIGH	NO
TEXTURED SOY PROTEIN	2–3	MODERATE	NO
PROTEIN ISOLATE (1 oz.)	38	MODERATE	NO
SOY MILK	1–4	MODERATE	NO
TOFU	1–4	MODERATE	YES
TEMPEH	8	LOW	YES
MISO	3–20	LOW	YES
FERMENTED BEAN CURD (NATTO)	18	LOW	YES
SOY HOT DOG	1–2	MODERATE	NO
TEMPEH BURGER	8	LOW	YES
SOY YOGURT	0.2	MODERATE	NO

Adapted from Wang and Murphy, 1994; Anderson and Wolf, 1995; Fukutake, 1996.

CHAPTER 17

HOW NUTRITION AFFECTS YOUR BREAST CANCER RISK

Making Good Choices Can Make the Difference

Each step of the way through the process of cancer growth—initiation, promotion, and progression—nutrients from healthful foods can play a role in stopping or slowing its advance. It's never too late to begin eating nourishing foods, since the start of breast cancer occurs eight to ten years before it has grown enough to be diagnosed. Each day the dietary choices you make can have an impact on whether you're ever diagnosed with this disease.

Experts agree that environmental risk factors, such as diet and exposure to toxins and pollutants, account for about 80 percent of breast cancers, and genetic factors account for about 20 percent. Among the environmental risk factors for breast cancer, diet is probably at least as important as exposure to toxins. Even those who happen to have a genetic predisposition can improve their chances of dodging a breast cancer diagnosis with hormone balance and a healthy diet.

Much research effort has been put forth to find which foods increase and which foods decrease breast cancer risk, and some findings have garnered more media attention than others. In this chapter we'll sort out what's hype and what's for real when it comes to diet and breast cancer risk.

Dietary Fat and Breast Cancer Risk

Much of the research on diet–breast cancer connections since the 1940s has encouraged the assumption that fat in the diet increases risk. Early population studies showed breast cancer incidence to be lower in nations where fat intake makes up 15 percent of daily calories and higher in nations where fat intake comprises 40 percent of daily calories. It is true that breast cancer incidence is highest in Western (North American and Western European) women, who eat more fat, and lowest in third-world women, who eat the least. The difference in breast cancer incidence between these two populations is as high as four- to sixfold. Because of this research, and other studies on animals and on other populations of women eating low- and high-fat diets, women were told that eating less fat would decrease their breast cancer risk. Newer research, however, has been shooting holes in this theory since at least 1996.

The problems with soy research we talked about in chapter 16 apply here as well. Women who eat a lot of fat tend to have diets radically different from those who eat little, especially when they live on different continents. A third-world diet generally consist of whole grains, legumes, vegetables, and moderate amounts of animal protein, while a typical Western diet includes more junk food, meats, refined grains, sugars, and not much in the way of vegetables or fruit. In nations where food is scarce, people might take in half the daily calories eaten by a Westerner and burn most of these calories off with exercise. Needless to say, the differences in diet between these two populations goes far beyond the amount of fat in it.

Today we're also learning that the type of fat you eat is an important consideration when it comes to disease risk. For a while saturated fats—the kind found in meats and dairy—were targeted as risky and undesirable, yielding the upsurge in popularity of margarines and polyunsaturated oils. Now we're finding that saturated fats, in moderation, aren't as dangerous as once thought, and the majority of studies show absolutely no connection between saturated fat intake and breast cancer risk. The latest research shows that trans-fats in margarines, and the polyunsaturated oils they're made from, are actually much more dangerous to your health than saturated fats. These fats affect the body in ways that appear to increase cancer and heart disease risk.

A March 1999 study, published in the *Journal of the American Medical Association*, tracked 88,795 women between the ages of 30 and 55 from 1980 to 1994. Their dietary habits were monitored with questionnaires. By the end of the study 2,956 of the women had been diagnosed with breast cancer, and it was found that breast cancer was no more common in women who ate high-fat diets. Women who kept their fat intake below 20 percent of total calories weren't any less likely to develop breast cancer. In fact, the group of less than 1,000 women who ate *less* than 20 percent of their calories as fat had 15 percent *more* breast cancer in this study!

In another study researchers found that women who ate more monounsaturated fats, such as those found in olive oil and canola oil, had lower breast cancer risk than those who ate more polyunsaturated fats, like those found in nut, seed, and vegetable oils. The authors of the study concluded that this was because monounsaturated fats are less subject to oxidation—the formation of free radicals—than polyunsaturated fats. Free radicals, in excess, are known to damage DNA and lead to mutations that cause cancerous changes in cells. Polyunsaturated fats are highly unstable and oxidize easily. When you open a bottle of oil and it smells rancid, it's because of oxidation. Rarely does a monounsaturated oil or saturated fat become rancid.

The processed food industry's answer to the rancidity problem was to bombard polyunsaturated oils with hydrogen atoms. This process, called hydrogenation, turns liquid oil into solid fat. While hydrogenation protects against oxidation and spoilage, it also creates trans–fatty acids, which are rarely found in nature.

These fake fats are found in margarine and in cakes, cookies, and other processed foods; they're more likely than natural fats to convert into dangerous oxidized lipids in the body, to damage cell membranes, and to induce cancerous changes in cells.

Fish oils are in the news these days almost as much as soy. They're recommended for prevention of heart disease and inflammatory diseases. The polyunsaturated oils found in fish are a rich source of omega-3 fatty acids, which newer research shows may help prevent cancer. Fish oils are prone to oxidation, like any other unsaturated fat, but if you get them directly from fish—rather than from fish oil capsules or liquid—they're safe, and they promote the proper balance of prostaglandins (which we'll discuss in more detail later in this chapter). If you use fish-oil supplements, be sure they are well preserved.

This explains why a woman in a Mediterranean country who eats a 40 percent fat diet rich in monounsaturated fats from olive oil and omega-3 fats from fish has quite a different breast cancer risk profile from a woman in Philadelphia eating her 40 percent fat in the form of cheese steak sandwiches and french fries!

The Role of Refined Carbohydrates

There's an inseparable connection between fat and estrogen, because fat cells are estrogen factories. Women become caught in a cycle in which increased body fat raises estrogen levels, and estrogen increases the tendency to accumulate body fat. It was once thought that the Western diet caused weight gain because of its high fat content, but today we know better. The evidence is everywhere: How many people do you know who jumped on the low-fat bandwagon, increased their consumption of low-fat carbohydrate-rich foods, and ended up heavier than they were to begin with? And how many people do you know who *lost* weight on a high-protein and -fat diet such as the one developed by Robert Atkins, M.D.? (We don't recommend either extreme.)

Dietary fat doesn't necessarily make you fat. In fact, the huge quantities of sugars and refined carbohydrates (breads, pastries, cookies, pastas, bagels) eaten by the typical Westerner have made a far more significant contribution to the expansion of American girths. The elimination of fats from the diet in the attempt to lose weight and improve health made way not for more vegetables and fruits but for packaged, processed, low-fat, high-carbohydrate products with lots of calories and little to no nutritive value.

An intracellular insulin-like growth factor called IGF-1 can, if excessive, interact with estrogen and increase the risk of greater human breast cancer cell replication rates. The levels of IGF-1 in a woman's body increase with insulin resistance, which is correlated with increased refined carbohydrate intake and body fat. A high-refined-carbohydrate diet sets up the body for weight gain and an increased estrogen burden more than does a diet with balanced amounts of fats from olive oil and whole foods.

Excess Calories, Not Just Excess Fat

The Western diet is relatively high in calories compared to energy needs. Almost every person in the Western world consumes more calories than he or she needs for fuel on a daily basis. The third-world diet is relatively high in fiber and is largely plant based, calorie intake is considerably lower, and exercise levels are considerably higher.

It's now clear that calories in excess of energy needs are stored as fat, which increases estrogen levels. When energy needs exceed calorie intake, total body fat and estrogen decline. When calorie intake exceeds energy needs, estrogen rises accordingly. This is one of nature's ways of reducing fertility during times when food is scarce and increasing fertility when it's abundant. Dr. Peter Ellison of Harvard, who has conducted worldwide assays of salivary hormone levels, believes that excessive calorie intake is the primary reason for the higher estrogen levels seen in premenopausal women in industrialized cultures.

One major source of excess calories in Western diets is refined carbohydrates from foods like breads, cakes, muffins, bagels, candy, cookies, pretzels, sodas, and other sweetened drinks. These foods are bad news—not only because they supply plentiful calories without any real nutritive value, but also because they keep blood sugars and insulin levels soaring and then dropping like a roller coaster, and predispose us to adult-onset diabetes. Recent research has shown that insulin resistance, a prediabetic condition caused primarily by excessive consumption of calories and a sedentary lifestyle, increases breast cancer risk.

Refined carbohydrates alter the balance of fatty acids in the body, raising levels of bad prostaglandins (see Good Fats and Bad Fats, below). Refined carbohydrate overconsumption has been linked to insulin resistance, and to disruption in the normal patterns of hormone production in the brain (LH and FSH) and ovaries. This leads to the polycystic ovaries and irregular menstrual cycles that are associated with overproduction of androgens and estrogens, and to the underproduction of progesterone. It is this state of persistent estrogen dominance in the absence of progesterone that predisposes the breast cells to overstimulation and risk of cancerous changes.

This doesn't mean you should avoid carbohydrates and eat lots of meat and dairy products, as many popular weight-loss diets suggest. Unrefined carbohydrates from whole foods such as vegetables and whole grains are a rich source of anticancer phytochemicals and are essential foods to include in a diet that reduces the risk of breast cancer.

Good Fats and Bad Fats

You need fat in your diet to build and maintain many parts of your body, including cell membranes, cholesterol, steroid hormones, and prostaglandins. Prostaglandins are a class of hormones produced within cells throughout the body. They affect a variety of bodily processes, including blood pressure, inflammation, and immune function. Some prostaglandins promote inflammation, whereas others inhibit it. However, the prostaglandins that promote inflammation are not necessarily bad, because your body needs all types of these hormones to function properly. What will cause problems is too much of any one type of prostaglandin. A healthy balance is a key to a healthy body.

The manufacture of prostaglandins is largely driven by the fats and oils we eat. Therefore, it's important to eat the fats that keep our prostaglandins in proper balance. Eating too much red meat, for instance, tends to increase the prostaglandins that are pro-inflammatory, which means that they increase vasoconstriction (narrowing of the blood vessels), platelet aggregation (sticky blood), and cellular proliferation, along with suppressing the immune system, thus increasing blood clotting and the risk of stroke. The oils that you get when you eat fresh vegetables and fish tend to be anti-inflammatory, meaning that they create vasodilation (opening of the blood vessels), inhibit platelet aggregation, control cell proliferation, and enhance the immune system.

Prostaglandins are yet another example of how the body's systems work to maintain a dynamic balance for good health. While the entire subject of fats and prostaglandin balance is quite complex, a major lesson to learn is that fresh, unprocessed natural fats common to human consumption for the past thousands of years are, in general, much more wholesome and healthy than are synthetic trans–fatty acids, such as those found in processed seed oils and deep-fat-fried foods so common these days. We recommend Dr. Mary Enig's book *Know Your Fats* and Andrew Stoll M.D.'s *The Omega-3 Connection* if you're looking for scientifically sound and detailed information on this topic. Suffice it to say that the categories of saturated, mono-, or polyunsaturated fats are less important to your health than the distinction between natural fats and synthetic trans–fatty acids. Learn to avoid trans–fatty acids, which most often show up on food labels as "hydrogenated" or "partially hydrogenated oils."

Research is giving us some guidance in choosing cancer-preventive fats. Women who eat more of their fat as olive oil (which is extracted from the olive without high pressure or high temperature) appear to enjoy decreased breast cancer risk compared to women who eat more of the trans-fats. Test tube and animal studies show that this could be explained by the effects of these fats on breast prostaglandin levels. Prostaglandin E_2, for example, which is increased by eating excessive quantities of red meat, increases the activity of aromatase, an enzyme that converts other steroids into estrogen in breast cells. Studies on rats show that too much of the omega-6 fats found in unsaturated oils such as corn and safflower can accelerate the promotion phase of breast cancer by enhancing the formation of pro-inflammatory prostaglandins, which may increase free-radical-mediated DNA damage and stimulate cell proliferation and higher free estrogen levels. In contrast, the omega-3s found in fish seem to promote anti-inflammatory prostaglandins that inhibit cell proliferation.

Again, we want to emphasize that this doesn't mean you should entirely give up red meat or corn oil; it means that you should eat these types of food in balance with a wide variety of other wholesome foods. Let's examine what this means more closely.

Practical Tips on Chewing the Fat

We don't think it's necessary for you to count fat grams or calories to find your ideal diet. Instead, think in terms of adjusting your diet according to these general guidelines until you find what works for you. If you generally choose good foods and avoid unhealthy ones, everything else has a way of falling into place.

Here's a general rule of thumb: The good fats are part of whole foods. This means fish, vegetables, nuts and seeds, free-range eggs, whole grains, and legumes. It doesn't mean that highly processed seed oils are good for you.

• *Olive oil* and modest amounts of butter for cooking and baking are part of a health-supporting diet. Wherever you can, substitute olive oil for other oils that require heavy processing. Look for dark green extra-virgin olive oils. They're expensive, but there's nothing better for you to spend your money on than a health-promoting diet. And they taste so good, you'll only need to use a small amount. Avocado oil is another monounsaturated fat that's rich in healthy essential fatty acids (EFAs).

• *Canola oil* is also monounsaturated, but it's highly processed for commercial uses and therefore less desirable. It's best to use canola oil only occasionally. If you love potato and corn chips and insist on having them, chips fried in canola oil are probably safer than chips fried in highly processed polyunsaturated oils like safflower, corn, sunflower, nut, or seed oils. Polyunsaturated oils are most likely rancid by the time you open the bottle to use them, so you can imagine how far gone they are when they've been sitting on the store shelf for a while, or when they've been heated to high temperatures and used for frying. It's best to completely avoid polyunsaturated or hydrogenated oils made from soy, corn, nuts, and seeds.

• *Saturated fats* such as butter, coconut oil, and lard are solid at room temperature and very stable. You can leave them sitting out and not worry that they'll spoil, and you can heat them up without creating free radicals. Unrefined coconut oil and butter are best for baking. Again, remember that these fats have gotten a bad name, but only because they've been eaten in excess; in moderate amounts they're beneficial to your health.

• *Hydrogenated oils* are the trans–fatty acids used to make everything from margarines to baked goods to potato chips to frozen desserts, and are now being linked to increased risk of artery disease. It seems that hydrogenated fats directly damage the delicate linings of blood vessels. They also throw off your hormone balance by blocking the actions of good fats.

• *Omega-3 fats* are found most abundantly in deep-water fish such as mackerel, herring, sardines, and cod. The FDA, however, has recently warned pregnant women away from eating mackerel due to high mercury content, so you can leave that one off the list. Albacore tuna is also a good source, but it too can accumulate mercury, although less than mackerel; just be moderate about how often you eat it. Salmon is also a good source of omega-3 fats, and if it's fresh it has a very mild flavor that even kids usually don't mind. Try to have omega-3-rich fish two or three times a week.

Green leafy vegetables and walnuts also contain omega-3s. Flaxseeds are especially rich in omega-3 fats. Flaxseed oil, however, spoils (becomes oxidized or rancid) easily; in fact, it's one of the most unstable oils known. It's better to buy whole flaxseeds and grind them at home (with a small coffee grinder) to sprinkle on cereal or salads. Although the omega-3s are beneficial oils, you don't need them in large amounts. Since oxidation overload in the body is a major factor in all types of chronic diseases and in cancer, please don't go overboard with the omega-3 oils.

• *Vegetable oils* contain omega-6 fatty acids, which are beneficial for you in small amounts. They go rancid easily and thus are best added to the diet by eating plenty of fresh vegetables.

Whole Foods Are Best

Of course, there's more to eating well than the types of fat you eat. Many popular diet books emphasize protein and carbohydrate intake; others focus on specific "superfoods" purported to have miraculous effects on health; still others focus on nutritional supplements or vitamins, minerals, and other nutrients from healthy foods. With all of the dietary advice that's available today, making the right choices can seem downright bewildering.

If we had to choose one single piece of advice to give you that would most improve your health, it would be to learn to eat modest amounts of fresh, whole, organic, unprocessed foods. They contain vitamins, minerals, and other nutrients you need, in abundance. They contain fiber, which is very important for proper digestion of food, intestinal transit, and hormone balance.

What does eating whole foods mean? It means eating whole grains such as brown rice, bulgur, millet, quinoa, and amaranth (really a seed), which are tasty and can be used by themselves or in casseroles. Look at the labels on store bread. It may be advertised as "whole wheat" or "whole rye," but the contents listed usually refer to flour made from these grains. In making flour, the outer fibrous, mineral-rich coat has been removed, as has the germ of the grain with its fat-soluble vitamins. Become a smart shopper. What you're looking for is "whole grain" bread. If your store doesn't sell good bread, ask the manager to get some in.

Eating whole foods means eating beans, including traditionally prepared soybean products. Beans won't cause gas in most people if they're introduced gradually into the diet. It's helpful if they're soaked overnight and the soaking water discarded. You can also use a product called Beano, which contains the enzyme necessary to digest beans, until your own body learns to make the enzymes. Just put a few drops of it onto the beans before you eat them. Most health food stores and pharmacies carry Beano.

Eating whole, unprocessed foods means emphasizing fresh vegetables. Vegetables contain dozens of natural cancer-fighting compounds (phytochemicals) that inhibit cancer initiation and promotion. The awful habit of boiling vegetables until they're mushy and tasteless has given them a bad name. Canning is equally hard on taste. Freezing is somewhat better, but you still lose important enzymes and vitamins when you freeze foods. Fresh vegetables are delicious raw or lightly steamed. Fresh root vegetables such as beets, carrots, turnips, onions, garlic, and potatoes are wonderful baked with some olive oil and fresh herbs. Experiment with some of the more exotic green leafy vegetables such as kale and bok choy. Broccoli, cauliflower, cabbage, and brussels sprouts—vegetables from the *Brassica* (cruciferous) genus—are especially potent cancer fighters, as are garlic, onions, and leeks (from the *Allium* genus). Once you become acquainted with these foods, you'll find that they're quick and simple to prepare and very tasty.

As we mentioned above in the section on fats, fish is a highly nutritious addition to a whole-foods diet. An excellent source of protein, fish also contains the omega-3 fatty acids eicosapentaenoic acid (EPA) and docosahexaenoic acid (DHA), which appear to offer some protection against breast cancer as well as heart disease.

And last but not least, eating whole, unprocessed foods means eating fresh fruit instead of desserts loaded with white sugar, fructose, or corn syrup. Before you balk at the idea of spending money on some expensive grapes or a papaya, stop and think how much you'd pay for a pie, cake, or ice cream. If you really have a sweet tooth, try sprinkling apples, pears, or peaches with cinnamon and baking them. Even then, your consumption of fruits shouldn't be overdone. They're primarily sugar, which will adversely affect your blood sugar balance if you eat too much. Remember that dried fruit contains all the sugar of the whole fruit, so be moderate about dried fruit too. If you like fruit juice, invest in a juicer and drink only freshly squeezed vegetable and fruit juices. Pasteurization and storage of packaged juices robs them of nutrients and enzymes.

The obvious opposite of eating whole foods is eating processed foods. While we don't advocate becoming extreme, it's best in general to avoid highly refined carbohydrates such as those containing white flour or sugar, as well as foods that contain additives, preservatives, or colorings. You'll find it's easier to maintain overall balance if you have that ice cream cone or chocolate chip cookie only now and then; eating sugary foods daily will set you up for a long list of health problems. But if having an ice cream cone is going to send you off on a binge of eating sugar, then don't do it; use your common sense here.

Eat Organic Foods Whenever Possible

Nonorganic farming leaves soil fallow, depleted of the minerals it needs to produce healthy, pest-resistant crops. Whatever plants can be eked out of this used-up soil need plenty of harsh fertilizers, herbicides, and pesticides to survive to market. The hybridization of crops—which is what makes those uniformly large, flawless-looking, and tasteless veggies you see in the supermarket produce section—means further exhaustion of nutrient content. Fruits and vegetables that are conventionally grown are low in nutrients, hybridized, sprayed, and fertilized with all manner of poisonous compounds, many of them with estrogenic properties, and they don't taste as good as organically grown produce. The pesticide residues left on that nice red apple may be small, but if you add them to all the other pesticides you're exposed to, the toxic load may be too much.

Organic produce is usually locally grown and fresher than conventional varieties. If you have a farmer's market in your area, take full advantage of it. You can usually find plenty of organic foods at reasonable prices because you're buying them directly from the grower. If you don't have a farmer's market, start one in your area! Or you can tell the produce manager at your local supermarket that you'd like organic produce. There are supermarkets springing up all around the country that feature hormone-free meat, whole foods, and organic produce in response to increased consumer demand for these items. If there's one in your area, it'll be worth the extra few dollars a week to shop there. Think of it as a long-term investment in your health.

Is Vegetarianism Protective?

Although we can't argue with those who are vegetarians for philosophical reasons, being a vegetarian isn't necessarily healthier, for most people. Some vegetarians may be healthier because they eat a lot of vegetables, but many have nutritional deficiencies caused by a lack of the nutrients supplied by meat and dairy products. In other words, you have to know what you're doing, and eat very carefully, if you're going to be a vegetarian. Eating only carrot sticks and bagels won't contribute to nutritional well-being!

None of the large, long-term studies looking at meat consumption and breast cancer has shown an increased risk. While there are good reasons not to overdo it with meat eating, there's no evidence that eating small portions of meat increases your risk of breast cancer. Poultry and beef are nutritious and satisfying accompaniments to vegetables and whole grains. If you don't go overboard with fast-food burgers or huge steaks, there's no reason you can't enjoy these foods as part of a balanced cancer-preventive diet. Rather than seeing meats as the main course, make vegetables the main course and use meat as a condiment.

The nutrients found in meats, eggs, and dairy products are important for methylation. In chapter 7 you learned that methylation is the addition of a methyl group to toxins, which neutralizes them and prepares them for removal from the body along with other wastes. Catechol estrogens—the bad estrogens that can be transformed into the really bad quinone estrogens—are tagged for safe excretion by the process of methylation. This happens mostly in your liver and kidneys. These organs need the amino acid cysteine to make methyl groups; cysteine is found in the most abundance in meat, eggs, and dairy products.

Opt for Free-Range Meats, Eggs, and Poultry

Range-raised cattle are naturally lean. The fats found in the meat of a cow that's grazed in open pasture are stable, saturated fats, while the meat of cattle raised in factory farms contains a conglomeration of polyunsaturated and saturated fats, chemicals, and hormones. Factory-farmed meat may come from cattle that are fed a mishmash of oils, grains, wastes from chemically fertilized crops, old newspapers urinated on by other cattle, and even unsalable parts of their slaughtered brethren. If you are what you eat, you're also what whatever you eat eats.

Many beef cattle are routinely injected with estrogen to fatten them up for market. This estrogen is still in the meat when it gets to your table; not in large quantities, but in measurable quantities, meat and eggs from conventionally raised chickens contain the antibiotics and petrochemical xenobiotics (pesticides) they're fed. Many of these toxins are concentrated in the fatty tissues of animal products, which means you're getting a far more potent dose with these foods than with vegetables.

The bottom line here is that you and your family are much better off eating organic meats and eggs. If you're on a tight budget and can afford to buy only some of your foods as organic, these are the ones you should choose: free-range, hormone-free eggs, meats, and chicken.

Cooking methods also make a difference when it comes to meats. Broiling meats at high heat yields substances that are known to initiate cancerous changes in cells. Baking and stir-frying are better alternatives than grilling or broiling over open flames, although grilling over lower heat should be fine.

Are Dairy Foods Right for You?

Most cultures in the world are allergic to cows' milk and do not have the enzymes to digest its lactose. Some Northern European cultures can tolerate milk to some degree, but for the most part there's no good reason for milk to be a staple of anybody's diet. Magnesium is necessary to utilize calcium for bone building, and milk has a poor magnesium-to-calcium ratio. Furthermore, dairy cows are forced to exist in intolerably unhealthy conditions and are loaded up with antibiotics and other drugs to compensate. When you drink milk or eat other dairy products, you're getting dosed with these drugs. The amount in any given glass of milk or piece of cheese may be minuscule, but added to other sources the effect can be cumulative.

If you want the complete story on why milk *doesn't* do a body good, read Dr. Lee's book *Optimal Health Guidelines Revised and Updated.*

Beware of BGH

Bovine growth hormone (BGH) or recombinant bovine growth hormone (rBGH) increases milk production in dairy cows. BGH-treated milk contains higher levels of insulin-like growth factor 1, which is identical in humans and cows. IGF-1 is a growth promoter that interacts with estrogen to make it more potent, and research is increasingly showing us that it could increase breast and colon cancer risk.

University of Illinois toxicologist Samuel Epstein, M.D., says that "all women from conception to death will now be exposed to an additional breast cancer risk due to milk from cows treated with recombinant bovine growth hormone." Despite these warnings from Dr. Epstein, which are based on solid research, the FDA still allows the use of BGH, and most dairy farmers use it. If you're sure that you and your family can tolerate milk, we recommend using organic brands.

Yogurt is the most beneficial way to eat dairy products. While it's usually made from cows' milk, the fermenting or culturing process used to make yogurt renders the offending lactose and proteins harmless. Some research has shown a decrease in cancer risk in populations that eat yogurt on a regular basis. Avoid yogurt that contains added sugar—this includes most flavored varieties. Choose organic, plain varieties and add your own fruit or granola.

Aged cheeses seem to be fairly well tolerated by many people;

try eating some on an empty stomach and wait an hour before eating anything else. If you feel fine, it's probably okay for you.

Eat Your Phytochemicals: Natural Defenses against Cancer

Phytochemicals are plant compounds, many of which have health-supporting effects on the body. It's estimated that there are more than 10,000 of these compounds in the plants we eat. Phytoestrogens are a family of plant phytochemicals that have weak estrogen-like activity. Though their chemical structure is unlike that of estrogen, they are able to bind to and activate estrogen receptors throughout the body. However, their binding is much weaker than estrogens such as estradiol, and their effects more subtle. At high levels they actually can displace estradiol from its receptors and in doing so act as weak anti-estrogens. They compete for estrogen receptors throughout the body, helping block the effects of excess or stronger estrogens. If you eat a variety of fresh vegetables and have fermented soy products a few times a week, you'll reap the benefits of these natural estrogen blockers. Some herbs, such as red clover, licorice root, anise, and fennel, contain phytoestrogens, but it's wise to consult with an herbalist or naturopathic doctor before using these plants medicinally over a long period of time.

As we discussed earlier, be wary of the hype around soy. While it does contain phytoestrogens than can help balance your hormones, it also contains other phytochemicals called phytates that block the absorption of needed nutrients such as zinc and iodine, and that disable enzymes your body needs to access other nutrients. Fermentation denatures these substances and thus reduces the nutrient-blocking effect of soy. Asian diets utilize mostly fermented soy products such as miso and tempeh in small amounts, and also adds seaweed, which is rich in minerals. Refer to chapter 16 for a detailed account of the pros and cons of soy foods, and how to enjoy their benefits without their liabilities.

Where to Find Your Phytochemicals

We've known for years that diets high in vegetables and fruits are protective against cancer, and studies on plant chemicals and their effects at the cellular level are showing us how they inhibit cancer initiation, promotion, and progression.

Let's look, for example, at the sulfated amino acids found in cruciferous vegetables such as broccoli, cauliflower, and cabbage. You'll recall from chapter 7 that when estrogens are transformed in the body to quinone estrogens, they can do damage to DNA that initiates cancer. Sulfated amino acids can quickly latch onto and neutralize quinone estrogens, preventing them from binding to and damaging DNA. Thus, by getting plenty of sulfated amino acids in your diet, you're helping prevent the initiation of cancer. If you're deficient in these amino acids, your cells are more vulnerable to chemical insults by these estrogens and by other toxins.

Remember, too, that estrogens can go down one of two pathways: the 4-hydroxy pathway or the 2-hydroxy pathway. The 4-hydroxy is the beginning of the cascade that ends up forming DNA-damaging catechol and quinone estrogens, while the 2-hydroxy is a safer pathway. Phytochemicals from *Brassica* (cruciferous) vegetables and *Allium* vegetables (garlic, onions, leeks) encourage estrogens down the 2-hydroxy pathway.

Here are a few other examples of phytochemicals that support your body's resistance against cancer:

SOME PHYTOCHEMICALS FOUND IN FOODS AND THEIR ANTI-CANCER ACTIONS

PLANT	CHEMICAL	ACTION IN BODY
Broccoli	Sulforaphane	Removes carcinogens from cells by boosting enzyme activity
Broccoli	Phenethyl isothiocyanate (PEITC)	Binds to enzymes that would otherwise bind carcinogens to DNA
Broccoli, cauliflower, cabbage	Indole-3-carbinol	Helps a precursor to estrogen break up into a benign rather than a cancer-causing form
Citrus fruits	Flavonoids	Prevents cancer-causing hormones from latching onto a cell
Onions and garlic	Allylic sulfide	Detoxifies carcinogens
Hot peppers	Capsaicin	Keeps toxic molecules from attaching to DNA
Tomatoes	P-coumaric acid Chlorogenic acid	Both disrupt the wedding between two common chemicals (e.g., nitrosamines) in cells—a union that can produce carcinogens
Soybeans	Genistein	Inhibits growth of blood vessels to cancer cells, which are needed for tumor growth (see chapter 16)

It's important to keep in mind when reading this table that each specific plant compound is only one factor out of thousands of other compounds in the same plant. These factors are simply the ones that we know about at this time. It's quite likely that some of the other compounds act synergistically to produce their full cancer-protective effect. Therefore, it's wiser to eat the actual plant than to isolate out just the single plant compound or some chemical patentable derivative or analogue of it.

Vitamins are also considered phytochemicals. Vegetables and fruits are very rich in vitamins C, E, and the carotenes, for example. Our primary source of vitamins and minerals should be our diet. Taking a multivitamin and mineral supplement is not the equivalent of eating a good vitamin- and mineral-rich diet. Consider your multivitamin and mineral supplement as a sort of insurance, not a substitute for a good diet. You'll find our guidelines later in this chapter.

You Have a Friend in Garlic

Garlic is one of the most delicious foods that Mother Nature has to offer. Any amateur chef can make a delicious dish with the help of garlic and olive oil or butter. And garlic isn't just tasty— it's now known to be protective against heart disease, cancer, and even colds and flu.

Regular garlic consumption gives us three lines of defense against cancer:

1. It inhibits the formation of cancer-causing chemicals. Garlic is a rich source of sulfur, which cells need to maintain high levels of glutathione—the anti-oxidant that works within all cells to rid the body of carcinogens and to prevent carcinogens from binding to and damaging DNA.
2. Garlic interferes with the promotion phase of cancer by directly suppressing the growth of newly formed cancer cells.

3. Garlic boosts immune function. Branched-chain carbohydrates found in garlic stimulate the activity of natural killer (NK) cells, which are the immune system's first line of defense against cancer cells. NK cells seek out and destroy cancer cells as they form.

In one Chinese city people eat as many as *six cloves* of garlic a day, and they have much lower rates of stomach cancer than residents of another Chinese city where garlic is rarely eaten. If you don't like the idea of eating garlic daily, you can still reap most of its benefits by taking an aged garlic extract. However, freshly crushed raw garlic is still your healthiest fare.

How about Alcohol?

High alcohol intake—more than two drinks a day—has been correlated with increased breast cancer risk. This is probably due to the fact that if your liver has to process a lot of alcohol every day, the resources left over to rid the body of estrogens and their metabolites are reduced.

If a glass of wine helps you relax, don't deprive yourself. One drink a day or a few times a week won't increase your cancer risk. In fact, red wine contains a phytochemical called resveratrol, which has been shown in test tube studies to inhibit breast cancer cell growth.

Eat More Fiber

Fiber is indigestible plant matter that passes all the way through the digestive tract. On its way through it has important "Roto Rooter" effects, and also absorbs waste products in the large intestine. People who eat plenty of fiber-rich food have lower rates of all types of cancer, especially colon cancer.

Adding supplemental fiber to an otherwise poor diet does not seem to be effective in preventing or slowing colon cancer—the lesson being, eat whole foods!

Plant cell walls are our only dietary sources of fiber. Fiber isn't just a rough broom that makes bowel movements easier; it also serves as a source of important nutrients for our bodies and for the friendly bacteria that live in our digestive tracts. Cellulose, found in most plant foods, binds water in the digestive tract, which makes for easier and more frequent elimination. Other varieties of fiber form gels within which excess dietary cholesterol is trapped and not absorbed. Mucilages are a type of fiber found in beans and around the moist inner layer of seeds, and they have potent cholesterol-lowering effects. Lignins (very small, indigestible fibers) are broken down into compounds that are protective against cancer.

The best possible way to get fiber into your diet is to eat whole, unprocessed foods. Whole grains, fresh fruits, vegetables, legumes, and nuts have plenty of fiber. If your diet presently consists mostly of processed foods, please introduce the fiber gradually, so your digestive system has time to adjust.

Dietary fiber carries excess estrogens out of the body. After estrogens have finished their work in the cells, activating growth and development in tissues such as the breast and uterus, they return to the bloodstream. They're carried in the blood to the liver, where they're metabolized to inactive estrogen conjugates. These conjugates are then incorporated into bile that carries them into the gastrointestinal tract. There, microbes convert the inactive estrogen conjugates back into active estrogens, which can be reabsorbed into the bloodstream. Fiber absorbs both active and inactive estrogen conjugates in the digestive tract, preventing them from being reabsorbed. Elimination of estrogens in feces helps decrease the body's estrogen load.

A plant-eating animal our size living in the wild would take in 30 to 90 grams of fiber a day. The average human gets only about 10 grams a day. Most omnivorous animals move their bowels more than once a day, after meals. (Follow a bear in the woods, if you dare.) As you follow our other dietary recommendations, you'll take in more fiber. An added bonus: On a high-fiber diet you'll feel satiated with less food than on a low-fiber diet. You'll eat less and probably lose a few pounds.

If you need to add even more fiber to your diet (due to constipation, for example), you can take 1 teaspoon of psyllium seed husk in 8 ounces of water or juice every morning. (You need to stir it vigorously and drink it right away.) The pure psyllium you find at your health food store is the same ingredient found in Metamucil and other similar products, without the sweeteners, preservatives, and food colorings.

Drink Plenty of Clean Water

Water is nature's inner cleanser. All metabolic actions require a water milieu in which to function. Most people in industrialized countries don't drink enough water and are chronically dehydrated. They drink coffee, tea, juice, and soda, but rarely water. Alcohol dehydrates tissues. Drinking clean water will help your body clear away wastes and toxins that can contribute to the development of cancer. Dehydration can create an imbalance of minerals, which can contribute to hormone imbalance.

Sadly, most water that comes out of your tap is now polluted beyond the point where it's truly safe to drink, and it generally tastes terrible because of the addition of chlorine. Since you can't always trust commercial bottled water to be clean, the best way to get clean water is to put a filter on your kitchen tap. A simple charcoal filter will *not* do the job. Be sure to get a type that filters out chlorine, heavy metals, benzene, and bacteria. You don't have to go to the expense of getting a reverse osmosis system—a ceramic or copper/zinc filter will do the job and takes just a few minutes to install. Check your Yellow Pages under "water."

Take Your Multivitamins

Our food crops today have half the nutrients of crops grown a century ago, and even though our consumption of food is greater than our need, we consume fewer nutrients than did our ancestors (who spent much of the day at hard physical labor). Factor in the fact that we tend to cook a lot of the nutrients out of our vegetables, add the large amounts of processed food that have replaced whole foods in most diets and generally poor digestion, and you see the dismal picture of the nutritional intake of the average modern American.

Because of these changes in our food supply, many people argue that we should take a good high-potency daily multivitamin. There is, however, little scientific evidence that taking isolated single nutrients, even in combination, is as nutritious as eating a good diet. Think of it as a sort of insurance against nutritional deficiencies.

Most quality multivitamins require you to take three to six tablets or capsules with each meal. If you can't tolerate taking that many pills, at least try to get some supplemental vitamin C and magnesium each day. Men should try to get 15 to 20 mg of zinc and selenium daily for prostate health. If you live in a cloudy climate, some supplemental vitamin D is a good idea. Women with fatigue problems should take a B-complex vitamin. If you're getting chronic infections, take a vitamin A supplement. (Now you're starting to see why it might be good to take a multivitamin.)

Although most multivitamins will contain it, we don't necessarily recommend beta-carotene or carotenoids. Green and yellow vegetables contain 600 different carotenes that work in synergy to create their antioxidant effects. Beta-carotene by itself does not have the potent effects of the vegetables.

Choosing a multivitamin can be difficult because there are so many out there, but we're going to try to make it a little easier by giving you some basic guidelines about which vitamins and minerals should be included. We recommend that you choose a multivitamin that contains the following:

Vitamins

• *Vitamin A*: 5,000–10,000 IU. This antioxidant is fat-soluble, and reserves can be stored in the liver for long periods. This means that it can have lasting positive effects. However, it also means that it can build up to toxic levels if more than 10,000 IU is taken daily for a long period of time. Fish and fish liver oils are naturally rich in vitamin A.

• *B vitamins*:
       Thiamine (B_1): 5 to 10 mg
       Riboflavin (B_2): 5 to 10 mg
       Niacin (B_3): 50 to100 mg
       Pantothenic acid (B_5): 10 to 50 mg
       Pyridoxine (B_6): 50 mg
       Vitamin B_{12}: 1,000 to 2,000 mcg (micrograms)
       Biotin: 100 to 300 mcg
       Choline: 50 to 100 mg
       Folic acid/folate/folacin: 400 to 800 mcg
       Inositol: 150 to 300 mg

The B vitamins play multiple roles in brain function, the transformation of food into energy within the cells, and neutralizing of a toxic by-product of protein metabolism called homocysteine. High levels of homocysteine are a newly emerging and very substantial risk factor for heart disease—the substance directly damages the walls of blood vessels. Pantothenic acid is essential for the healthy functioning of your adrenal glands, and vitamin B_{12} is necessary for the proper absorption of some vitamins. B vitamins are found in whole grains, fruits, vegetables, and meats. It's best to take the B vitamins together, as their effects are synergistic.

- *Vitamin C*: 1,000 to 2,000 mg. This super-antioxidant nutrient has been making news for decades, since Linus Pauling and Ewan Cameron began researching its amazing immunity-boosting effects. Vitamin C also helps in the building of collagen, the basic building block of connective tissue. It's water-soluble, so you eliminate what you don't need. The adrenal glands are dependent on adequate vitamin C: They concentrate vitamin C over 100-fold in the adrenal gland. When you're sick or stressed, vitamin C is used up at a much faster rate. It's a good idea to keep a bottle of vitamin C around so that you can take more when you're coming down with a cold or flu bug, or are under stress. One or two grams (1,000 to 2,000 mg) a day should suffice when you're feeling your best. Good food sources include citrus fruits, tomatoes, mangoes, kiwi, and red peppers. Remember, heat destroys vitamin C, so you don't get it in cooked foods.

- *Vitamin D*: 100 to 400 IU. We make some vitamin D when we go out into the sunshine, but a little extra is a good idea, especially for women. Vitamin D interacts with calcium and phosphorus to build strong, healthy bones. It's fat-soluble and can build up to toxic levels if doses higher than 400 IU are taken for long. Fish and fish liver oil contain vitamin D.

- *Vitamin E*: 100 to 500 IU. The many roles of this fat-soluble antioxidant are the subject of a great deal of research these days. It stops free radicals from damaging cells and repairs other spent antioxidant and B vitamins. It helps prevent the blood from being too sticky, relieves edema (accumulation of excess fluid), and strengthens blood vessel walls. Vitamin E is found in the germ of all grains and nuts.

- *Other antioxidants*. Powerful, newly discovered antioxidants are showing promise as cancer preventives. Especially promising are proanthocyanidins (PCOs) from grapeseed extract; resveratrol from purple grape juice and red wine; bioflavonoids such as quercetin, hesperidin, and rutin; and phytochemicals found in green tea. Coenzyme Q-10 (CoQ-10) is also a powerful antioxidant that has been shown in some studies to help prevent breast cancer growth.

Minerals

The passage of minerals in and out of cells is a delicately balanced operation, dependent on the health of the membrane around each cell. Too-high levels of estrogen coupled with synthetic progestins actually impair the action of cell membranes, while natural progesterone heals cell membranes and allows normal mineral balance to be restored. Make sure that your multivitamin contains optimal amounts of the following minerals:

- *Boron*: 1 to 5 mg. This mineral plays a role in the maintenance of healthy bones.
- *Calcium*: up to 300 mg. Total daily calcium intake should be around 600 to 800 mg per day, which is easily accomplished by any good diet, even without milk. A cupful of spinach contains 300 mg, and a tablespoon of cheese contains 300 mg, for example. Taking up to 300 mg of calcium daily should be fine, as long as you're also taking magnesium.

Calcium is well known for its role as a bone and tooth builder, and that's the role of 99 percent of the calcium in the body. The 1 percent left over is an indispensable player in nerve conduction, muscle contraction, heartbeat and blood pressure regulation, clotting of blood, and functioning of the thyroid gland. Tofu, black-eyed peas, leafy green vegetables, dairy products, and broccoli are good sources of calcium in the diet.

- *Chromium*: 200 to 400 mcg (as chromium picolinate). This trace mineral helps keep blood sugars steady so you can fight off cravings for sugar and refined flour. It also helps manufacture needed nutrients such as cholesterol and fatty acids. It's found naturally in mushrooms, beef, beets, liver, whole wheat, brewer's yeast (used often as a nutritional supplement), and molasses made from beet sugar. Low-fat, processed-food diets often result in chromium deficiency.

• *Copper*: 1 to 5 mg. Copper has many roles in the body, including wound healing, transport of oxygen through the blood (it's a component of the body's oxygen-carrying molecule, hemoglobin), and maintaining the integrity of nerves, skin, and bones. Seafood, beans, almonds, whole grains, and green leafy vegetables are good sources of this mineral.

• *Magnesium*: 300 to 400 mg. This mineral is involved in just about every aspect of our physiology. It makes up 0.05 percent of our body weight, and is incorporated into bones as well as being distributed throughout our other tissues. Calcium and magnesium need each other to fulfill their roles. Intravenous magnesium has been used to treat heart arrhythmias, high blood pressure, heart failure, and asthma with great success. It's also an effective laxative.

Because of soil depletion, our plant food is deficient in magnesium. Most Americans are sorely deficient in magnesium. It's found in nuts, seeds, figs, corn, apples, milk, soybeans, and wheat germ. Just as iron is what makes hemoglobin red, magnesium makes chlorophyll green.

If you have asthma, chronic muscle cramps, or high blood pressure, or are at high risk of osteoporosis or heart disease, take 300 mg in the morning and evening for a total of 600 mg daily. Reduce the dose if it causes diarrhea.

• *Manganese*: 10 mg. The B vitamins and vitamin C need manganese to do their jobs. This mineral also helps the thyroid gland and ovaries make their hormones and participates in the synthesis of carbohydrates, fatty acids, cholesterol, and protein. It's an important one for hormone balance as well as for prevention of heart disease and diabetes. Egg yolks, green veggies, seeds, whole grains, and nuts contain generous amounts of manganese.

• *Selenium*: 60 to 100 mcg. This mineral behaves like an antioxidant in the body. Selenium and vitamin E work together to prevent the oxidation of polyunsaturated fats in the bloodstream. Prostaglandins can't be produced without selenium. It plays a role in cellular energy production, has great potential as a cancer fighter, and has antiviral properties. Those parts of the world where the soil is depleted of selenium tend to have higher rates of cancer.

• *Vanadyl sulfate*: 10 to 25 mcg. Vanadyl is another blood-sugar-balancing mineral that works cooperatively with chromium.

• *Zinc*: 10 to 20 mg. Zinc aids the immune system, works in synergy with vitamin A, and is required for healthy prostate function.

Note the absence of iron in this recommendation. Unless you have a documented iron deficiency or anemia, there's no reason for you to take extra iron. Excess iron can be very harmful, sparking the formation of free radicals. Iron is the only mineral that isn't excreted by urine. Its absorption is determined by an intestinal transfer factor. Excessive iron increases the risk of heart disease, liver and colon cancer, and rheumatoid degeneration of joints. More than 4 percent of the population has hemochromatosis (absorbs too much iron), and about 40 percent of the population carries the recessive gene for this disease.

Your Ideal Diet

Although you now have some guidelines to follow if you want to eat for breast cancer prevention, a regimented, written-in-stone plan is not what we have set out to create. We don't want to tell every woman to eat the same way, because every woman's body is different and will thrive on a different combination of foods. You don't have to rigidly adhere to a specific number of fat grams and carbohydrate grams; nor do you have to eat foods that don't agree with you. Learn to listen to your body; it will tell you what's good for you.

For example: While some women do quite well on a diet rich in soy, others get terrible indigestion when they eat soy foods. While some women thrive on a nice cut of red meat a couple of times a week, others feel red meat is too heavy and feel sluggish after eating it. Some women choose a vegetarian diet and find it's the right thing for their bodies, while other women always feel hungry if they don't eat protein-rich foods with most meals. Many people are allergic to certain foods, especially wheat, soy, and dairy, and feel better when they eliminate these foods from their diets.

Each woman's ideal diet may change over the years. Foods that agreed with you as a 20-year-old may not cut it when you're pushing 50. The point isn't to eat exactly the same diet everyone else is eating, but to find the combination that includes cancer-fighting foods, excludes cancer-causing foods, and works best for your particular physiological makeup.

DOS AND DON'TS OF THE
ANTI-CANCER DIET

DON'T eat lots of meat; use it as a condiment rather than a main course.

DON'T eat meat, eggs, or dairy products from conventionally raised animals.

DON'T use hydrogenated or otherwise trans-fats and -oils.

DON'T eat refined grain products or foods with added sugar.

DON'T drink too much alcohol, but don't deprive yourself if you can be moderate about it.

DO eat plenty of a wide variety of vegetables, especially of the *Brassica* (cruciferous) and *Allium* genera.

DO eat whole fruits when you want something sweet.

DO eat deep-water fish two to three times a week.

DO eat whole grains and legumes.

DO take a daily multivitamin and mineral supplement.

DO drink eight to ten glasses of clean water a day.

DO use small amounts of olive oil or butter for cooking.

DO eat plenty of garlic.

DO choose organic whenever possible.

DO eat a high-fiber diet. (If you don't move your bowels at least once a day, add extra fiber to your diet in supplement form, drink more water, and get more exercise.)

CHAPTER 18

PROTECTING THE PRESENT
AND THE FUTURE

*Creating an Environment Where
Cancer Can't Get Started*

Back in the early 1990s when Dr. Lee wrote his first book about natural progesterone, the suggestion that pollutants and chemicals could affect human reproductive organs, and could affect an embryo in ways that could cause reproductive damage that would show up later in life, was met with much scorn and skepticism by his colleagues. Now, just a decade later, this fact is no longer even arguable; there are thousands of studies showing the hormonal effects of petrochemical pollutants, also known as xenohormones (*xeno* means "foreign"), or endocrine disruptors (the endocrine system includes the glands that make brain hormones, reproductive system hormones, adrenal hormones, insulin, and thyroid hormone, for example). Congressional committees have been formed to fund and direct research on the subject, and new findings are coming out almost weekly.

Xenohormones can have a variety of negative hormonal effects. For example, a xenoestrogen can block or oppose the action of your own estrogen; it can mimic your own estrogen but with a stronger or weaker effect; or it can even send different messages to your cells than your own estrogen would, altering the production and breakdown of your own estrogen.

Xenohormones can also affect the production and function of your hormone receptors. While there are some petrochemical pollutants that have androgenic or male hormone effects (or antieffects), the majority of them have estrogenic effects.

There are now quite a number of studies showing that exposure to xenohormones suppresses the immune system, in particular hampering T-lymphocyte function and lowering the proportions and numbers of natural killer cells. These are two of your immune system's most important defenses. The latest studies are showing even more widespread damage to the immune system. Infants of women who have been chronically exposed to xenohormones seem to be particularly susceptible to immune system damage through exposure in breast milk, and children are more susceptible than adults.

Many of the xenobiotics activate the CYP-1B1 enzyme, which converts estrogens to 4-catechols—the bad estrogens that can damage DNA and lead to breast cancer. Progesterone inhibits activity of CYP-1B1, which would suggest that progesterone may protect against xenobiotic-activated estrogen metabolite formation.

The conclusion is the same as it was a decade ago: We are awash in a sea of pollutants with estrogenic effects that are pervasively affecting the reproductive systems of all living creatures, including humans. Since estrogen is the hormone that has feminizing effects on living creatures, you could say that life on planet earth is being feminized.

To understand how xenohormones influence your body, think of your cells as having many unique combination locks that open doors to specific genes. Once these doors are open and the genes are activated, the cells are given instructions to carry out very specific functions such as replication. Throughout the millions of years of human evolution there have been a very restricted number of substances that have the combination to each lock; your genes are very selective about "whom" they will allow to give them instructions. One of these combination locks is opened by the estrogens, including your own natural estrogens like estradiol and a few phytoestrogens found in foods you eat. Overall, this system worked fine for millennia, until the twentieth century came along and introduced countless numbers of new synthetic petrochemicals that mimic estrogen in some way—and thus have the combination to the estrogen lock.

Petrochemical pollutants and products are those made from petroleum oil. All plastics, virtually all pesticides and herbicides, solvents, glues, detergent breakdown products, many cosmetic ingredients, gasoline and diesel fuel and their resulting exhaust, and many industrial chemicals such as PCBs and dioxins are petrochemically based. Alcohols and formaldehyde are also petrochemically based.

Virtually all petrochemical products have the potential to have xenohormonal effects on living creatures; the question is, how potent are they, and how prevalent are they? For example, dioxins can have hormonal effects in minute amounts: Parts per million can cause permanent damage to an embryo. If you want to conceptualize parts per million, think of a few grains of sand in a bathtub full of sand.

A single dose of dioxin at 0.064 µg/kg given to a pregnant female rat can result in the inhibition of masculinization in the male rat offspring. One gram is about the weight of a pencil eraser (an ordinary paper clip is about half a gram). If you cut that into 20,000 pieces of equal size, each piece would be 0.05 µg—about like a speck of dust. Although in general xenohormones are weaker than your own hormones, unlike your own hormones they accumulate in the body.

The nonylphenols—xenohormones that are the breakdown products of detergents—are relatively weak in their effects, and are less potent than your own hormones. However, when they're present in sewage treatment or industrial plant discharge that's pouring into a river by the thousands of gallons every day, it's more than enough to affect the fish in that river.

By far the most susceptible cells to the effects of xenohormones are those in a developing embryo; when you're in the womb you are exquisitely sensitive to the effects of hormones. The parts of an embryo that are most susceptible (as far as we know now) are the reproductive organs. (There's a good chance that down the road we'll discover that the brain is equally sensitive to the effects of these substances.) Every day millions of pregnant women unknowingly expose their unborn children to damaging substances that can cause a lifetime of reproductive problems and abnormal reproductive development, and short of living in a bubble, there's no escape. It could be dioxins in that fish you just ate, or the pesticides just sprayed in the elevator or airplane you're riding in, or the new carpet that's off-gassing fumes in your office, or in the nail polish you're using to paint your toenails, or the paint you're using to decorate the new baby's bedroom.

It's likely that the class of pesticides known as organochlorines (of which DDT is the most notorious) are the most widely pervasive *and* potent form of estrogenic pollutants on the planet. According to the book *The Truth about Breast Cancer,* by Claire Hoy, "Greenpeace found that the one country that banned organochlorine pesticides—Israel—quickly went from breast cancer rates that were among the highest in the world to rates in keeping with those of other industrialized nations. It also found that U.S. counties with waste sites were 6.5 times more likely to have elevated breast cancer rates than those without waste sites, and that women with breast cancer tend to have higher levels of organochlorine pesticides and PCBs in their tissues than women without breast cancer." Organochlorines have since been shown repeatedly to cause mammary cancers in laboratory animals, but they remain a fundamental part of U.S. agriculture. Thus does perceived economic necessity take the life of tens of thousands of women in the United States alone every year.

Awareness can go a long way toward avoidance of xenohormones, but ultimately it will take political action at the grassroots level to change the big picture.

COMMON SOURCES OF XENOHORMONES

- Petrochemically derived pesticides, herbicides, and fungicides.
- Car exhaust.
- Solvents and adhesives such as those found in nail polish, paint remover, and glues.
- Emulsifiers and waxes found in soaps and cosmetics.
- Dry-cleaning chemicals.
- Nearly all plastics.
- Phthalates, synthetic compounds that add flexibility to plastics, such as the plastic tubes and bags used in storing and delivering IV fluids to patients, and the rubbery toys children play with. Exposure to phthalates during embryo and perinatal life will also damage testes and ovaries just as the pesticides and solvents do. *Do not* let your infants and toddlers chew on soft plastic toys.
- Industrial waste such as PCBs and dioxins.
- Meat from livestock animals fed estrogenic drugs to fatten them up.
- Waste from sewage treatment plants that contains nonylphenols, estrogenic breakdown products of detergents.
- Synthetic estrogens and progestins found in the urine of millions of women taking birth control pills and hormone replacement therapy that is flushed down the toilet and eventually works its way into the food chain.

The first evidence that petrochemical pollutants could affect the endrocrine systems of living creatures was found in wildlife. Decades ago we discovered that DDT made bird eggs so fragile that they couldn't sustain life. Rachel Carson alerted the world to the dangers of pesticides to current and future generations of life in her courageous book *Silent Spring,* which was published in 1962. The public awareness generated by Carson's book created a firestorm of attacks against her by the chemical companies, but it resulted in the banning of DDT. However, thousands of new chemicals have been produced and put on the market since then, many of them untested and more dangerous than DDT.

In the early 1990s environmental scientist Theo Colborn began putting together material for a book she coauthored, *Our Stolen Future,* which details in a rigorously scientific detective story how synthetic chemicals have already done widespread damage to all types of wildlife and are in the process of damaging humans. Most of the xenohormone damage done to wildlife occurs as a result of exposure during the embryo stage, and has resulted in the near extinction of a number of species. *Our Stolen Future* was all but ignored by the media, but not by a U.S. Congress that began listening to testimonials from scientists that human male sperm counts are half of what they were a few decades ago, thanks to petrochemical pollutants, and that children exposed to PCBs in utero have lower IQ levels than normal.

Since that time other excellent books on the topic of xenohormones and reproductive damage have been published, and if you're interested in delving further into this topic, we highly recommend reading them. They include:

• *Generations at Risk: Reproductive Health and the Environment,* by Ted Schettler, M.D., Gina Solomon, M.D., et al., which explains reproductive and developmental physiology, describes how toxins affect this physiology, and then gives guidelines for investigating possible exposure to toxins and for creating change in your community and workplace.

- *Hormonal Chaos: The Scientific and Social Origins of the Environmental Endocrine Hypothesis,* by Sheldon Krimsky, focuses more on how the endocrine disruptor theory emerged, and examines the ethics of a scientific, economic, and political community that has been trying to ignore these findings for decades, as well as the social and medical consequences of continuing to allow these substances to be dumped into the environment.

- *Pandora's Poison,* by Joe Thornton, focuses most on the issue of organochlorines (products made using chlorine gas, including pesticides, plastics, paper, PCBs, and dioxins) as the key substances most seriously affecting human physiology. Thornton specifically proposes ways that we can change chemical testing and environmental protection policies to—in effect—save ourselves.

- *Living Downstream,* by Sandra Steingraber, combines meticulous science and lucid writing with the author's personal experience of fighting bladder cancer. The book will open your eyes to the ubiquity of petrochemical toxins accumulating in our environment.

Miners used to take canaries in cages down into coal mines to help detect the presence of dangerous gases. If the canary stopped singing or fell off its perch dead, the miners knew they were next. We can consider the widespread reproductive damage, birth defects, and brain changes showing up in fish, reptiles, amphibians, birds, and mammals all over the United States and Canada to be our equivalent of a canary warning us of danger. To the extent that we fail to get ourselves out of this situation, we will be physically and reproductively crippled and cancer-prone nations.

The Effects of Xenohormones
on the Human Body

As could be expected, the chemical industry has mounted a vigorous campaign to try to discredit researchers working on endocrine disruptors and their effects on animal and human populations. One of its arguments has been that phytoestrogens, plant estrogens found in a variety of foods that humans regularly consume, are much more potent than xenohormones, and yet the human race has successfully dealt with them for millennia.

However, this argument doesn't help the chemical company cause, because phytoestrogens are easily metabolized and excreted by the body within a matter of hours. Petrochemically derived xenohormones are nonbiodegradable, so they'll continue to accumulate in the environment for as long as they are being manufactured. Xenohormones are fat-soluble, so they pass easily through the skin, and they're cumulative, meaning they accumulate in the body over time. This is why even though a dose of pesticide may not affect a normal healthy adult immediately in the same way that it does an embryo in the womb, many exposures over time can eventually cause cellular damage that can lead to cancer.

While the levels of xenohormones in the blood may be lower than that of the more powerful phytoestrogens, it's a whole different story when researchers begin to look at the fatty tissues of the body (such as the breasts), where they find relatively high concentrations of xenohormones such as DDT and PCBs. Mary Wolff of Mount Sinai Medical Center in New York City brought world attention to her clinical study on the relationship of pollutants to breast cancer, published in the *Journal of the National Cancer Institute*. In this study she provided the strongest evidence to date that pesticides mimicking the action of estrogens increased the incidence of breast cancer by 400 percent in those women with the highest levels of organochlorine contamination in their breast tissue.

The effects that xenohormones have on tissues are also different from those of the phytoestrogens. Phytoestrogens tend to support the body in regulating and balancing hormones. In contrast, xenoestrogens tend to move down harmful biochemical pathways that ultimately lead to the types of damage to DNA that can lead to cancer. Xenohormones can accumulate and profoundly affect the functioning of the glands that manufacture hormones, such as the ovaries, testes, thyroid, and adrenal glands. For example, a chemical called hexachlorobenzene (HCB) has been shown to suppress progesterone synthesis in cynomolgus monkeys. As you know by now, suppression of progesterone synthesis leads to estrogen dominance, which can lead to breast cancer.

As we know from our experience with diethylstilbesterol (DES), the synthetic estrogen given to thousands of pregnant women in the 1950s and 1960s, and from long-term animal studies, xenohormone toxicity may not show up until the midlife of the generation born after the generation exposed. In other words, if your mother is exposed to a xenohormone while you're in the womb, you and possibly your children could be affected. Chemical safety testing has only just begun to routinely test for these types of effects at the extremely low doses that can cause them.

Further, the large number of petrochemical xenohormones released into the environment, combined with their known persistence and lipophilic nature (they're fat loving, so they easily absorb through the skin and easily accumulate in fatty tissue), makes it inevitable that multiple endocrine disrupters accumulate in target tissues over time. It's common to find PCBs, dioxins, DDT, and a number of other organochlorine pesticides together in human breast tissue. This, of course, raises concern about their additive and synergistic effects. Researchers at Johns Hopkins University are finding that toxins such as PCBs selectively activate the enzyme that favors 4- over 2-hydroxylation of estradiol. As you learned in chapter 7, 4-hydroxy estrogens are the ones that can damage DNA and lead to breast cancer.

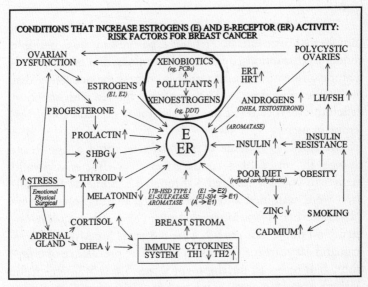

It's likely that xenohormones (or xenobiotics) play a large role in the high rate of breast cancer in Westernized countries.

This may explain why not all animals equally exposed to a given xenohormone produce offspring with similar effects. The damage that becomes evident is subject to at least three factors:

1. The environmental dose
2. The genetic predisposition
3. The age at the time of the exposure

Exposure to xenohormones during the embryo stage, or chronic exposure as an adult, can result in functional loss of ovarian follicles in females. The ultimate consequence of this is decreased progesterone production, which results in estrogen dominance, PMS, endometriosis, and miscarriages, and probably contributes to many types of ovarian dysfunction. The damage to a woman's developing follicle and corpus luteum may result in lower progesterone production during pregnancy, which in turn could cause impaired brain development in the fetus.

It's likewise recognized that xenohormones can have more complicated toxic effects. Prenatal exposure can cause multiple endocrine disruptions, anatomic deformities, and even intellectual impairment. We must seriously address the possibility that the profound increase in the number of children with attention deficit disorders could be due to inadequate exposure to progesterone in utero.

The April 1997 issue of *Pediatrics* reported a significant change in onset of secondary sexual characteristics and menses in young girls aged 3 through 12. Some 17,077 children were examined and their pubertal maturation rated by 225 clinicians. It was found that mean ages of breast development and pubic hair growth were 8.8 years for African American and 10 years for Caucasian girls. The prevalence of either pubic hair or breast development at age 5 was 5.7 percent for African American and 1.9 percent for Caucasian girls. By age 11 menses is established in 28 percent of African American and 13.4 percent of Caucasian girls. Taken together, these figures show that puberty is starting two years earlier now than standards of just 10 to 20 years ago. Early onset of menstruation is a known risk factor for breast cancer, likely because it creates a longer lifetime exposure to estrogen during menstrual cycles.

It's interesting—and odd—that the conclusion in the authors' abstract merely advises practitioners to recognize the new norms and revise their criteria for referral of girls with precocious puberty. Referring to the premature pubertal changes as a new "norm" rather than an abnormality seems to miss the point.

Since it's extremely unlikely that the change found is independent of some external cause such as environmental xenohormones, it would be more appropriate that the study should call for deeper investigation into the cause of the early pubertal changes.

It's likely that xenohormones are also causing the epidemic of endometriosis we're seeing in young women. Gerhard and Runnebaum (1992) first brought attention to the link between the high levels of dioxins in blood and endometriosis. Scientific research with female rhesus monkeys fed different amounts of dioxin-laden foods supports epidemiological studies suggesting that endometriosis in humans is caused by xenohormones. Monkeys were given different amounts of dioxin in their diet for four years. One group of seven animals was fed as usual without dioxin in their food, a second group had 5 parts per trillion dioxin, and the third group was fed 25 parts per trillion dioxin. Ten years following dioxin administration, five of seven animals (71 percent) given the high dose of dioxin developed moderate or severe endometriosis. In the group receiving the intermediate dose three of seven animals (43 percent) developed endometriosis. And in the group receiving no dioxin only about 33 percent developed any level of endometriosis, which is consistent with the expected frequency of endometriosis in rhesus monkeys in captivity.

COMPARISON OF SEVERAL XENOESTROGENS WITH ESTRADIOL

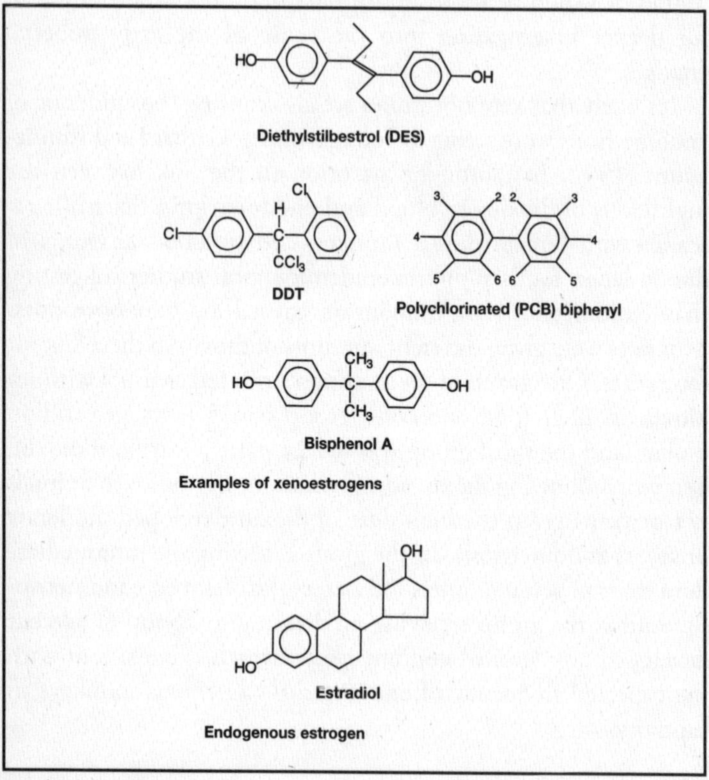
HO
OH
Diethylstilbestrol (DES)
Cl
H
C
Cl
CCl3
DDT
3
2 2
3
4
4
5
6 6
5
Polychlorinated (PCB) biphenyl
CH3
HO
C
OH
CH3
Bisphenol A
Examples of xenoestrogens
OH
HO
Estradiol
Endogenous estrogen

Structurally, xenoestrogens have enough in common with estrogen to have estrogen-like effects on the body.

Should we not be calling for a meaningful reduction in the use of petrochemical xenohormones that are now threatening not only our health but also the normal development of humankind? Xenohormones are ubiquitous in our diet and environment, and already are recognized as the likely cause of the threatened die-off of a number of animal species in areas exposed to these toxic compounds. The fate of future generations of humanity may hinge on our ability to substantially decrease environmental contamination by the petrochemical xenohormones.

Getting Pesticides Out of Your Life

The truth is that if you live in a Western nation, you can't get pesticides entirely out of your life. They're pervasive in the air, soil, water, and food. They're thoughtlessly sprayed on crops, lawns, gardens, homes, and in public buildings. Planes spray known carcinogenic pesticides on crops situated right next to schools and crowded office buildings. Homeowners have their houses "tented" and filled with pesticide-laden gas. Not only do the pesticides linger, but their by-products stick around as well, creating at least as much biochemical havoc in the body as the identified pesticide. Thus, your strategy in handling pesticide exposure has to be first to take all the personal steps that you can to minimize your exposure to pesticides, and second to maintain your hormone balance as best you can despite the pesticide exposure. (This is why progesterone is needed by women today even postmenopausally when nature drops it so low.)

SOME OF THE MOST COMMON
XENOHORMONE PESTICIDES

We recommend that you throw away your pesticides in general, but check the labels of any that you might still have around to see if they contain any of the following ingredients (including insecticides, herbicides, and fungicides):

- Alachlor
- Aldicarb
- Aldrin
- Atrazine
- Benomyl
- Chlordane
- Dibromochloropropane
- Dieldrin
- Dichlorvos
- Dicofol
- Endosulfan
- Kepone
- Mancozeb
- Methoxychlor
- Nitrofen
- O,p'-DDT (a breakdown product of DDT)
- Phthalates
- Toxaphene
- Tributyl tin

Just because a pesticide isn't on this list doesn't mean it's not harmful. Pesticides remain largely untested and unregulated, and their unlisted inert ingredients may be just as harmful as the listed pesticide. Given the government's inability to control pesticide manufacture, distribution, and use, the only reasonable course of action is to assume that *all* pesticides are harmful and avoid them as much as possible.

The Hidden Solvents in Your Life

A common source of potent xenohormones is the type of chemicals called solvents. All organic solvents are volatile liquids at room temperature and are lipophilic (fat loving). They enter the body extremely easily through the skin, and they accumulate in lipid-rich tissues such as the brain, myelin (nerve sheath), and adipose (fat). In combination they may be additive, synergistic, or potentiated, meaning that their effects on the body could be vastly more potent and toxic in combination than separately.

Industries in which exposure to solvents is well known include automotive manufacturing and repair, paint and varnish manufacturing, the electronics industry, industrial cleaning, metal-part degreasing, and dry cleaning. In addition to the work environment, exposure via hobbies must be considered. The use of most glues and fiberglass involves exposure to solvents.

One of the most insidious routes of solvent exposure and toxicity is through fingernail polish and fingernail polish remover. Young girls are especially susceptible to the toxic and xenohormonal effects of solvents, and yet they're the ones most likely to have a dozen different shades of fingernail polish in the bedroom.

Some of the immediate effects of exposure to solvents include central nervous system (CNS) depression (which would look like fatigue or depression), psychomotor or attention deficits (which would look like incoordination and inability to focus), brain swelling (headaches), CNS capillary damage, and oxygen deprivation in the brain, with possible permanent brain damage resulting in lowered cognitive abilities.

Long-term exposure to solvents can cause mood disturbances such as depression, irritability, fatigue, anxiety, inability to focus, incoordination, and short-term memory loss.

Solvents in very small amounts can also damage a developing fetus and should be studiously avoided in any amount by pregnant women. It should be required by law that nail polish labels contain warnings to pregnant women, and that beauty salons display warning signs in areas where nail polish is applied and removed.

SOME GENERAL CLASSES OF ORGANIC SOLVENTS

Check product labels for the following (you might find them in cosmetics, nail polish and nail polish remover, glues, paints, varnishes and other types of finishes, cleaning products, pesticides and herbicides, carpet, fiberboard and other processed woods, and even in clothing and mattresses):

- Alcohols (e.g., methanol)
- Aldehydes (e.g., acetaldehyde)
- Aliphatic hydrocarbons (e.g., n-hexane)
- Aromatic hydrocarbons (e.g., benzene)
- Cyclic hydrocarbons (e.g., cyclohexane)
- Esters (e.g., ethyl acetate)
- Ethers (e.g., ethyl ether)
- Glycols (e.g., ethylene glycol)
- Halogenated hydrocarbons (e.g., carbon tetrachloride, trichlorethylene)
- Ketones (e.g. acetone, methylethylketone)
- Nitrohydrocarbons (ethyl nitrate)

CLEANING UP YOUR HOUSE

- Throw away all pesticides, herbicides, fungicides. Take a class in organic gardening and read up on natural pest control. *Do not* tent your house and fumigate it with pesticides, or "bomb" it, or have your lawn sprayed with chemicals.
- Check your cosmetics for toxic ingredients and try as much as possible to use "clean" cosmetics. It's unlikely that there's any truly nontoxic hair spray on the market. Throw away the nail polish and nail polish remover; they're toxic both when you breathe them and when you put them on your nails. There is no safe nail polish at this time.
- Don't use fabric softeners; this puts petrochemicals directly onto your skin, which as you know by now is quite capable of absorbing all kinds of substances.
- Most scented products and perfumes are petrochemically based, and when you inhale them they go directly to your brain. Don't use petrochemically based perfumes or air fresheners. Try some of the natural aromatic oils and combinations if you want to change the way you, your house, or your car smell. In the same vein, use unscented laundry soaps and naturally scented shampoos and conditioners.
- Don't use tap or bottled water as a source of drinking water; get a good-quality filter for your whole house or for taps that are used for drinking and cooking water.
- Be aware that all plastics leach into the environment; some leach faster and some are more potent. The soft plastics such as are found in many baby toys and in some water bottles leach the most. *Do not* let your child chew on plastic toys.

- *Do not* microwave food in plastic containers, and especially avoid microwaving food covered by plastic wrap.
- Eliminate or decrease consumption of foods most likely to be contaminated with petrochemicals. If you eat red meat, poultry, eggs, other meat, and fish, they should be organic and hormone- and antibiotic-free. A primarily plant-based diet of fresh, unprocessed organically grown plants of all sorts is a foundation for good health and longevity for us and for the environment.
- Avoid surfactants such as nonoxonyl (spermicides) found in many condoms and diaphragm gels.
- A new home or office can be a toxic soup of noxious gases coming from glues, fiberboard, new carpet, and new paint. If your new home makes you feel sick, it's probably *not* all in your head; have the air tested. Chances are it's loaded with formaldehyde and solvent fumes. When you're pregnant or have an infant, it's not a good idea to move into a newly built home, to remodel, or even to paint. This can be challenging for a pregnant woman when the nesting instinct kicks in, but first consider the future health of your baby.

CLEANING UP YOUR OFFICE

- Be aware that new carpeting can give off noxious fumes.
- Be aware that any type of fiberboard can give off noxious fumes, especially when it's new. Most office furniture is made out of fiberboard.
- Copiers and printers that use toner and inks give off noxious fumes.
- If you work in an office building, be sure there's a firm policy in place that requires notification of building

occupants when pesticides of any kind are being used. Take an active interest in exactly what is being used, and why, and what the alternatives might be.

- Be aware that the air quality in office buildings can be a source of a wide range of toxins, from fungi to xenohormones.

- Computers, monitors, printers, and other electronic office equipment can give off very high levels of electromagnetic fields (EMFs). While we haven't covered EMFs in detail in this book, we believe there's enough scientific evidence to justify avoiding them. The good news is that EMFs coming from electronic equipment tend to drop off within a few feet. Never sit right next to a computer hard drive or right behind a computer monitor. It's wise to invest in a handheld gauss meter and test both your office and your house for EMFs. (Search the Web or see Resources at the end of this book for how to find a gauss meter.)

MEDICAL SOURCES OF BREAST CANCER

- Hormone replacement therapy
- Birth control pills
- X rays

Your Liver, the Great Detoxifier

Just as it's important to keep your home and office clean, it's important to keep your body clean. Your liver is your most important cleansing organ. In Chinese medicine the relative strength or weakness of the liver plays a central role regarding health and disease. This is appropriate, since every system in the body is affected by your liver health, albeit sometimes in subtle ways. In conventional Western medicine the liver has been relegated to a back shelf because problems don't show up in standard blood tests until your liver has actually been damaged. In contrast, Chinese medicine has numerous diagnostic methods for determining liver health, including examining your eyes, tongue, and urine, taking your pulse, and finding combinations of other symptoms that point to liver trouble. Here in the West we would do well to pay more attention to liver function.

A recent study in the medical journal *The Lancet* about Wilson's disease reminds us of the importance of good liver health. Wilson's disease is a genetic disorder in which copper accumulates in the liver and brain, with dire consequences. It's clinically characterized by peculiar whitish rings around the iris in the eye (Kayser-Fleischer rings) and leads to liver failure and Parkinson-like dystonia (a muscle disorder). The researchers found that the copper accumulation caused enzyme defects, suggesting free-radical formation and oxidative damage, particularly of mitochondrial function.

While Wilson's disease is relatively rare (occurring in 1 in 30,000 people), it can range from severe to very mild, suggesting that many subclinical cases may go unrecognized. To us, the importance of the study is the focus on oxidative damage and the potential benefit of antioxidants in preventing liver failure from oxidative problems, regardless of underlying causes.

Health problems associated with compromised liver function tend to be nonspecific ailments that baffle conventional physicians. These people are the walking wounded who struggle with low energy, poor sleep, digestive problems, obscure aches and pains, chronic fatigue, mental lethargy, and increased susceptibility to infections. Such symptoms may signify accumulation of toxins, which are chemical agents that impair metabolic functions throughout the body.

Toxins, Oxidants, and Antioxidants

The liver is the largest metabolically active organ in the body. It occupies a good deal of the space under your rib cage on the right side, and it enlarges when it's overtaxed. Your liver is the organ that's most important in protecting your body against toxins.

Exotoxins originate from outside the body, and endotoxins originate from metabolic processes within the body. Examples of exotoxins are alcohol, cigarette smoke, carbon monoxide, pesticides, drugs, and fluoride. Some endotoxins are perfectly normal—they're by-products of bodily functions, and your liver is perfectly capable of eliminating them. Others are not normal and can originate from poor diet, sedentary lifestyle, stress, trauma, impaired digestion (dysbiosis), genetic predisposition, allergies, and food sensitivities. Regardless of the source, the accumulation of toxins over time leads to impaired functioning of various organ systems. The approach of treating the symptoms is doomed to failure. The only successful treatment involves avoiding exotoxins, optimizing your body's ability to metabolize and excrete endotoxins, and supporting your body with a healthy lifestyle.

The classic example of biological toxins involves various reactive oxygen forms known as free radicals that are produced in the body through normal metabolic processes or as a result of exposure to radiation, pollutants, viruses or other infections, and prescription drugs. These oxygen radicals are highly reactive and can damage cell membranes, fats (making them rancid), proteins and enzymes (altering their structure, impairing their function), and DNA (leading to gene mutations).

Fortunately, the body has an antioxidant system designed to protect us against these oxygen radicals. It includes the compounds superoxide dismutase, catalase and glutathione peroxidase, and coenzyme Q-10 (CoQ-10), in addition to amino acids (glycine, glutamine, taurine, methionine, cysteine, and glutathione) that help neutralize oxygen radicals for safe excretion. The body also uses a variety of antioxidant nutrients to help neutralize oxygen radicals. These include vitamins A, C, E, and B_2 (riboflavin), bioflavonoids, carotenes, polyphenols, quinones, anthocyanidins (pigments in berries, especially blueberries and grapes), selenium, zinc, copper, and manganese. Good health requires minimizing the formation of exposure to free radicals and maximizing all aspects of your antioxidant system.

An Elegant Toxic Waste Disposal System

While all body cells must engage in fighting toxins, the main battlefield is in the liver cells. The liver uses two strategies— detoxification (breaking down toxins) and conjugation (combining them safely to other products for excretion in bile or via the kidney).

Credit for elucidating these two phases and the factors that influence them should go to Jeffrey Bland, Ph.D. (We recommend his book *The 20-Day Rejuvenation Diet Program*.) The battle against toxins mainly involves two intracellular factors, the cytochrome p450 system and the mitochondria. People differ greatly in the functioning of these two important factors, probably as a function of genetics, environmental exposures, concurrent drugs and medications, stress, and nutrition.

Mitochondria are small inclusions within our cells, meaning they operate somewhat independently from the rest of the cell. Their importance, however, is great. They are the power plants of cellular metabolism, converting the food we eat into adenosine triphosphate (ATP) energy units. If mitochondrial function is hindered, sugar, for example, is converted into fat for storage rather than into energy for the body. Cholesterol levels rise, energy is low, and muscles and connective tissue gradually disintegrate. Mitochondrial function can be impaired by radiation, heavy metals such as mercury, lead, and cadmium, excess or unopposed estrogen, lack of vitamin B_2, lack of progesterone and testosterone, various toxins including fluoride, and oxidative damage.

In your liver the cytochrome p450 system changes the molecular structure of potentially toxic substances so that they can be safely excreted from the body. The p450 system is made up of a group of enzymes, some of which metabolize estrogens, others specific families of pesticides, and so forth. The enzymes work by recognizing unique structures on the molecules they metabolize. Excess estrogens, for example, must be converted by enzymes to a form that's recognized by the organs of elimination, the liver (bile), kidneys (urine), and sweat glands (sweat). The types of molecule that change estrogen to make it safe for excretion are found abundantly in foods such as broccoli, cauliflower, and garlic. If the p450 system is hindered in its function, then estradiol will not be excreted and will instead accumulate to undesirable concentrations in the bloodstream.

What Clogs the System

Any substance that overuses the p450 system will tax the liver and clog the system. Medications are likely the most common cause of liver dysfunction in Westerners; many of them block or overtax the p450 system. Selective serotonin inhibitors such as Prozac inhibit parts of the p450 system. In response, estrogen levels rise, leading to water retention, weight gain, brain cell excitability, crazy dreams, and, often, panic reactions. Similarly, the drug cimetidine (Tagamet) inhibits hydrochloric acid production in the stomach but also inhibits liver detoxification of many other agents, thus increasing their toxic effects. Many other examples of this problem exist with prescription drugs. The book *Prescription Alternatives* by Earl Mindell and Virginia Hopkins has more detailed descriptions of these kinds of interactions.

In addition to the above, genetic variations in the p450 system can result in different detoxification abilities. It's wise, therefore, to avoid factors that inhibit its ability to function. Unfortunately, conventional medicine generally ignores this important factor.

The Liver Protection Plan

To keep your liver in optimal health, your best course is a good diet of fresh unprocessed fruit and vegetables, pure water, and exercise in unpolluted air. You should also avoid sugar, and highly refined starches, soft drinks, artificial sweeteners, colorings, flavorings, preservatives, and trans–fatty acids. (Read chapter 17 for details.) If you know your liver function is compromised, you can avoid gluten-rich wheat and spelt.

To specifically support your liver choose foods high in

carotenes (carrots, sweet potato, spinach, cantaloupe, pumpkin, kale, winter squash) and vitamin C (citrus fruit, broccoli, strawberries, tomatoes, melons, bell peppers, brussels sprouts, and cabbage). Nutritional supplements should include antioxidant vitamins (A, C, E, B_2) and a multimineral formulation containing magnesium, zinc, copper, manganese, chromium, and molybdenum. Supplementation of coenzyme Q-10 is also often helpful (30 to 90 mg daily), as is alpha lipoic acid (500 mg twice daily).

One of the best ways to rid the body of toxins is through sweating, which bypasses the liver. Your skin is your largest route for excreting toxins, and sweating helps it do this job. Aerobic exercise stimulates sweating, as does a sauna or steam room.

In Short

Xenohormones can increase the risk of developing breast cancer by:

- Direct, persistent stimulation of breast ductal cells by xenoestrogens in the absence of progesterone (xenoestrogen dominance). These xenoestrogens are concentrated in fat tissue adjacent to normal breast cells.
- Damaging the ovaries, which can result in increased estrogen and decreased progesterone production (estrogen dominance).
- Increasing the enzyme 1B1, which leads to higher levels of catechol estrogens. (See chapter 7 for details on catechol estrogens.)
- Suppression of the immune system, which hampers its ability to fight cancer.

While it's impossible to avoid all xenobiotics, we must learn how to minimize our exposure to the best of our abilities. We must learn how to control pests in our homes and gardens without the use of pesticides. We must demand organic food from our markets. We can choose home and office furnishings that avoid petrochemical toxins. Further, we must learn how to keep our natural defenses in the best working order. We are the victims of an insidious and ubiquitous poisoning, now a major health issue for which finding a solution has become imperative.

The Bottom Line

We have many deeply held hopes for the readers of this book, and particularly those of you who have been affected in some way by breast cancer. First and foremost, we hope that you'll be able to use this book to take better care of yourselves and your loved ones, and to achieve optimal health. Although we know that some of the information you have read could cause feelings of anger, sadness, and even outrage, we hope that ultimately you'll use these emotions to bring attention, awareness, and education about breast cancer to others. Few forces on this planet are more powerful than a grassroots movement of caring people reaching out to help others.

If you have breast cancer, we hope that you'll work in partnership with your doctor, but at the same time that you won't accept treatments that you know—through education and/or intuition—aren't going to help you heal. We hope this book has been simple and straightforward enough to give you a good basic education about how breast cancer is created and promoted, yet technical enough to help you wade through the scientific literature if you or a loved one has breast cancer and you want to find out more about it.

We hope you'll remember that progesterone isn't a magic pill; you're a complex human with a body, emotions, a mind, and a soul, and it may be time to pay more attention to what's going on with some or all of these aspects of yourself.

On a nitty-gritty level we hope that you'll get your hormone levels tested, keep your hormones balanced, eat your broccoli and cauliflower, and avoid trans–fatty acids and xenoestrogens.

Please keep us in touch and let us know how you're doing. We're constantly getting new information and giving out new information through talks, newsletters, and revisions of our books. Although we're not able to answer you personally, when you keep us in touch, you're keeping all the millions of people who read our books and newsletters in touch.

RESOURCES

More Information on Cancer

One of the best Web sites we've found on the topic of cancer, including solid, reliable scientific information, detailed information on alternative treatments, and supplements, is www. canceroption.com.

Cancer tumor cells are dependent on insulin, and an alternative treatment taking advantage of this is insulin potentiation therapy. You can find out more about this at the Web site www.IPTQ.com.

Dr. Lee's Web Site

www.johnleemd.com

Dr. Zava's Web Site

www.salivatest.com

Dr. Lee's Newsletter

The John R. Lee, M.D., Medical Letter. If you want to know what's on Dr. Lee's mind every month and keep up with the latest in women's health research, this is the way to do it. A subscription is $49.95 per year in the United States. For more information visit Dr. Lee's Web site at www.johnleemd.com, call (800) 528-0559 or (602) 252-4477, write to P.O. Box 84900, Phoenix, AZ, 85071 or e-mail info@ johnleemd.com for more information.

Dr. Lee's Online Newsletter for Doctors

John R. Lee M.D.'s Online Letter for Doctors is an online-only newsletter written by Dr. Lee for doctors. It includes essays, reviews, and commentary on studies, letters, and information from doctors and other health professionals, as well as the text of the *Medical Letter*. A one-year subscription costs $195 U.S. For more information, visit www.johnleemd.com.

How to Find Natural Progesterone Cream

You can find progesterone creams in most health food stores these days, but many contain little to no real progesterone—buyer beware. If you have any doubt, call the company and ask how many milligrams of progesterone per ounce the cream contains.

Regardless of the source, please be sure you're getting the real thing. If the label says "wild yam extract," don't buy the product without confirming that it contains progesterone and not the so-called precursors such as diosgenin. The following are progesterone creams that we know contain real progesterone.

None of the authors endorses any one progesterone cream or company, or makes any money from the sale of any progesterone cream.

Many natural progesterone creams contain ingredients other than progesterone that may be active, including wild yam extract—usually diosgenin, a variety of herbs, and aromatic oils. We don't know which are active and which aren't, or what biochemical effects these ingredients may or may not have, nor do we know what effect they may have when used by women who are pregnant or nursing.

This list changes regularly. Please visit Dr. Lee's Web site (www.johnleemd.com) for the most up-to-date list.

AIM International, Inc.
3904 East Flamingo Avenue
Nampa, ID 83687
(208) 465-5116
Renewed Balance progesterone cream (contains 750 mg of progesterone per ounce of cream).

Arbonne International, Inc.
P.O. Box 2488
Laguna Hills, CA 92654
(800) ARBONNE
www.arbonne.com
customerservice@arbonne.com
They make PhytoProlief and Prolief Natural Balancing Creams.

Awakening Vital Life
601 16th Street, #C–#105
Golden, CO 80401
toll-free (877) 753-5424
www.altmednetwork.net
sales@altmednetwork.net
They make Awakening Woman Natural Progesterone Cream which contains only progesterone as its active ingredient.

Better Health Naturally by Helen Pensanti, M.D.
P.O. Box 5033
Irvine, CA 92616
(877) 880-0170
www.askdrhelen.com, www.doctortodoctor.com
info@askdrhelen.com
Dr. Pensanti has developed ProHELP natural progesterone creme and Menopause Relief Creme.

Bio-Nutritional Formulas
106 E. Jericho Turnpike
P.O. Box 311
Mineola, NY 11501
(800) 950-8484
Fem-Gest cream.

Broadmoore Labs, Inc.
3875 Telegraph Road/294
Ventura, CA 93003
(800) 822-3712
Makers of Natra-Gest progesterone creams.

Easy Way International
5340 Commerce Circle, #E
Indianapolis, IN 46237
(800) 267-4522
They make Gentle Changes progesterone cream.

Elan Vitale
P.O. Box 13990
Scottsdale, AZ 85267
(800) 527-5898, (602) 483-5650
They make BioBalance progesterone cream.

Emerita
621 SW Alder, Suite 900
Portland, OR 97205-3627
(503) 226-1010 or (800) 648-8211
www.transitionsforhealth.com and www.progest.com
The original natural progesterone cream, Pro-Gest cream. A
Division of Transitions For Health, Inc.

The Health and Science Research Institute
661 Beville Road, Suite 101
Daytona Beach, FL 32119
(888) 222-1415
fax (904) 267-9005
www.health-science.com
Serenity for Women progesterone cream.

HM Enterprises
5215 Wexford Lane
Norcross, GA 30071
(800) 742-4773
www.awomansneeds.com or
www.paulbunyan.net/users/mlzeller
They make Happy PMS progesterone cream.

International Health
8704 E. Mulberry St.
Scottsdale, AZ 85251
(800) 481-9987 or (480) 874-1419
nopms@doitnow.com
Makers of EssPro'Leve Plus Progesterone Creme with Essential
Oils.

Kevala, a division of Karuna
42 Digital Drive, #7
Novato, CA 94949
(888) 749-8643
www.kevalahealth.com
info@kevalahealth.com
They make PureGest Lotion which is free from additional hormones, herbs and alcohols.

Kokoro, LLC.
P.O. Box 597
Tustin, CA 92781
(800) 599-9412, (714) 836-7749
www.kokorohealth.com
They offer Kokoro Women's Balance Crème.

Life Extension
Hollywood, FL
(800) 544-4440
www.lef.org
Makers of Pro Fem Progesterone Creme.

Life-flo Health Care Products
8146 North 23rd Avenue, Suite E
Phoenix, AZ 85021
(888) 999-7440
care@life-flo.com
www.life-flo.com, www.sheld.com/lifeflo/
They make Progestacare cream.

Matol
Botanical International
Quebec, Canada
(514) 639-3347
www.matol.com
Makers of Botanelle Progesterone Cream.

Neways
150 E. 400 North
P.O. Box 651
Salem, UT 84653
(801) 423-2800
They make Endau cream.

Products of Nature
54 Danbury Road
Ridgefield, CT 06877
(800) 665-5952
www.pronature.com - Connecticut
www.prodnature.com - Texas
Maker of Natural Woman progesterone cream.

Pure Essence Labs
1999 Whitney Mesa Drive, Suite A
Henderson, NV 89014
(800) 264-8000
Makers of Femcream.

Restored Balance, Inc.
42 Meadowbridge Drive SW
Cartersville, GA 30120
(800) 865-7499
www.restoredbalanceusa.com
restoredbalance@adelphia.net
They make Restored Balance PMS/Menopausal progesterone cream.

Springboard
3115 Stoney Oak Drive
Spring Valley, CA 91978
toll free (866) 882-6868 or (619) 670-3860
fax (619) 670-4149
www.springboard4health.com, www.naturalprogesterone.com
They make ProBalance progesterone cream.

Sarati International
Route 3, Box 385, Ted Hunt Road
Los Fresno, TX 78566
(800) 900-0701
www.sarati.com
Online distributors: www.sunrisewd.com or
www.progestnet.com
They make Natural Progesterone Cream.

Vitality Lifechoice
Carson City, NV
(800) 423-8365
They make Balance Cream.

Vitamin Research Products, Inc.
3579 Highway 50 East
Carson City, NV 89701
(775) 884-1300, (800) 877-2447
www.vrp.com
Makers of HerBalance Cream.

Woman to Woman
625 Dara Road
Goleta, CA 93117
(888) 267-5032
www.womantowomanco.com
Woman to Woman cream.

Women's Medicine, Inc.
toll free (866) 628-6337
www.womensmedicine.com
This is Dr. Randy Randolph's cream, Natural Balance Progesta-Fem Progesterone Cream, which contains only progesterone as its active ingredient, and no chemicals (600 mg of progesterone per ounce of creme).

Compounding Pharmacists

If your doctor is interested in natural hormones but hesitant about prescribing an over-the-counter cream, you can put him/her in touch with a compounding pharmacist skilled in the use of natural hormone supplements, who can educate your physician and provide dosing guidelines. For a referral in your area contact IACP (International Academy of Compounding Pharmacists), (800) 927-4227, ext 300, or go online to www.iacprx.org.

RECOMMENDED READING

(In addition to the books mentioned in the text.)

Breast Cancer

Berkson, D. Lindsey. *Hormone Deception: How Everyday Foods and Products Are Disrupting Your Hormones—and How to Protect Yourself and Your Family.* Chicago: Contemporary Books, 2000.

Epstein, Samuel S. *The Breast Cancer Prevention Program.* New York: Macmillan, 1997.

Keuneke, Robin. *Total Breast Health: Power Foods for Protection and Wellness.* New York: Kensington Books, 1998.

Creating a Toxin-Free Environment

Schultz, Warren. *The Chemical-Free Lawn: The Newest Varieties and Techniques to Grow Lush, Hardy Grass with No Pesticides, No Herbicides, No Chemical Fertilizers.* Emmaus, Pa.: Rodale Press, 1989.

Steinman, David, and Michael R. Wisner. *Living Healthy in a Toxic World.* New York: Perigee, 1996.

Steinman, David. *Diet for a Poisoned Planet: How to Choose Safe Foods for You and Your Family.* New York: Ballantine Books, 1990.

Women's Health

The Boston Women's Health Collective. *The New Our Bodies, Ourselves.* New York: Simon & Schuster, 1992.

Love, Susan, M.D. *Dr. Susan Love's Breast Book.* Reading, Mass.: Addison Wesley, 1990.

Northrup, Christiane, M.D. *Women's Bodies, Women's Wisdom.* Rev. ed. New York: Bantam Books, 1998.

Peat, Raymond. *From PMS to Menopause: Female Hormones in Context.* Eugene, Ore.: Raymond Peat, 1997.

Alternative Medicine and Nutrition

Batmanghelidj, F., M.D. *Your Body's Many Cries for Water.* Falls Church, Va.: Global Health Solutions, 1995.

D'Adamo, Peter. *Eat Right 4 Your Type.* New York: Putnam, 1996.

Fallon, Sally. *Nourishing Traditions.* San Diego: ProMotion Publishing, 1995.

Galland, Leo, M.D. *The Four Pillars of Healing.* New York: Random House, 1997.

Golan, Ralph, M.D. *Optimal Wellness.* New York: Ballantine Books, 1995.

Jahnke, Roger. *The Healer Within.* San Francisco: HarperCollins, 1997.

Lee, John R., *Optimal Health Guidelines.* Rev. ed. Phoenix: BLL Publishing, 1999.

Mindell, Earl, and Virginia Hopkins. *Prescription Alternatives.* Chicago: Keats Publishing, 1998.

Mindell, Earl, and Virginia Hopkins. *Dr. Earl Mindell's Secrets of Natural Health.* Chicago: Keats Publishing, 2000.

Pizzorno, Joseph N. *Total Wellness.* Roseville, Calif.: Prima Publishing, 1996.

Robbins, John. *Reclaiming Our Health.* Tiburon, Calif.: HJ Kramer, 1996.

Rose, Marc, M.D., and Michael Rose, M.D. *Save Your Sight.* New York: Warner Books, 1998.

Sears, Barry. *The Zone.* New York: HarperCollins, 1996.

Todd, Gary Price, M.D. *Nutrition, Health and Disease.* West Chester, Pa.: Whitford Press, 1985.

Hormones

Broda Barnes. *Hypothyroidism: The Unsuspected Illness.* New York: Harper and Row, 1976.

Khalsa, Dharma Singh, M.D. *Brain Longevity.* New York: Warner Books, 1997.

Lee, John R. *Natural Progesterone: The Multiple Roles of a Remarkable Hormone.* Rev. ed. Phoenix: BLL Publishing, 2000.

Lee, John R., M.D., and Virginia Hopkins. *What Your Doctor May Not Tell You about Menopause: The Breakthrough Book on Natural Progesterone.* New York: Warner Books, 1996.

Lee, John R., M.D., and Virginia Hopkins. *What Your Doctor May Not Tell You about Premenopause: Balance Your Hormones and Your Life from Thirty to Fifty.* New York: Warner Books, 1999.

Sahelian, Ray. *DHEA: A Practical Guide.* Garden City Park, N.Y.: Avery Publishing, 1996.

Sahelian, Ray. *Pregnenolone: A Practical Guide.* Marina del Rey, Calif.: Melatonin/DHEA Research Institute, 1996.

Drugs

Breggin, Peter. *Talking Back to Prozac.* New York: St. Martin's Press, 1994.

Fried, Stephen. *Bitter Pills: Inside the Hazardous World of Legal Drugs.* New York: Bantam Books, 1998.

Lappé, Marc. *When Antibiotics Fail: Restoring the Ecology of the Body.* Berkeley, Calif.: North Atlantic Books, 1995.

Schmidt, Michael, Lendon Smith, and Keith Sehnert. *Beyond Antibiotics.* Berkeley, Calif.: North Atlantic Books, 1994.

Exercise

Andes, Karen. *A Woman's Book of Strength.* New York: Perigee, 1995.

Protugues, Gladys, and Joyce Vedral. *Hard Bodies.* New York: Dell Paperbacks, 1997.

REFERENCES

General References

The following is a general list of references that apply to more than one chapter in the book. It's followed by a list of references that apply to specific chapters. Some of the references may appear in both lists.

Andrews, R. V. "Influence of Adrenal Gland on Gonadal Function." In *Advances in Sex Hormone Research,* edited by R. A. Thomas and R. L. Singhal. *Volume 3* of *Regulatory Mechanisms Affecting Gonadal Hormone Action* (Baltimore: University Park, 1976): 197–215.

Arafat, E. S., and J. T. Hargrove. "Sedative and Hypnotic Effects of Oral Administration of Micronized Progesterone May Be Mediated through Its Metabolites." *Am J Obstet Gynecol* 159 (1988): 1203–1209.

Asch, R. H., and R. Greenblatt. "Steroidogenesis in the Postmenopausal Ovary." *Clin Obstet Gynecol* 4(1) (1977): 85.

Ashcroft, G. S., et al. "Estrogen Accelerates Cutaneous Wound Healing Associated with an Increase in TGF-beta 1 Levels." *Nature Med* (1997): 11.

Aufrere, M. B., et al. "Progesterone: An Overview and Recent Advances." *J Pharmaceut Sci* 65 (1976): 783.

Backstrom, T. "Epileptic Seizure in Women Related to Plasma Oestrogen and Progesterone during the Menstrual Cycle." *Acta Neurol Scand* 54 (1976): 321–347.

Backstrom, T., et al. "Estrogen and Progesterone in Plasma in Relation to Premenstrual Tension." *J Steroid Biochem Mol Biol* 5 (1974): 257–260.

Backstrom, T., et al. "Effects of Ovarian Steroid Hormones on Brain Excitability and Their Relation to Epilepsy Seizure Variation during the Menstrual Cycle." *Advances in Epileptology, Fifteenth Epilepsy International Symposium.* New York: Raven Press, 1993.

Beumont, P. J. L., et al. "Luteinizing Hormone and Progesterone Levels after Hysterectomy." *Brit Med J* 836 (1972): 363.

Beynon, H. I. C., N. D. Garbett, and P. J. Barnes. "Severe Premenstrual Exacerbations of Asthma: Effect of Intramuscular Progesterone." *The Lancet* (1988): 370–371.

Bloom, T., A. Ojanotko-Harri, M. Laine, I. Huhtaniemi. "Metabolism of Progesterone and Testosterone in Human Parotid and Submandibular Salivary Glands in Vitro." *J Steroid Biochem Mol Biol* 44(1) (1993): 69–76.

Bourgain, C., et al. "Effects of Natural Progesterone on the Morphology of the Endometrium in Patients with Primary Ovarian Failure." *Hum Reprod* 5 (1990): 537–543.

Bower, B. "Stress Hormones May Speed Up Brain Aging." *Sci News* 153(17) (1998): 263.

Businco, L., et al. "Allergenicity and Nutritional Adequacy of Soy Protein Formulas." *J Pediatr* 121 (1992): S21–S28.

Campbell, B. C., and P. T. Ellison. "Menstrual Variation in Salivary Testosterone among Regularly Cycling Women." *Horm Res* (Switzerland) 37(4–5) (1992): 132–136.

Campbell, W. W., et al. "Increased Energy Requirements and Changes in Body Composition with Resistance Training in Older Adults." *Am J Clin Nutr* 60(2) (1994): 167–175.

Cavalieri, E. L., D. E. Stack, P. D. Devanesan, R. Todorovic, et al. "Molecular Origin of Cancer: Catechol Estrogen-3,4-quinones as Endogenous Tumor Initiators." *Proc Nat Acad Sci* 94 (1997): 10937–10942.

Centerwall, B. S. "Premenopausal Hysterectomy and Cardiovascular Disease." *Am J Obstet Gynecol* 139 (1981): 58–61.

Chang, K. J., T. T. Y. Lee, G. Linares-Cruz, S. Fournier, and B. de Lingieres. "Influences of Percutaneous Administration of Estradiol and Progesterone on Human Breast Epethial Cell Cycle in Vivo." *Fertil Steril* 63 (1995): 785–791.

Christ, J. E., et al. "The Residual Ovary Syndrome." *Obstet Gynecol* 46 (1975): 551–556.

Clark, G. M., and W. L. McQuire. "Progesterone Receptors and Human Breast Cells." *Breast Cancer Res Treat* 3 (1983): 157–163.

Corvol, P., et al. "Effect of Progesterone and Progestins on Water and Salt Metabolism." In *Progesterone and Progestins* (New York: Raven Press, 1983).

Cowan, L. D., L. Gordis, J. A. Tonascia, and G. S. Jones. "Breast Cancer Incidence in Women with a History of Progesterone Deficiency." *Am J Epidemiol* 114 (1981): 209–217.

Cranton, E., and W. Fryer. *Resetting the Clock.* New York: M. Evans, 1996.

Cummings, S. R., et al. "Risk Factors for Hip Fracture in White Women." *N Eng J Med* 332 (1995): 767–773.

Dalton, K. "The Aetiology of Premenstrual Syndrome Is with the Progesterone Receptors." *Med Hyp* 31 (1987): 321–327.

Dalton, K. "Erythema Multiforme Associated with Menstruation." *J Roy Soc Med* 78 (1985): 787–788.

Dalton, K. "Influence of Menstruation on Glaucoma." *Brit J Ophthal* 51(10) (1967): 692–695.

Dalton, K. *Premenstrual Syndrome and Progesterone Therapy,* 2d ed. London: Heinemann, 1984.

Dalton, K. "Progesterone Suppositories and Pessaries in the Treatment of Menstrual Migraine." *Headache* 12(4) (1973): 151–159.

Darcy, K. M., S. F. Shoemaker, P. H. Lee, B. A. Ganis, and M. Margot. "Hydrocortisone and Progesterone Regulation of the Proliferation, Morphogenesis, and Functional Differentiation of Normal Rat Mammary Epithelial Cells in Three Dimensional Primary Culture." *J Cell Physiol* 163 (1995): 365–379.

Davis, D. L., H. L. Bradlow, M. Wolff, T. Woodruff, D. G. Hoel, and H. Anton-Culver. "Medical Hypothesis: Xenohormones as Preventable Causes of Breast Cancer." *Env Health Perspectives* 101 (1993): 372–377.

DeBold, J. F., and C. A. Frye. "Progesterone and the Neural Mechanisms of Hamster Sexual Behavior." *Psychoneuroendocrinology* 19 (1994): 563–579.

Dennerstein, L., C. Spencer-Gardner, J. B. Brown, M. A. Smith, and G. D. Burrows. "Premenstrual Tension—Hormone Profiles." *J Psychosomat Obstet Gynaec* 3 (1984): 37–51.

Dennerstein, L., et al. "Progesterone and the Premenstrual Syndrome: A Double Blind Crossover Trial." *Brit Med J* 290 (1985): 1017–1021.

Devroey, P., G. Palermo, et al. "Progesterone Administration in Patients with Absent Ovaries." *Int J Fertil* 34 (1990): 188–193.

Eliasson, O., and H. H. Scherzer. "Recurrent Respiratory Failure in Premenstrual Asthma." *Connecticut Med* 48(12) (1984): 777–778.

Ellison, P. T. "Measurements of Salivary Progesterone." *Ann NY Acad Sci* 694 (1993): 161–176.

Ellison, P. T., S. F. Lipson, M. T. O'Rourke, G. R. Bentley, A. M. Harrigan, C. Painter-Brick, and V. J. Vizthum. "Population Variation in Ovarian Function" (letter). *The Lancet* 342(8868) (1993): 433–434.

Ellison, P. T., C. Painter-Brick, S. F. Lipson, and M. T. O'Rourke. "The Ecological Context of Human Ovarian Function." *Hum Reprod Dec* 8(12) (1993): 2248–2258.

Fallon, S. W., and M. G. Enig. "Soy Products for Dairy Products? Not So Fast." *Health Freedom News* (September 1995).

Ferguson, E. L., et al. "Dietary Calcium, Phytate, and Zinc Intakes and the Calcium, Phytate, and Zinc Molar Ratios of the Diets of a Selected Group of East African Children." *Am J Clin Nutr* 50(6) (1989): 1450–1456.

Formby, B., and T. S. Wiley. "Progesterone Inhibits Growth and Induces Apoptosis in Breast Cancer Cells: Inverse Effect on Expression of p53 and Bcl-2." *Ann Clin Lab Sc.* 28(6) (1998): 360–9.

Gambrell, R. D. "Use of Progestogens in Post-menopausal Women." *Int J Fertil* 34 (1989): 315–321.

Garcia, C. R., and W. Cutler. "Preservation of the Ovary: A Reevaluation." *Fertil Steril* 42(4) (1985): 510–514.

Gibbs, C. J., I. I. Coutts, R. Lock, O. S. Finnegan, and R. J. White. "Premenstrual Exacerbation of Asthma." *Thorax* 39 (1984): 833–836.

Gillet, J. Y. "Induction of Amenorrhea during Hormone Replacement Therapy: Optimal Micronized Progesterone Doses: A Multicenter Study." *Maturitas* 19 (1994): 103–116.

Gompel, A., C. Malet, P. Spritzer, J.-P. La Lardrie, et al. "Progestin Effect on Cell Proliferation and 17β-hydroxysteroid Dehydrogenase Activity in Normal Human Breast Cells in Culture." *J Clin Endocrinol Metab* 63 (1986): 1174.

Gompel, A., J. C. Sabourin, A. Martin, H. Yaneva, et al. "Bcl-2 Expression in Normal Endometrium during the Menstrual Cycle." *Am J Path* 144 (1994): 1196–1202.

Gray, L. A. "The Use of Progesterone in Nervous Tension States." *South Med J* 34 (1941): 1004.

Greene, R., and K. Dalton. "The Premenstrual Syndrome." *Brit Med J* 1 (1953): 1007–1011.

Hammond, C. B., and W. S. Maxson. *Physiology of the Menopause.* New York: Upjohn, 1983.

Hanley, S. P. "Asthma Variations with Menstruation." *Brit J Dis Chest* 75 (1981): 306–308.

Harris, B., L. Lovett, R. G. Newcombe, G. F. Read, R. Walker, and D. Riad-Fahmy. "Maternity Blues and Major Endocrine Changes: Cardiff Puerperal Mood and Hormone Study II (Wales)." *Brit Med J,* April 9, 1994.

Harris, S., et al. "Influence of Body Weight on Rates of Change in Bone Density of the Spine, Hip, and Radius in Post-menopausal Women." *Calcif Tissue Int* 50 (1992): 19–23.

Herman-Giddens, M. E., E. J. Slora, R. C. Wasserman, C. J. Bourdony, et al. "Secondary Sexual Characteristics and Menses in Young Girls Seen in Office Practice: A Study from the Pediatric Research in Office Settings Network." *Pediatrics* 99 (1997): 505–512.

Herzog, A. G. "Intermittent Progesterone Therapy and Frequency of Complex Partial Seizures in Women with Menstrual Disorders." *Neurology* 36 (1986): 1607–1610.

Hreshchyshn, M. M., et al. "Effects of Natural Menopause, Hysterectomy, and Oophorectomy on Lumbar Spine and Femoral Neck Bone Densities." *Obstet Gynecol* 72 (1988): 631–638.

Hrushesky, W. J. M. "Breast Cancer, Timing of Surgery, and the Menstrual Cycle: Call for Prospective Trial." *J Women's Health* 5 (1996): 555–566.

Inoh, A., K. Kamiya, Y. Fujii, and K. Yokoro. "Protective Effects of Progesterone and Tamoxifen in Estrogen-induced Mammary Carcinogenesis in Ovariectomized W/Fu Rats." *Jpn J Cancer Res* 76 (1985): 699–704.

Jacobson, J. L., and S. W. Jacobson. "Intellectual Impairment in Children Exposed to Poly-chlorinated Biphenyls in Utero." *N Eng J Med* 335 (1996): 783–789.

Kandouz, M., M. Siromachkova, D. Jacob, B. C. Marquet, et al. "Antagonism between Estradiol and Progestin on Bcl-2 Expression in Breast Cancer Cells." *Int J Cancer* 68 (1996): 120–125.

Kushi, L. H. "Physical Activity and Mortality in Postmenopausal Women." *JAMA* 277(16) (1997): 1287–1292.

LaPierre, A., et al. "Exercise and Psychoneuroimmunology." *Med Sci Sports Exer* 26(2) (1994): 182–190.

Leis, H. P. "Endocrine Prophylaxis of Breast Cancer with Cyclic Estrogen and Progesterone." *Intern Surg* 45 (1966): 496–503.

Liener, I. E. "Implications of Antinutritional Components in Soybean Foods." *Crit Rev Food Sci Nutr* 34 (1994): 31–67.

Lipsett, M. P. "Steroid Hormones." In *Reproductive Endocrinology, Physiology, and Clinical Management,* edited by S. S. C. Yen and R. B. Jaffe (Philadelphia: W. B. Saunders, 1978): 80.

Lipson, S. F., and P. T. Ellison. "Reference Value for Lutal 'Progesterone' Measured by Salivary Radioimmunoassay." *Fertil Steril* 61(3) (1994): 448–454.

Lydon, J. P., F. J. DeMayo, O. M. Conneely, and B. W. O'Malley. "Reproductive Phenotypes of the Progesterone Receptor Null Mutant Mouse." *J Steroid Biochem Molec Biol* 56 (1996): 67–77. Dept. of Cell Biology, Baylor College of Medicine, Houston, Tex.

Magill, P. J. "Investigation of the Efficacy of Progesterone Pessaries in the Relief of Symptoms of Premenstrual Syndrome." *Brit J Gen Prac,* November 1995, 598–593.

Mahesh, V. B., D. W. Brann, and L. G. Hendry. "Diverse Modes of Action of Progesterone and Its Metabolites." *J Steroid Biochem Molec Biol* 56 (1996): 209–219. Dept. of Physiology and Endocrinology, Medical College of Georgia, Augusta.

Majewska, M. D. "Steroid Hormone Metabolites Are Barbituratelike Modulators of GABA System." *Science* 232 (1986): 1004–1007.

Matthews, K. A., et al. "Prior to Use of Estrogen Replacement Therapy, Are Users Healthier than Nonusers?" *Am J Epidemiol* 143(10) (1996): 971–978.

McKinlay, S. M., et al. "The Normal Menopause Transition." *Maturitas* 14 (1992): 103–114.

Miles, R. A. "Pharmacokinetics and Endometrial Tissue Levels of Progesterone after Administration by Intramuscular and Vaginal Routes: A Comparative Study." *Fertil Steril* 62 (1994): 485–490.

Miyagawa, K., J. Rosch, F. Stanczyk, and K. Hermsmeyer. "Medroxyprogesterone Acetate Interferes with Ovarian Steroid Protection Against Coronary Vasospasm." *Nature Medicine* 3 (1997) 324–327.

Mohr, P. E., D. Y. Wang, W. M. Gregory, M. A. Richards, and I. S. Fentiman. "Serum Progesterone and Prognosis in Operable Breast Cancer." *Brit J Cancer* 73 (1996): 1552–1555.

Moyer, D. L., et al. "Prevention of Endometrial Hyperplasia by Progesterone during Long Term Estradiol Replacement: Influence of Bleeding Pattern and Secretory Changes." *Fertil Steril* 59 (1993): 992–997.

Munday, M. R., et al. "Correlations between Progesterone, Oestradiol and Aldosterone Levels in the Premenstrual Syndrome." *Clin Endocrinol* 14 (1981): 1–9.

Nash, M. S. "Exercise and Immunology." *Med Sci Sports Exer* 26(2) (1994): 125–127.

Nillius, S. J., et al. "Plasma Levels of Progesterone after Vaginal, Rectal or Intramuscular Administration of Progesterone." *Am J Obstet Gynecol* 110 (1971): 470–477.

Novak, E. R., et al. "Enzyme Histochemistry of the Menopausal Ovary Associated with Normal and Abnormal Endometrium." *Am J Obstet Gynecol* 93 (1965): 669.

O'Brien, P. M. S., C. Selby, and E. M. Symonds. "Progesterone, Fluid and Electrolytes in Premenstrual Syndrome." *Brit Med J* 1 (1980): 1161–1163.

O'Rourke, M. T., and P. T. Ellison. "Age and Prognosis in Pre-monopausal Breast Cancer" (letter; comment). *The Lancet* 342(8862) (1993): 60.

Painter-Brick, C., D. S. Lotstein, and P. T. Ellison. "Seasonality of Reproductive Function and Weight Loss in Rural Nepali Women." *Hum Reprod* 8(5) (1993): 684–690.

Pate, R. R., et al. "Physical Activity and Public Health: A Recommendation from the Centers for Disease Control and Prevention and the American College of Sports Medicine." *JAMA* 273(5) (1995): 402–407.

Petrakis, N. L., et al. "Stimulatory Influence of Soy Protein Isolate on Breast Secretion in Pre- and Postmenopausal Women." *Cancer Epidemiol Biomarkers Prev* 5 (1996): 785–794.

Pujol, P., S. G. Hilsenbeck, G. C. Chamness, and R. M. Elledge. "Rising Levels of Estrogen Receptor in Breast Cancer over 2 Decades." *Cancer* 74 (1994): 1601–1606.

Rannevik, G., et al. "A Longitudinal Study of the Perimenopausal Transition: Altered Profiles of Steroid and Pituitary Hormones, SHBG and Bone Mineral Density." *Maturitas* 21 (1995): 103–113.

Ranney, B., et al. "The Future Function and Fortune of Ovarian Tissue which Is Retained in Vivo during Hysterectomy." *Am J Obstet Gynecol* 128 (1977): 626–634.

Reid, I. R. "Determinants of Total Body and Regional Bone Mineral Density in Normal Postmenopausal Women—A Key Role for Fat Mass." *J Clin Endocrinol Metab* 75 (1992): 45–51.

Reidel, H. H., et al. "Ovarian Failure Phenomena after Hysterectomy." *J Reprod Med* 31 (1986): 597–600.

Rodriguez Macias, K. A. "Catamenial Epilepsy: Gynecological and Hormonal Implications. Five Case Reports." *Gynecol Endocrinol* 10 (1996): 139–142.

Rodriquez, C., E. E. Calle, R. J. Coates, H. L. Miracle-McMahill, M. J. Thun, and C. W. Heath. "Estrogen Replacement Therapy and Fatal Ovarian Cancer." *Am J Epidemiol* 141 (1995): 828–834.

Rubinow, D. R., M. C. Hoban, G. N. Grover, D. S. Galloway, P. Roy-Byrne, R. Andersen, and G. R. Merriam. "Changes in Plasma Hormones across the Menstrual Cycle in Patients with Menstrually Related Mood Disorders and in Control Subjects." *Am J Obstet Gynec* 158(1) (1988): 5–11.

Rylance, P. B., et al. "Natural Progesterone and Antihypertensive Action." *Brit Med J* 290 (1985): 13–14.

Sabourin, J. C., A. Martin, J. Baruch, J. B. Truc, et al. "Bcl-2 Expression in Normal Breast Tissue during the Menstrual Cycle." *Int J Cancer* 59 (1994): 1–6.

Sampson, G. A. "Premenstrual Syndrome: A Double Blind Controlled Trial of Progesterone and Placebo." *Brit J Psychiat* 135 (1979): 209.

Sandstrom, B., et al. "Absorption of Zinc from Soy Protein Meals in Humans." *J Nutr* 117 (1987): 321–327.

Santell, R. C., et al. "Dietary Genistein Exerts Estrogenic Effects upon the Uterus, Mammary Gland and the Hypothalamic/Pituitary Axis in Rats." *J Nutr* 127(2) (1997): 263–269.

Seppa, N. "Even Fraternal Twins May Share Cancer Risk." *Sci News* 152 (20 and 27 December 1997): 389.

Shi-Zhong Bu, De-Ling Yin, Xiu-Hai Ren, Li-Zhen Jiang, et al. "Progesterone Induces Apoptosis and Up-regulation of p53 Expression in Human Ovarian Carcinoma Cell Lines." *Am Cancer Soc* (1997): 1944–1950.

Siddle, N., et al. "The Effect of Hysterectomy on the Age at Ovarian Failure: Identification of a Subgroup of Women with Premature Loss of Ovarian Function and Literature Review." *Fertil Steril* 47 (1987): 94–100.

Simon, J. A., "Micronized Progesterone: Vaginal and Oral Uses." *Clin Obstet Gynecol* 38(4) (1995): 902–914.

Sitruk-Ware, R., et al. "Oral Micronized Progesterone." *Contraception* 36 (1987): 373.

Snow-Harter, C. M. "Bone Health and Prevention of Osteoporosis in Active and Athletic Women." *Clinics in Sports Med* 13(2) (1994): 389–404.

Stinberg, K. K., et al. "Sex Steroids and Bone Density in Premenopausal and Perimenopausal Women." *J Clin Endocrinol Metab* 69 (1989): 553–559.

Stone, S. C., et al. "The Acute Effect of Hysterectomy on Ovarian Function." *Am J Obstet Gynecol* 121 (1975): 193–197.

Sulak, P. J. "The Perimenopause: A Critical Time in a Woman's Life." *Int J Fertil* 41(2) (1996): 85–89.

Thompson, H. J. "Effects of Physical Activity and Exercise on Experimentally-induced Mammary Carcinogenesis." *Breast Cancer Res Treat* 46(2–3) (1997): 135–141.

Tzourio, Christophe, et al. "Case-Controlled Study of Migraine and Risk of Ischemic Stroke in Young Women." *Brit Med J* 310 (1995): 830–833.

Vitzthum, V. J., M. von Dornum, and P. T. Ellison. "Brief Communication: Effect of Coca-leaf Chewing on Salivary Progesterone Assays." *Am J Phys Anthropol* 92(4) (1993): 539–544.

Watson, N. R., and J. W. W. Studd. "Bone Loss Following Hysterectomy with Ovarian Conservation." *Eur J Obstet Gynecol Reprod Biol* 49 (1993): 87.

Weinberg, R. A. "How Cancer Arises." *Scientific American* (September 1996): 62–70.

Wen, X. L., et al. "Effects of Adrenocorticotropic Hormone, Human Chorionic Gonadotropin, and Insulin on Steroid Production by Human Adrenocortical Carcinoma Cells in Culture." *Cancer Res* 45(8) (1985): 3974–3978.

White, R. F., and S. P. Proctor. "Solvents and Neurotoxicity." *The Lancet* 349 (1997): 1239–1243.

Wilgus, H. S., Jr., et al. "Goitrogenicity of Soybeans." *J Nutr* 22 (1941): 43–52.

Witt, D. M., J. Young, and D. Crews. "Progesterone and Sexual Behavior in Males." *Psychoneuroendocrinology* 19 (1994): 553–562.

Wojnarowska, F., M. W. Greaves, R. D. Peachey, P. I. Drury, and G. M. Besser. "Progesterone-induced Erythema Multiforme." *J Roy Soc Med* 78 (1987): 407–481.

The Writing Group for the PEPI Trial. "Effects of Estrogen or Estrogen/Progestin Regimens on Heart Disease Risk Factors in Postmenopausal Women: The Postmenopausal Estrogen/Progestin Interventions." *JAMA* 273 (1995): 199–208.

Bibliography: General

Estrogens and Progestogens in Clinical Practice. Edited by Ian S. Fraser, R. P. S. Jansen, R. A. Lobo, and M. I. Whitehead. London: Churchhill Livingstone, 1998.

Jefferies, W. McK. *Safe Uses of Cortisone.* Springfield, Ill.: Charles C. Thomas, 1981.

Novak's Textbook of Gynecology, 12th ed. Edited by Howard W. Jones, III, Anne Colston Wentz, and Lonnie S. Burnett. Philadelphia: Williams & Wilkins, 1996.

Textbook of Clinical Chemistry. Edited by Norbert W. Tietz. Philadelphia: W. B. Saunders, 1986.

Thomas, J. Hywel, and Brian Gillham. *Will's Biochemical Basis of Medicine,* 2d ed. London: Wright, 1989.

Bibliography: Breast Cancer

Clorfene-Casten, Liane. *Breast Cancer: Poisons, Profits and Prevention.* Monroe, Maine: Common Courage Press, 1996.

Epstein, Samuel S. *The Politics of Breast Cancer Revisited.* Fremont Center, N.Y.: Eastridge Press, 1998.

Hoy, Claire. *The Truth about Breast Cancer.* Toronto: Stoddard, 1995.

Keon, Joseph. *The Truth about Breast Cancer.* Mill Valley, Calif.: Parissound Publishing, 1999.

Phillips, Robert H., and Paula Goldstein. *Coping with Breast Cancer.* Garden City Park, N.Y.: Avery Publishing, 1998.

Rinzler, Carol Ann. *Estrogen and Breast Cancer: A Warning to Women.* New York: Macmillan, 1993.

Stabiner, Karen. *To Dance with the Devil: The New War on Breast Cancer.* New York: Delta, 1997.

Bibliography: Xenohormones

Colborn, Theo, et al. *Our Stolen Future.* New York: Penguin Books, 1997.

Krimsky, Sheldon. *Hormonal Chaos: The Scientific and Social Origins of the Environmental Endocrine Hypothesis.* Baltimore, Md.: Johns Hopkins University Press, 2000.

Schettler, Ted, Gina Solomon, Maria Valenti, and Annette Huddle. *Generations at Risk: Reproductive Health and the Environment.* Cambridge, Mass.: MIT Press, 1999.

Thornton, Joe. *Pandora's Poison: Chlorine, Health and a New Environmental Strategy.* Cambridge, Mass.: MIT Press, 2000.

References by Chapter

Chapter 1

THE HISTORY AND POLITICS OF THE BREAST CANCER INDUSTRY
Why We Can't Seem to Prevent or Cure Breast Cancer

American Cancer Society. "1999–2000 Breast Cancer Facts and Figures." www.cancer.org/statistics.

Armstrong, B. "Chemoprevention." Cancer Control Information Center, New South Wales, Australia, 1985.

Bailar, J. C., III. "Mammographic Screening: A Reappraisal of Benefits and Risks." *Clin Obstet Gynecol* 21(1) (1978): 1–14.

Bailar, J. C., III. "Mammography: A Contrary View." *Ann Intern Med* 84(1) (1976): 77–84.

Bailar, J. C., III. "Mammography—A Time for Caution." *JAMA* 237(10) (1977): 997–998.

Bailar, J. C., III. "Mammography before Age 50 Years?" *JAMA* 259(10) (1988): 1548–1549.

Bailar, J. C., III. "Radiation Hazards of X-ray Mammography." Monograph: 251–261.

Bailar, J. C., III. "Randomization in the Canadian National Breast Screening Study: A Review for Evidence of Subversion." *CMAJ* 156(2) (1997): 193–199.

Bailar, J. C., III. "Screening for Early Breast Cancer: Pros and Cons." *Cancer* 39(6 Suppl) (1977): 2783–2795.

Bailar, J. C., III, et al. "Diagnostic Drift in the Reporting of Cancer Incidence." *J Nat Cancer Inst* 90(11) (1998): 863–864.

Bailar, J. C., III, and S. R. Thomas. "What Are We Doing When We Think We Are Doing Risk Analysis?" *Basic Life Sci* 33 (1985): 65–76.

Bergman, E. "Risk and Prognosis of Endometrial Cancer after Tamoxifen for Breast Cancer." *The Lancet* 356 (2000): 881.

Cancer Rates and Risks, 4th ed. National Cancer Institute, 1996.

Cauchon, Dennis. "FDA Advisers Tied to Industry." *USA Today* (25 September 2000).

Citizens for Health. "Use Your Consumer Power to Fight Breast Cancer." *Natural Activist* 6(6) (1998).

Cuzick, J., H. Stewart, L. Rutqvist, et al. "Cause-specific Mortality in Long-term Survivors of Breast Cancer Who Participated in Trials of Radiotherapy." *J Clin Oncol* 12 (1994): 447–453.

"Drug-company Influences on Medical Education in USA" (editorial). *The Lancet* 356 (2000).

Early Breast Cancer Trialists' Collaborative Group. "Effects of Radiotherapy and Surgery in Early Breast Cancer: An Overview of the Randomized Trials." *N Eng J Med* 333 (1995).

Early Breast Cancer Trialists' Collaborative Group. "Favourable and Unfavourable Effects on Long-term Survival of Radiotherapy for Early Breast Cancer: An Overview of the Randomized Trials." *The Lancet* 355 (2000): 1757.

Gelmon, K. "One Step Forward or One Step Back with Tamoxifen?" *The Lancet* 356 (2000): 868.

Getzsche, P. C., and O. Olsen. "Is Screening for Breast Cancer with Mammography Justifiable?" *The Lancet* 355 (2000): 129–134.

Greenlee, R. T., et al. "Cancer Statistics 2000." *Cancer J Clinicians* 50(1) (2001): 7–33.

Hojris, I., M. Overgaard, J. J. Christensen, and J. Overgaard. "Morbidity and Mortality of Ischaemic Heart Disease in High-risk Breast Cancer Patients after Adjuvant Postmastectomy Systemic Treatment with or without Radiotherapy: Analysis of DBCG 82b and 82c Randomised Trials." *The Lancet* 354 (1999): 1425–1430.

Kurtz, J. M., "Radiotherapy for Early Breast Cancer: Was a Comprehensive Overview of Trials Needed?" *The Lancet* 355(9217) (2000): 1739–1740.

Mitchell, G. H., et al. "Weighing the Risks and Benefits of Tamoxifen Treatment for Preventing Breast Cancer." *J Nat Cancer Inst* 91(21) (1999).

Napoli, M. "Breast Cancer Awareness Month: Fear Mongering Sells Drugs." Center for Medical Consumers, *Health Facts* 24(10) (1999).

Overgaard, M., M.-B. Jensen, J. Overgaard, et al. "Postoperative Radiotherapy in High-risk Postmenopausal Breast Cancer Patients Given Adjuvant Tamoxifen." *The Lancet* 353 (1999): 1641–1648.

Peto, R., et al. "UK and USA Breast Cancer Deaths Down 25% in Year 2000 at Ages 20–69 Years." *The Lancet* 355 (2000): 1822–1830.

Powles, T., R. Eeles, S. Ashley, D. Easton, et al. "Interim Analysis of the Incidence of Breast Cancer in the Royal Marsden Hospital Tamoxifen Randomized Chemoprevention Trial." *The Lancet* 352 (1998): 98–101.

Pritchard, K. I. "Is Tamoxifen Effective in Prevention of Breast Cancer?" *The Lancet* 352(9122) (1998): 80–81.

Reinhardt, U. E. "Academic Medicine's Financial Accountability and Responsibility." *JAMA* 284(9) (2000).

Seer Cancer Statistics Review, 1973–1997.

Sjonell, G., and L. Stahle. "Halsokontroller med mammografi minskar inte dodligheten i brostcancer." *Lakartidningen* 96 (1999): 904–913.

Veronesi, U., P. Maisonneuve, A. Costa, V. Sacchini, et al. "Prevention of Breast Cancer with Tamoxifen: Preliminary Findings from the Italian Randomized Trial among Hysterectomized Women." *The Lancet* 352 (1998): 93–97.

Whelan, T. J., et al. "Does Locoregional Radiation Therapy Improve Survival in Breast Cancer? A Meta-analysis." *J Clin Oncol* 18 (2000): 1220–1229.

Chapter 2

RISK FACTORS FOR BREAST CANCER
Why It All Points to Estrogen

Hulka, B., et al. "Steroid Hormones and Risk of Breast Cancer." *Cancer Supp* 73 (1994): 3.

Longnecker, M., et al. "Alcohol Intake and Cancer . . . ," *J Nat Cancer Inst* 87 (1995): 923–929.

McPherson, K., et al. "ABC of Breast Diseases: Breast Cancer—Epidemiology, Risk Factors, and Genetics." *Brit Med J* 321 (2000).

Phillips, K., et al. "Putting the Risk of Breast Cancer in Perspective." *N Eng J Med* 340 (1999): 2.

Pollan, M., et al. "High-risk Occupations for Breast Cancer in the Swedish Female Working Population." *Am J Pub Health* 89 (1999): 875–881.

Rockhill, B., et al. "A Prospective Study of Recreational Physical Activity and Breast Cancer Risk." *Arch Int Med* 159 (1999): 2290–2296.

Sinha, R., et al. "Alcohol and Cancer." *J Nat Cancer Inst* 92 (2000): 1352–1354.

Chapter 3

THE NATURE OF CANCER
Normal Cells That Refuse to Grow Up

Ernster, V. L., et al. "Incidence and Treatment for Ductal Carcinoma in Situ of the Breast." *JAMA* (March 27, 1996).

Ernster, V. L., et al. "Mortality among Women with Ductal Carcinoma in Situ of the Breast in the Population-based Surveillance, Epidermiology and End Results Program." *Arch Intern Med* 160 (2000).

Euhus, D. M., et al. "Increased Microsatellite Abnormalities in Breast Epithelial Cells from Women at Increased Risk for Breast Cancer." Program and abstracts of the Twenty-second Annual San Antonio Breast Cancer Symposium, December 1999, San Antonio, Tex. Abstract 31.

"Have Our Pathologists Run Amok" (editorial). *The Lancet* 347 (1996).

Schwartz, G. F., et al. "Subclinical Ductal Carcinoma in Situ of the Breast. Treatment by Local Excision and Surveillance Alone." *Cancer* 70(10) (1992): 2468–2474.

Silverstein, M. J. "Ductal Carcinoma in Situ of the Breast." *Brit Med J* 317 (1998): 734–739.

Silverstein, M. J., et al. "The Influence of Margin Width on Local Control of Ductal Carcinoma in Situ of the Breast." *N Eng J Med* 340 (1999): 1455–1461.

Sledge, G. "Trying to Be a Real Cancer: Ductal Carcinoma in Situ (DCIS) and Other Premalignant States." Twenty-second Annual San Antonio Breast Cancer Symposium.

Stoll, B. A. "Biological Mechanisms in Breast Cancer Invasiveness: Relevance to Preventive Interventions." *Eur J Cancer Prev* 9(2) (2000): 73–79.

Waisman, J. R., et al. "Breast Cancer Mortality after Local Invasive Recurrence in Patients with Ductal Carcinoma in Situ (DCIS) of the Breast." Twenty-second Annual San Antonio Breast Cancer Symposium. Abstract 36.

Waldman, F. M., et al. "Related Genetics Aberrations in Primary DCIS and Their DCIS Recurrences." Twenty-second Annual San Antonio Breast Cancer Symposium. Abstract 35.

Welch, Gilbert H., and W. C. Black. "Using Autopsy Series to Estimate the Disease 'Reservoir' for Ductal Carcinoma in Situ of the Breast: How Much More Breast Cancer Can We Find?" *Ann Int Med* 127 (1997): 11.

Chapter 4

OTHER FACTORS THAT INCREASE BREAST CANCER RISK
Insulin Resistance, Birth Control Pills, Early Puberty, DHEA, Prolactin, Melatonin, Thyroid

Arafah B. M. "Increased Need for Thyroxine in Women with Hypothyroidism During Estrogen Therapy." *N Engl J Med* 344(23) (2001): 1743–1749.

Bhatavdekar, J. M., et al. "Prolactin as a Local Growth Promoter in Patients with Breast Cancer: GCRI Experience." *Eur J Surg Oncol* 26(6) (2000): 540–547.

Binart, N., et al. "Mammary Gland Development and the Prolactin Receptor." *Adv Exp Med Biol* 480 (2000): 85–92.

Ciampelli, M., et al. "Insulin and Polycystic Ovary Syndrome: A New Look at an Old Subject." *Gynecol Endocrinol* 12(4) (1998): 277–292.

Clevenger, C. V., and T. L. Plank. "Prolactin as an Autocrine/Paracrine Factor in Breast Tissue." *J Mammary Gland Biol Neoplasia* 2(1) (1997): 59–68.

Cos, S., et al. "Melatonin and Mammary Pathological Growth." *Front Neuroendocrinol* 21(2) (2000): 133–170.

Del Giudice, M. E., et al. "Insulin and Related Factors in Premenopausal Breast Cancer Risk." *Breast Cancer Res Treat* 47(2) (1998): 111–120.

Fernandez, R. "Melatonin Effects on Intercellular Junctional Communication in MCF-7 Human Breast Cancer Cells." *J Pineal Res* 29(3) (2000): 166–171.

Hankinson, S. E. "Circulating Concentrations of Insulin-like Growth Factor-I and Risk of Breast Cancer." *The Lancet* 351(9113) (1998): 1393–1396.

Herman-Giddens, M. E., et al. "Secondary Sexual Characteristics and Menses in Young Girls Seen in Office Practice: A Study from the Pediatric Research in Office Settings Network." *Pediatrics* 99 (1997): 505–512.

Hill, S. M., et al. "The Modulation of Oestrogen Receptor-alpha Activity by Melatonin in MCF-7 Human Breast Cancer Cells." *Eur J Cancer* 36(Suppl 4) (2000): 117–118.

Jones, B. A., S. V. Kasi, M. G. Curnen, P. H. Owens, and R. Dubrow. "Severe Obesity as an Explanatory Factor for the Black/White Difference in Stage at Diagnosis of Breast Cancer." *Am J Epidemiol* 146 (1997): 394–404.

Li, C. I., K. E. Malone, E. White, and J. R. Daling. "Age When Maximum Height Is Reached as a Risk Factor for Breast Cancer among Young U.S. Women." *Epidemiology* 8 (1997): 559–565.

Limanova, Z., et al. "Frequent Incidence of Thyropathies in Women with Breast Carcinoma." *Vnitr Lek* 44(2) (1998): 76–82.

Maestroni, G. J. "Therapeutic Potential of Melatonin in Immunodeficiency States, Viral Diseases, and Cancer." *Adv Exp Med Biol* 467 (1999): 217–226.

Nagata, C., et al. "Relations of Insulin Resistance and Serum Concentrations of Estradiol and Sex Hormone-binding Globulin to Potential Breast Cancer Risk Factors." *Jpn J Cancer Res* 91(9) (2000): 948–953.

Ram, P. T., et al. "Differential Responsiveness of MCF-7 Human Breast Cancer Cell Line Stocks to the Pineal Hormone, Melatonin." *J Pineal Res* 28(4) (2000): 210–218.

Ramamoorthy, P., et al. "In Vitro Studies of a Prolactin Antagonist, hPRL-G129R, in Human Breast Cancer Cells." *Int J Oncol* 18(1) (2001): 25–32.

Shering, S. G., et al. "Thyroid Disorders and Breast Cancer." *Eur J Cancer Prev* 5(6) (1996): 504–506.

Smyth, P. P. "The Thyroid and Breast Cancer: A Significant Association?" *Ann Med* 29(3) (1997): 189–191.

Stoll, B. A. "Adiposity as a Risk Determinant for Postmenopausal Breast Cancer." *Int J Obes Relat Metab Disord* 24(5) (2000): 527–533.

Stoll, B. A. "Dietary Supplements of Dehydroepiandrosterone in Relation to Breast Cancer Risk." *Eur J Clin Nutr* 53(10) (1999): 771–775.

Stoll, B. A. "Western Nutrition and the Insulin Resistance Syndrome: A Link to Breast Cancer." *Eur J Clin Nutr* 53(2) (1999): 83–87.

Talamini, R. "Selected Medical Conditions and Risk of Breast Cancer." *Brit J Cancer* 75(11) (1997): 1699–1703.

Walsh, P. V., I. W. McDicken, R. D. Bulbrook, J. W. Moore, W. H. Taylor, W. D. George. "Serum Oestradiol-17 Beta and Prolactin Concentrations During the Luteal Phase in Women with Benign Breast Disease." *Eur J Cancer Clin Oncol* 20(11) (1984): 1345–1351.

Welch, Gilbert H., and W. C. Black. "Using Autopsy Series to Estimate the Disease 'Reservoir' for Ductal Carcinoma in Situ of the Breast: How Much More Breast Cancer Can We Find?" *Ann Int Med* 127(11) (1997): 1023–1027.

Chapter 6

THE NATURE OF ESTROGENS
Angels of Life, Angels of Death

Also see General References.

Brincat, M. P. "Hormone Replacement Therapy and the Skin." *Maturitas* 35(2) (2000): 107–117.

Castelo-Branco, C., et al. "Skin Collagen Changes Related to Age and Hormone Replacement Therapy." *Maturitas* 15(2) (1992): 113–119.

Maheux, R., et al. "A Randomized, Double-blind, Placebo-controlled Study on the Effect of Conjugated Estrogens on Skin Thickness." *Am J Obstet Gynecol* 170(2) (1994): 642–649.

Rodriguez, C., E. E. Calle, R. J. Coates, et al. "Estrogen Replacement Therapy and Fatal Ovarian Cancer." *Am J Epidemiol* 141 (1995): 828–834.

Schairer, C., et al. "Menopausal Estrogen and Estrogen-Progestin Replacement Therapy and Breast Cancer Risk." *JAMA* 283 (2000): 485–491.

Uzuka, M., et al. "Induction of Hyaluronic Acid Synthetase by Estrogen in the Mouse Skin." *Biochem Biophys Acta* 673(4) (1981): 387–393.

Vaillant, L., et al. "Hormone Replacement Therapy and Skin Aging." *Therapie* 51(1) (1996): 67–70.

ALLOPREGNANOLONE AND PMS

Bicikova, M., et al. "Serum Levels of Neurosteroid Allopregnenolone in Patients with Premenstrual Syndrome and Patients after Thyroidectomy." *Endocrinol Regul* 32(2) (1998): 87–92.

Monteleone, P., et al. "Allopregnanolone Concentrations and Premenstrual Syndrome." *Eur J Endocrinol* 142(3) (2000): 269–273.

Rapkin, A. J., et al. "Progesterone Metabolite Allopregnanolone in Women with Premenstrual Syndrome." *Obstet Gynecol* 90(5) (1997): 709–714.

Sundstrom, I., et al. "Endocrine Response to Pregnanolone." *Gynecol Endocrinol* 13(5) (1999): 352–360.

Chapter 7

HOW ESTROGEN TALKS TO YOUR CELLS
The Right Communication Is Everything

Adlercreutz, H., S. L. Gorbach, B. R. Goldin, M. N. Woods, J. T. Dwyer, and E. Hamalainen. "Estrogen Metabolism and Excretion in Oriental and Caucasian Women." *J Nat Cancer Inst* 86(14) (1994): 1076–1082.

Adlecreutz, H., S. L. Gorbach, B. R. Goldin, M. N. Woods, J. T. Dwyer, K. Hockerstedt, K. Wahala, T. Hase, E. Hamalainen, and T. Fotsis. "Estrogen and Metabolite Levels in Women at Risk for Breast Cancer." *Cancer Res* 35 (1994): 703.

Akanni, A., K. Tabakovic, and Y. J. Abul-Hajj. "Estrogen–Nucleic Acid Adducts: Reaction of 3,4-estrone o-Quinone with Nucleic Acid Bases." *Chem Res Toxicol* 10(4) (1997): 477–481.

Bolton, J. L., and L. Shen. "p-Quinone Methides Are the Major Decomposition Products of Catechol Estrogen o-Quinones." *Carcinogenesis* 17(5) (1996): 925–929.

Cavalieri, E. L., D. E. Stack, P. D. Devanesan, R. Todorovic, I. Dwivedy, S. Higginbotham, S. L. Johansson, K. D. Patil, M. L. Gross, J. K. Gooden, R. Ramanathan, R. L. Cerny, and E. G. Rogan. "Molecular Origin of Cancer: Catechol Estrogen-3, 4-Quinones as Endogenous Tumor Initiators." *Proc Nat Acad Sci USA* 94 (1997): 10937–10942.

Han, X., and J. G. Liehr. "Microsome-mediated 8-Hydroxylation of Guanine Bases of DNA by Steroid Estrogens: Correlation of DNA Damage by Free Radicals with Metabolic Activation to Quinones." *Carcinogenesis* 16(10) (1995): 2571–2574.

Iverson, S. L., L. Shen, N. Anlar, and J. L. Bolton. "Bioactivation of Estrone and Its Catechol Metabolites to Quinoid-glutathione Conjugates in Rat Liver Microsomes." *Chem Res Toxicol* 9(2) (1996): 492–499.

Jellinck, P. H., J. J. Michnovicz, and H. L. Bradlow. "Influence of Indole-3-carbinol on the Hepatic Microsomal Formation of Catechol Estrogens." *Steroids* 56(8) (1991): 446–450.

Kirschner, M. A. "The Role of Hormones in the Etiology of Human Breast Cancer." *Cancer* 39(6) (1977): 2716–2726.

Liehr, J. G. "Catechol Estrogens as Mediators of Estrogen-induced Carcinogenesis." *Cancer Res* 35 (1994): 704.

Liehr, J. G. "Genotoxic Effects of Estrogens." *Mutat Res* 238(3) (1990): 269–276.

Liehr, J. G. "Mechanisms of Metabolic Activation and Inactivation of Catecholestrogens: A Basis of Genotoxicity." *Polycyclic Aromatic Compounds* 6 (1994): 229–239.

Liehr, J. G., M. J. Ricci, C. R. Jefcoate, E. V. Hannigan, J. A. Hokanson, and R. T. Zhu. "4-Hydroxylation of Estradiol by Human Uterine Myomerium and Myoma Microsomes: Implications for the Mechanism of Uterine Turmorigenesis." *Proc Nat Acad Sci* 92 (1995): 1229–1233.

MacLusky, N. J., F. Naftolin, L. C. Krey, and S. Franks. "The Catechol Estrogens." *J Steroid Biochem* 15 (1981): 111–124.

Nutter, L. M., Y. Y. Wu, E. O. Ngo, E. E. Sierra, P. L. Gutierrez, and Y. J. Abul-Hajj. "An o-Quinone Form of Estrogen Produces Free Radicals in Human Breast Cancer Cells: Correlation with DNA Damage." *Chem Res Toxicol* 7(1) (1994): 23–28.

Osborne, M. P., H. L. Bradlow, G. Y. C. Wong, and N. T. Telang. "Upregulation of Estradiol C16-alpha-hydroxylation in Human Breast Tissue: A Potential Biomarker of Breast Cancer Risk." *J Nat Cancer Inst* 85(23) (1993): 1917–1993.

Reed, M. J., and A. Purohit. "Breast Cancer and the Role of Cytokines in Regulating Estrogen Synthesis: An Emerging Hypothesis." *Endocrine Rev* 18 (1997): 701–715.

Shen, L., E. Pisha, Z. Huang, J. M. Pezzuto, E. Krol, Z. Alam, R. B. van Breemen, and J. L. Bolton. "Bioreductive Activation of Catechol Estrogen-ortho-quinones: Aromatization of the B Ring in 4-Hydroxyequilenin Markedly Alters Quinoid Formation and Reactivity." *Carcinogenesis* 18(5) (1997): 1093–1101.

Shen, L., E. Pisha, Z. Huang, D. E. Stack, J. Byun, M. L. Gross, E. G. Rogan, and E. L. Cavalieri. "Molecular Characteristics of Catechol Estrogen Quinines in Reactions with Deoxyribonucleosides." *Chem Res Toxicol* 9 (1996): 851–859.

Theron, C. N., V. A. Russell, and J. J. F. Taljaard. "Estrogen-2/4-Hydroxylase Activities in Rat Brain and Liver Microsomes Exhibit Different Substrate Preferences and Sensitivities to Inhibition." *J Steroid Biochem* 28(5) (1987): 533–541.

Chapter 8

ESTRIOL, A SAFER REPLACEMENT ESTROGEN
Mother Nature's Designer Estrogen

ESTRIOL: REVIEWS

Diczfalusy, E. "The Early History of Estriol." *J Steroid Biochem* 20(4B) (1984): 945–953.

Head, K. A. "Estriol: Safety and Efficacy." *Alt Med Rev* 3(2) (1998): 101–113.

Smith, G. V. S., and O. W. Smith. "Internal Secretions and Toxemia of Late Pregnancy." *Am Physiol Soc* 28(1) (1948): 1–22.

Wolf, A. S. "Hormonal Changes in Aging from the Viewpoint of the Gynecologist." *Fortschr Med* 109(18) (1991): 374–378.

ESTRIOL: ALTERNATIVE ESTROGEN REPLACEMENT THERAPY

Henriksson, L., M. Stjernquist, L. Boquist, U. Alander, and I. Selinus. "A Comparative Multicenter Study of the Effects of Continuous Low-dose Estradiol Released from a New Vaginal Ring versus Estriol Vaginal Pessaries in Postmenopausal Women with Symptoms and Signs of Urogenital Atrophy." *Am J Obstet Gynecol* 171(3) (1994): 624–632.

Kim, S., S. M. Liva, M. A. Dalal, M. A. Verity, and R. R. Voskuhl. "Estriol Ameliorates Autoimmune Demyelination Disease: Implications for Multiple Sclerosis." *Neurology* 52(6) (1999): 1230–1238.

Lauritzen, C., and S. Velibese. "Clinical Investigations of a Long-acting Oestriol (Polyoestriol Phosphate)." *Acta Endocrinologica* 38 (1961): 73–87.

Raz, R., and W. E. Stamm. "A Controlled Trial of Intravaginal Estriol in Postmenopausal Women with Recurrent Urinary Tract Infections." *N Eng J Med* 329(11) (1993): 753–756.

Schiff, I., B. Wentworth, B. Koos, K. J. Ryan, and D. Tulchinsky. "Effect of Estriol Administration on the Hypogonadal Woman." *Fertil Steril* 30(3) (1978): 278–282.

Staland, B. "Continuous Treatment with Natural Oestrogens and Progestogens: A Method to Avoid Endometrial Stimulation." *Maturitas* 3 (1981): 141–156.

Tzingounis, V. A., M. F. Aksu, and R. B. Greenblatt. "The Significance of Oestriol in the Management of the Postmenopause." *Acta Endocrinologica* 235 (1980): 45–50.

Utian, W. H. "The Place of Oestriol Therapy after Menopause." *Acta Endocrinologica* 235 (1980): 51–56.

Weiderpass, E., J. A. Baron, H. O. Adami, C. Magnusson, A. Lindgren, R. Bergstrom, N. Correia, and I. Persson. "Low-potency Oestrogen and Risk of Endometrial Cancer: A Case-control Study." *The Lancet* 353 (1999): 1824–1828.

Yang, T. S., S. H. Tsan, S. P. Chang, and H. T. Ng. "Efficacy and Safety of Estriol Replacement Therapy for Climacteric Women." *Chung Hua I Shueh Tsa Chih* (Taipei) 55(5) (1995): 386–391.

ESTRIOL: BONE

Melis, G. B., A. Cagnacci, V. Bruni, L. Falsetti, V. M. Jasonni, C. Nappi, F. Polatti, and A. Volpe. "Salmon Calcitonin Plus Intravaginal Estriol: An Effective Treatment for the Menopause." *Maturitas* 24(1–2) (1996): 83–90.

Minaguchi, H., et al. "Effect of Estriol on Bone Loss in Postmenopausal Japanese Women: A Multicenter Prospective Open Study." *J Obstet Gynaecol Res* 22(3) (1996): 259–265.

Nishibe, A., S. Morimoto, K. Hirota, O. Yasuda, H. Ikegami, T. Yamamoto, K. Fukuo, T. Onishi, and T. Ogihara. "Effect of Estriol and Bone Mineral Density of Lumbar Vertebrae in Elderly and Postmenopausal Women." *Nippin Ronen Igakkai Zassi* 33(5) (1996): 353–359.

Nozaki, M., K. Hashimoto, Y. Inoue, M. Sano, and H. Nakano. "Usefulness of Estriol for the Treatment of Bone Loss in Postmenopausal Women." *Nippon Sanka Fujinka Gakkai Zasshi* 48(2) (1996): 83–88.

Yang, T. S., S. H. Tsan, S. P. Chang, and H. T. Ng. "Efficacy and Safety of Estriol Replacement Therapy for Climacteric Women." *Chung Hua I Shueh Tsa Chih* (Taipei) 55(5) (1995): 386–391.

ESTRIOL: CARDIOVASCULAR

Blanosz, S., B. Lisiecka, T. Wesolowska, G. Sycz, K. Goertz, D. Kuligowiski, and B. Kosciuszkiewicz. "The Influence of Modified Sequential Therapy on Lipid Metabolism in Post-menopausal Women." *Ginekol Pol* 66(5) (1995): 284–288.

Campagnoli, C., L. P. Tousijn, P. Belforte, L. Ferruzzi, A. M. Dolfin, and G. Morra. "Effects of Conjugated Equine Oestro-gens and Oestriol on Blood Clotting, Plasma Lipids and En-dometrial Proliferation in Post-menopausal Women." *Maturitas* 3(2) (1981): 135–144.

Christiansen, C., M. S. Christensen, P. Grande, and I. Transbol. "Low-risk Lipoprotein Pattern in Post-menopause Women on Sequential Oestrogen/Progestogen Treatment." *Maturitas* 5(3) (1984): 193–199.

Ottoson, U. B. "Oral Progesterone and Estrogen/Progestogen Therapy: Effects of Natural and Synthetic Hormones on Sub-fractions of HDL Cholesterol and Liver Proteins." *Acta Obstet Gynecol Scand* 127 (1984): 1–37.

Punnonen, R., and L. Rauramo. "Effect of Castration and Long-term Oral Oestrogen Therapy with Oestriol Succinate on Serum Lipids." *Ann Chir Gynaecol* 65(3) (1976): 216–219.

Samsioe, G. "Cardioprotection by Estrogens: Mechanisms of Action—The Lipids." *Int J Fertil Menopausal Stud* 39(Suppl) (1994): 43–49.

ESTRIOL: PHARMACOKINETICS, ENDOGENOUS SYNTHESIS, RECEPTOR/TISSUE BINDING

Haaften, M. V., J. Poortman, G. H. Donker, M. A. H. M. Wiegerinck, A. A. Haspels, and J. H. H. Thijssen. "Effects of Oestriol: Preliminary Results on Receptor Kinetics in Target Tissues of Postmenopausal Women." *J Steroid Biochem* 20(4B) (1984): 1015–1019.

Katzenellenbogen, B. S. "Biology and Receptor Interactions of Estriol and Estriol Derivatives in Vitro and in Vivo." *J Steroid Biochem* 20(4B) (1984): 1033–1037.

Longcope, C. "Estriol Production and Metabolism in Normal Women." *J Steroid Biochem* 20(4B) (1984): 959–962.

Ojasso, T., J. P. Raynaud, and J. C. Dore. "Affiliations among Steroid Receptors as Revealed by Multivariate Analysis of Steroid Binding Data." *J Steroid Molec Biol* 48 (1994): 31–46.

Stormshak, F., R. Leake, N. Wertz, and J. Gorski. "Stimulatory and Inhibitory Effects of Estrogen on Uterine DNA Synthesis." *Endocrinology* 99(6) (1976): 1501–1511.

Thijssen, J. H. H., M. A. H. M. Wiegerinck, G. H. Donker, and J. Poortman. "Uptake and Metabolism of Oestriol in Human Target Tissues." *J Steroid Biochem* 20(4B) (1984): 955–958.

ESTRIOL: SKIN

Kainz, C., G. Gitsch, J. Stani, G. Breitenecker, M. Binder, and J. B. Schmidt. "When Applied to Facial Skin, Does Estrogen Ointment Have Systemic Effects?" *Arch Gynecol Obstet* 253(2) (1993): 71–74.

Punnonen, R., and L. Rauramo. "The Effect of Long-term Oral Oestriol Succinate Therapy on the Skin of Castrated Women." *Ann Chir Gynaecol* 66(4) (1977): 214–215.

Punnonen, R., P. Vaajalahti, and K. Teisala. "Local Oestriol Treatment Improves the Structure of Elastic Fibers in the Skin of Postmenopausal Women." *Ann Chir Gynaecol* 201 (1987): 39–41.

Punnonen, R., S. Vilska, and L. Rauramo L. "Skinfold Thickness and Long-term Post-menopausal Hormone Therapy." *Maturitas* 5(4) (1984): 259–262.

Schmidt, J. B., M. Binder, G. Demschik, C. Bieglmayer, and A. Reiner. "Treatment of Skin Aging with Topical Estrogens." *Int J Dermatol* 35(9) (1996): 669–674.

Schmidt, J. B., M. Binder, W. Macheiner, C. H. Kainz, G. Gitsch, and C. H. Bieglmayer. "Treatment of Skin Aging Symptoms in Perimenopausal Females with Estrogen Compounds: A Pilot Study." *Maturitas* 20 (1994): 25–30.

Schmidt, J. B., and J. Spona. "Estriol Skin Effects—Clinical, Hormonal and Sebum Parameters in Female Acne Patients." *Z Hautkr* 58(17) (1983): 1228–1241.

Schrock, A., K. Kofler, K. Baumgarten, J. Endl, J. Schmidt, and S. Tatschl. "Intravaginal Treatment of Colpitis Maculosa with an

Oestriol-containing Vaginal Cream." *Wien Klin Wochenschr* 93(23) (1981): 713–716.

Wendker, H., H. Schaefer, and A. Zesch. "Penetrations Kinetic and Distribution of Topically Applied Estrogens." *Arch Dermatol Res* 256(1) (1976): 67–74.

ESTRIOL: BREAST CANCER

Lemon, H. M. "Estriol Prevention of Mammary Carcinoma Induced by 7, 12-Dimethylbenzanthracene and Procarbazine." *Cancer Res* 35 (1975): 1341–1353.

Lemon, H. M., P. F. Kumar, C. Peterson, J. F. Rodriguez-Sierra, and K. M. Abbo. "Inhibition of Radiogenic Mammary Carcinoma in Rats by Estriol or Tamoxifen." *Cancer* 63(9) (1989): 1685–1691.

Chapter 9

THE NATURE OF PROGESTERONE
The Great Protector

Also see General References.

Barengolts, E. I., D. J. Curry, J. Botsis, and S. C. Kukreja. "Comparison of the Effects of Progesterone and Estrogen on Established Bone Loss in Ovariectomized Aged Rats." *Cells Mat Supp* 1 (1991): 105–111.

Burry, K. A., P. E. Patton, and K. Hermsmeyer. "Percutaneous Absorption of Progesterone in Postmenopausal Women Treated with Transdermal Estrogen." *Am J Obstet Gynecol* 180 (1999): 1504–1511.

Chang, K. J., T. T. Y. Lee, G. Linares-Cruz, S. Fournier, and B. de Lignieres. "Influences of Percutaneous Administration of Estradiol and Progesterone on Human Breast Epithelial Cell Cycle in Vivo." *Fertil Steril* 63 (1995): 785–791.

Cowan, L. D., L. Gordis, J. A. Tomascia, and G. S. Jones. "Breast Cancer Incidence in Women with a History of Progesterone Deficiency." *Am J Epidemiol* 114 (1981): 209–217.

Cummings, S. R., W. S. Browner, D. Bauer, K. Stone, et al. "Endogenous Hormones and the Risk of Hip and Vertebral Fractures among Older Women." *N Eng J Med* 339 (1998): 733–738.

Foidart, J.-M., C. Colin, X. Denoo, J. Desroux, et al. "Estradiol and Progesterone Regulate the Proliferation of Human Breast Epithelial Cells." *Fertil Steril* 69 (1998): 963–969.

Formby, B., and T. S. Wiley. "Progesterone Inhibits Growth and Induces Apoptosis in Breast Cancer Cells: Inverse Effects on Bcl-2 and p53." *Ann Clin Lab Sci* 28 (1998): 360–369.

Hrushesky, W. J. "Menstrual Cycle Timing of Breast Cancer Resection: Prospective Study is Overdue." *J Natl Cancer Inst.* 87(2) (1995): 143–4.

Leonetti, H. B., S. Longo, and J. N. Anasti. "Transdermal Progesterone Cream for Vasomotor Symptoms and Postmenopausal Bone Loss." *Obstet Gynecol* 94 (1999): 225–228.

Levine, H., and N. Watson. "Comparison of the Pharmacokinetics of Crinone 8% Administered Vaginally versus

Prometrium Administered Orally in Postmenopausal Women." *Fertil Steril* 73 (2000): 516–521.

Mohr, P. E., D. Y. Wang, W. M. Gregory, M. A. Richards, and I. S. Fentiman. "Serum Progesterone and Prognosis in Operable Breast Cancer." *Brit J Cancer* 73 (1996): 1552–1555.

Monteleone, P., S. Louisi, A. Tonetti, F. Bernardi, et al. "Allopregnanolone Concentrations and Premenstrual Syndrome." *Eur J Endocrinol* 142(3) (2000): 269–273.

Prior, J. C. "Perimenopause: The Complex Endocrinology of the Menopause Transition." *Endocrine Rev* 19 (1998): 397–428.

Radwnaska, E., G. S. Berger, and J. Hammond. "Luteal Deficiency among Women with Normal Menstrual Cycles, Requesting Reversal of Tubal Sterilization." *Obstet Gynecol* 54 (1979): 189–192.

Schairer, C., J. Lubin, R. Troisi, S. Sturgeon, et al. "Menopausal Estrogen and Estrogen-Progestin Replacement Therapy and Breast Cancer Risk." *JAMA* 283 (2000): 485–491.

Chapter 10

THE NATURE OF THE ANDROGENS
The Part "Male" Hormones Play in a Woman's Hormonal Orchestra

Grattarola, R., and G. Secreto. "Breast Cancer Years after Hysterectomy and Bilateral Ovariectomy and Increased Androgenic Activity." *Oncology* 37(1) (1980): 37–40.

Grattarola, R., G. Secreto, and C. Recchione. "Androgens in Breast Cancer. III. Breast Cancer Recurrences Years after Mastectomy and Increased Androgenic Activity." *Am J Obstet Gynecol* 121(2) (1975): 169–172.

Greenblatt, R. B. "The Use of Androgens in the Menopause and Other Gynecic Disorders." *Obstet Gynecol Clin N Am* 14(1) (1987): 251–268.

Le Bail, J. C., et al. "Dehydroepiandrosterone Sulfate Estrogenic Action at Its Physiological Plasma Concentration in Human Breast Cancer Cell Lines." *Anticancer Res* 18(3A) (1998): 1683–1639.

Lissoni, P., et al. "Dehydroepiandrosterone Sulfate (DHEAS) Secretion in Early and Advanced Solid Neoplasms: Selective Deficiency in Metastatic Disease." *Int J Biol Markers* 13(3) (1998): 154–157.

Preda, F., and G. Pizzocaro. "Correlation between Clinical Response to Bilateral Oophorectomy, Estrogen Receptors and Urinary Androgen Excretion in 49 with Advanced Breast Cancer." *Tumori* 65(3) (1979): 325–330.

Secreto, G., and B. Zumoff. "Abnormal Production of Androgens in Women with Breast Cancer." *Anticancer Res* 14(5B) (1994): 2113–2117.

Stoll, B. A. "Dietary Supplements of Dehydroepiandrosterone in Relation to Breast Cancer Risk." *Eur J Clin Nutr* 53(10) (1999): 771–775.

Zeleniuch-Jacquotte, A., et al. "Relation of Serum Levels of Testosterone and Dehydroepiandrosterone Sulfate to Risk of

Breast Cancer in Postmenopausal Women." *Am J Epidemiol* 145(11) (1997): 1030–1038.

Zumoff, B. "Hormonal Profiles in Women with Breast Cancer." *Obstet Gynecol Clin N Am* 21(4) (1994): 751–772.

Chapter 11

THE PROBLEM OF ERT AND HRT
How Hormone Replacement Therapy Causes Cancer

Anasti, J. N., H. B. Leonetti, and K. J. Wilson. "Topical Progesterone Cream Has Anti-proliferative Effect on Estrogen-Stimulated Endometrium." *Obstet Gynecol* 97 (2001): S10.

Bernstein, L., and R. K. Ross. "Endogenous Hormones and Breast Cancer Risk." *Epidemiol Rev* 15(1) (1993): 48–65.

Bernstein, L., R. K. Ross, M. C. Pike, et al. "Hormone Levels in Older Women: A Study of Post-menopausal Breast Cancer Patients and Healthy Population Controls." *Brit J Cancer* 61(2) (1990): 298–302.

Chen, W., and G. Colditz. "Estrogen Replacement Therapy and the Risk of Breast Cancer." Medscape UpToDate, 1 August 2000.

Colditz, G. A. "Hormones and Breast Cancer: Evidence and Implications for Consideration of Risks and Benefits of Hormone Replacement Therapy." *J Women's Health* 8(3) (1999): 347–357.

Colditz, G. A. "Hormone Replacement Therapy Increases the Risk of Breast Cancer." *Ann NY Acad Sci* 833 (1997): 129–136.

Colditz, G. A. "Relationship between Estrogen Levels, Use of Hormone Replacement Therapy, and Breast Cancer." *J Nat Cancer Inst* 90(11) (1998): 814–823.

Colditz, G. A., K. M. Egan, and M. J. Stampfer. "Hormone Replacement Therapy and Risk of Breast Cancer: Results from Epidemiologic Studies." *Am J Obstet Gynecol* 168(5) (1993): 1473–1480.

Colditz, G. A., B. Rosner, and Nurses Health Study Research Group. "Use of Estrogen Plus Progestin Is Associated with Greater Increase in Breast Cancer Risk Than Estrogen Alone." *Am J Epidemiol* 147(Suppl) (1998): 645.

Colditz, G. A., M. J. Stampfer, W. C. Willett, et al. "Prospective Study of Estrogen Replacement Therapy and Risk of Breast Cancer in Postmenopausal Women." *JAMA* 264(20) (1990): 2648–2653.

Colditz, G. A., et al. "The Use of Estrogens and Progestins and the Risk of Breast Cancer in Postmenopausal Women." *N Eng J Med* 332(24) (1995): 1589–1593.

Collaborative Group on Hormonal Factors in Breast Cancer. "Breast Cancer and Hormone Replacement Therapy: Collaborative Reanalysis of Data from 51 Epidemiological Studies of 52,705 Women with Breast Cancer and 108,411 Women without Breast Cancer." *The Lancet* 350(9084) (1997): 1047–1059.

Hofseth, L. J., A. M. Raafat, et al. "Hormone Replacement Therapy with Estrogen or Estrogen Plus Mexdroxyprogesterone Acetate Is Associated with Increased Epithelial Proliferation in the Normal Postmenopausal Breast." *J Clin Endocrinol Metab* 84(12) (1999): 4559–4565.

Jacobs, H. S., "Controversies in Management: Not for Everybody." *Brit Med J* 313 (1996): 351–352.

Jacobs, H. S. "Hormone Replacement Therapy and Breast Cancer." *Endocrinol Relat Cancer* 7(1) (2000): 53–61.

Key, T. J., and M. C. Pike. "The Role of Oestrogens and Progestagens in the Epidemiology and Prevention of Breast Cancer." *Eur J Cancer Clin Oncol* 24(1) (1988): 29–43.

Laidlaw, I. J. "The Proliferation of Normal Human Breast Tissue Implanted into Athymic Nude Mice Is Stimulated by Estrogen but Not Progesterone." *Endocrinology* 136(1) (1995): 164–171.

Lower, E. E., et al. "The Effect of Estrogen Usage on the Subsequent Hormone Receptor Status of Primary Breast Cancer." *Breast Cancer Res Treat* 58(3) (1999): 205–211.

Moerman, C. J., et al. "Postmenopausal Hormone Therapy: Less Favourable Risk-Benefit Ratios in Healthy Dutch Women." *J Intern Med* 248(2) (2000): 143–150.

Persson, I., et al. "Risks of Breast and Endometrial Cancer after Estrogen and Estrogen-Progestin Replacement Therapy." *Cancer Causes Control* 10 (1999): 253–260.

Pike, M. C., et al. "Problems Involved in Including Women with Simple Hysterectomy in Epidemiologic Studies Measuring the Effects of Hormone Replacement on Breast Cancer Risk." *Am J Epidemiol* 147 (1998): 718–721.

Ross, R. K., A. Paganini-Hill, P. C. Wan, and M. C. Pike. "Effect of Hormone Replacement Therapy on Breast Cancer Risk: Estrogen versus Estrogen Plus Progestin." *J Nat Cancer Inst* 92(4) (2000): 328–332.

Schairer, C., et al. "Estrogen Replacement Therapy and Breast Cancer Survival in a Large Screening Study." *J Nat Cancer Inst* 91 (1999): 264–270.

Schairer, C., et al. "Menopausal Estrogen and Estrogen-Progestin Replacement Therapy and Breast Cancer Risk." *JAMA* 283 (2000): 485–491.

Schairer, C., et al. "Menopausal Estrogen and Estrogen-Progestin Replacement Therapy and Risk of Breast Cancer (United States)." *Cancer Causes Control* 5 (1994): 491–500.

Stephens, M. B. "Estrogen-Progestin Increases Breast Cancer Risk." *J Fam Pract* 49(4) (2000): 301–302.

Chapter 12

TAMOXIFEN AND RALOXIFENE
Why Synthetic Drugs Create New Problems

Also see General References.

Bergman, L., et al. "Risk and Prognosis of Endometrial Cancer after Tamoxifen for Breast Cancer." *The Lancet* 356 (2000): 881–887.

Burger, H. G. "Selective Oestrogen Receptor Modulators." *Horm Res* 53(Suppl 3) (2000): 25–29.

Early Breast Cancer Trialists' Collaborative Group. "Tamoxifen for Early Breast Cancer: An Overview of the Randomised Trials." *The Lancet* 351 (1998): 1451–1467.

Erlandsson, M. C. "Effects of Raloxifene, a Selective Estrogen Receptor Modulator, on Thymus, T Cell Reactivity, and Inflammation in Mice." *Cell Immunol* 205(2) (2000): 103–109.

Fisher, B. "Tamoxifen in Treatment of Intraductal Breast Cancer: National Surgical Adjuvant Breast and Bowel Project B-24 Randomised Controlled Trial." *The Lancet* 353 (1999).

Gelmon, K. "One Step Forward, One Step Back with Tamoxifen?" *The Lancet* 356 (2000): 868–869.

Graham, J. D., et al. "Thoughts on Tamoxifen Resistant Breast Cancer: Are Coregulators the Answer or Just a Red Herring?" *J Steroid Biochem Mol Biol* 74(5) (2000): 255–259.

Hozumi, Y. "In Vitro Study of the Effect of Raloxifene on Lipid Metabolism Compared with Tamoxifen." *Eur J Endocrinol* 143(3) (2000): 427–430.

Katzenellenbogen, B. S. "Molecular Mechanisms of Estrogen Action: Selective Ligands and Receptor Pharmacology." *J Steroid Biochem Mol* 74(5) (2000): 279–285.

Mitchell, G. H., et al. "Weighing the Risks and Benefits of Tamoxifen Treatment for Preventing Breast Cancer." *J Nat Cancer Inst* 91(21) (1999).

Powles, T., R. Eeles, S. Ashley, D. Easton, et al. "Interim Analysis of the Incidence of Breast Cancer in the Royal Marsden Hospital Tamoxifen Randomized Chemoprevention Trial." *The Lancet* 352 (1998): 98–101.

Thomas, T., et al. "Estrogen and Raloxifene Activities on Amyloid-beta-Induced Inflammatory Reaction." *Microvasc Res* 61(1) (2001): 28–29.

van Leeuwen, F. E., et al. "Risk of Endometrial Cancer after Tamoxifen Treatment of Breast Cancer." *The Lancet* 343(8895) (1994): 448–452.

Veronesi, U., P. Maisonneuve, A. Costa, V. Sacchini, et al. "Prevention of Breast Cancer with Tamoxifen: Preliminary Findings from the Italian Randomized Trial among Hysterectomized Women." *The Lancet* 352 (1998): 93–97.

Chapter 13

HOW AND WHEN TO USE PROGESTERONE
The Guardian Angel of Breast Cancer

de Lignieres, B., L. Dennerstein, and T. Backstrom. "Influence of Route of Administration on Progesterone Metabolism." *Maturitas* 21(3) (1995): 251–257.

Levine, H., and N. Watson. "Comparison of the Pharmacokinetics of Crinone 8% Administered Vaginally versus Prometrium Administered Orally in Postmenopausal Women." *Fertil Steril* 73(3) (2000): 516–521.

Nahoul, K., and D. de Ziegler. "'Validity' of Serum Progesterone Levels after Oral Progesterone." *Fertil Steril* 60(1) (1993): 26–33.

O'Leary, P., P. Feddema, K. Chan, M. Taranto, M. Smith, and S. Evans. "Salivary, but Not Serum or Urinary Levels of Progesterone Are Elevated after Topical Application of Progesterone Cream to Pre- and Postmenopausal Women." *Clin Endocrinol* 53 (2000): 615–620.

Wren, B. G., K. McFarland, L. Edwards, et al. "Effect of Sequential Transdermal Progesterone Cream on Endometrium, Bleeding Pattern, and Plasma Progesterone Levels in Postmenopausal Women." *Climacteric* 3 (2000): 155–160.

Chapter 14

HOW AND WHEN TO USE OTHER HORMONES
Estrogen, DHEA, Pregnenolone, the Corticosteroids, Testosterone, and Androstenedione

Bonanni, B., and U. Veronesi. "The Italian Tamoxifen Prevention Trial." *Dis Markers* 15(1–3) (1999): 199–200.

Bone, H. G., et al. "Alendronate and Estrogen Effects in Postmenopausal Women with Low Bone Mineral Density." *J Clin Endocrinol Metab* 85(2) (2000): 720–726.

Cauley, J. A. "Elevated Serum Estradiol and Testosterone Concentration Associated with a High Risk for Breast Cancer; Study of Osteoporotic Fractures Research Group." *Ann Intern Med* 130(4 Pt 1) (1999): 270–277.

Cummings, S. R., W. S. Browner, D. Bauer, K. Stone, et al. "Endogenous Hormones and the Risk of Hip and Vertebral Fracture among Older Women." *N Eng J Med* 339 (1998): 733–738.

Decensi, A., B. Bonanni, A. Guerrieri-Gonzaga, R. Torrisi, L. Manetti, C. Robertson, G. De Palo, F. Formelli, A. Costa, and U. Veronesi. "Chemoprevention of Breast Cancer: The Italian Experience." *J Cell Biochem Suppl* 34 (2000): 84–96. Review.

Dorgan, J. F. "Relationship of Serum Dehydroepiandrosterone (DHEA), DHEA Sulfate, and 5-Androstene-3 Beta, 17 Beta-diol to Risk of Breast Cancer in Postmenopausal Women." *Cancer Epidemiol Biomarkers Prev* 6(3) (1997): 177–178.

Lee, S. H. "Androgen Imbalance in Premenopausal Women with Benign Breast Disease and Breast Cancer." *Clin Biochem* 32(5) (1999): 375–380.

Lee, S. H., and P. Lissoni. "Dehydroepiandrosterone Sulfate (DHEAS) Secretion in Early and Advanced Solid Neoplasms: Selective Deficiency in Metastatic Disease." *Int J Biol Markers* 13(3) (1998): 154–157.

Maggiolini, M. "Adrenal Androgens Stimulate the Proliferation of Breast Cancer Cells as Direct Activators of Estrogen Receptor Alpha." *Cancer Res* 59(19) (1999): 4864–4869.

Ribeiro, G., and R. J. Swindell. "The Christie Hospital Adjuvant Tamoxifen Trial." *Natl Cancer Inst Monogr* 11 (1992): 121–125.

Shifren, J. L. "Transdermal Testosterone Treatment in Women with Impaired Sexual Function after Oophorectomy." *N Eng J Med* 343(10) (2000): 682–688.

Stoll, B. A. "Dietary Supplements of Dehydroepiandrosterone in Relation to Breast Cancer Risk." *Eur J Clin Nutr* 53(10) (1999): 771–775.

Tanaka, Y., et al. "Gonadotropins Stimulate Growth of MCF-7 Human Breast Cancer Cells by Promoting Intracellular Conversion of Adrenal Androgens to Estrogens." *Oncology* 59(Suppl 1) (2000): 19–23.

Valentini, M., E. Mari, M. Belfiglio, and A. Nicolucci. "Is Adjuvant Tamoxifen Used Optimally in the Treatment of Breast Cancer? Results of an Italian Survey." *Ann Oncol* 10(7) (1999): 789–793.

Zeleniuch-Jacquotte, A. "Relation of Serum Levels of Testosterone and Dehydroepiandrosterone Sulfate to Risk of Breast Cancer in Postmenopausal Women." *Am J Epidemiol* 145(11) (1997): 1030–1038.

Chapter 15

TESTING AND SYMPTOMS
How to Determine Your Hormone Balance

Chang, K. J., T. T. Y. Lee, et al. "Influences of Percutaneous Administration of Estradiol and Progesterone on Human Breast Epithelial Cell Cycle in Vivo." *Fertil Steril* 63 (1995): 785–791.

Devenuto, F., et al. "Human Erythrocyte Membrane: Uptake of Progesterone and Chemical Alterations." *Biochim Biophys Acta* 193 (1969): 36–47.

Dollbaum, C. M., and G. F. Duwe. "Absorption of Progesterone after Topical Applications: Serum and Saliva Levels." Presented at the Seventh Annual Meeting of the American Menopause Society.

Johnson, M. E., et al. "Permeation of Steroids through Human Skin." *J Pharm Sci* 84 (1995): 1144–1146.

Koefoed, P., and J. Brahm. "The Permeability of the Human Red Cell Membrane to Steroid Sex Hormones." *Biochim Biophys Acta* 1195 (1994): 55–62.

Saliva Hormone Testing: Applications

Aardal-Eriksson, E., B. Karlberg, and A. Holm. "Salivary Cortisol—An Alternative to Serum Cortisol Determinations in Dynamic Function Tests." *Clin Chem Lab Med* 36 (1998): 215–222.

Barrou, Z., D. Guiban, A. Maroufi, C. Fournier, M. Dugue, J. Luton, and P. Thomopoulos. "Overnight Dexamethasone Suppression Test: Comparison of Plasma and Salivary Cortisol Measurement for the Screening of Cushing's Syndrome." *Eur J Endocrinol* 134 (1996): 93–96.

Belkien, L., J. Bordt, P. Moller, R. Hano, and E. Nieschlag. "Estradiol in Saliva for Monitoring Follicular Stimulation in an in Vitro Fertilization Program." *Fertil Steril* 44 (1985): 322.

Booth, A., D. Johnson, D. Granger, A. Crouter, and S. McHale. "Testosterone and Child and Adolescent Adjustment: The Moderating Role of Parent-Child Relationships." October 2000. Unpublished manuscript.

Castro, M., P. Elias, A. Quidute, F. Halah, and A. Moreira. "Out-patient Screening for Cushing's Syndrome: The Sensitivity of the Combination of Circadian Rhythm and Overnight Dexamethasone Suppression Salivary Cortisol Tests." *J Clin Endocrinol Metab* 84 (1999): 878–882.

Christiansen, K., and R. Knussmann. "Androgen Levels and Components of Aggressive Behaviour in Men." *Horm Behav* 21 (1987): 170–180.

Christiansen, K., and R. Knussmann. "Sex Hormones and Cognitive Functioning in Men." *Neuropsychobiology* 18 (1987): 27–36.

Dabbs, J. "Salivary Testosterone Measurements: Reliability Across Hours, Days and Weeks." *Phys Behav* 48 (1990): 83–86.

Davies, R., B. Harris, R. Thomas, N. Cook, G. Read, and D. Riad-Fahmy. "Salivary Testosterone Levels and Major Depressive Illness in Men." *Brit J Psych* 161 (1992): 629–632.

Duclos, M., J. Corcuff, L. Arsac, F. Moreau-Gaudry, et al. "Corticotroph Axis Sensitivity after Exercise in Endurance-trained Athletes." *Clin Endocrinol* 48 (1998): 493–501.

Filaire, E., and G. Lac. "Dehydroepiandrosterone (DHEA) Rather Than Testosterone Shows Saliva Androgen Responses to Exercise in Elite Female Handball Players." *Int J Sports Med* 21 (2000): 17–20.

Goodyer, I., J. Herbert, P. Altham, J. Pearson, S. Secher, and H. Shiers. "Adrenal Secretion During Major Depression in 8- to 16-year-olds, Altered Diurnal Rhythms in Salivary Cortisol and Dehydroepiandrosterone (DHEA) at Presentation." *Psychol Med* 26 (1996): 245–256.

Granger, D., E. Schwartz, A. Booth, M. Curran, and D. Zakaria. "Assessing Dehydroepiandrosterone in Saliva: A Simple Radioimmunoassay for Use in Studies of Children, Adolescents and Adults." *Psychoneuroendocrinology* 24 (1999): 567–579.

Granger, D., J. Weisz, and D. Kauneckis. "Neuroendocrine Reactivity, Internalizing Behavior Problems, and Control-related Cognitions in Clinic-referred Children and Adolescents." *J Abn Psychol* 103 (1994): 267–276.

Granger, D., J. Weisz, J. McCracken, S. Ikeda, and P. Douglas. "Reciprocal Influences among Adrenocortical Activation, Psychosocial Processes, and the Behavioral Adjustment of Clinic-referred Children." *Child Dev* 67 (1996): 3250–3262.

Harris, B., L. Lovett, R. Newcombe, G. F. Read, R. Walker, and D. Riad-Fahmy. "Maternity Blues and Major Endocrine Changes: Cardiff Puerperal Mood and Hormone Study II." *Brit Med J* 308 (1994): 949–953.

Heim, C., U. Ehlert, J. Hanker, and D. Hellhammer. "Abuse-related Posttraumatic Stress Disorder and Alterations of the Hypothalamic-Pituitary-Adrenal Axis in Women with Chronic Pelvic Pain." *Psychosom Med* 60 (1998): 309–318.

Heine, R., J. McGregor, and V. Dullien. "Accuracy of Salivary Estriol Testing Compared to Traditional Risk Factor Assessment in Predicting Preterm Birth." *Am J Obstet Gynecol* 180 (1999): S214–218.

Kudielka, B., A. Schmidt-Reinwald, D. Hellhammer, and C. Kirschbaum. "Psychological and Endocrine Responses to Psychosocial Stress and Dexamthasone/Corticotropin-releasing Hormone in Healthy Postmenopausal Women and Young Controls: The Impact of Age and a Two-week Estradiol Treatment." *Neuroendocrinology* 70 (1999): 422–430.

Lac, G., P. Marquet, P. Chassain, and F. Galen. "Dexamethasone in Resting and Exercising Men. II. Effects on Adrenocortical Hormones."

Lachelin, G., and H. McGarrigle. "A Comparison of Saliva, Plasma Unconjugated and Plasma Total Oestriol Levels throughout Normal Pregnancy." *Brit J Obstet Gynaecol* 91 (1984): 1203–1209.

Lipson, S., and P. Ellison. "Comparison of Salivary Steroid Profiles in Naturally Occurring Conception and Non-conception Cycles." *Hum Reprod* 11 (1996): 2090–2096.

Lipson, S. F., and P. T. Ellison. "Normative Study of Age Variation in Salivary Progesterone Profiles." *J Biosoc Sci* 24 (1992): 233–244.

Lo, M., M. Ng, B. Azmy, and B. Khalid. "Clinical Applications of Salivary Cortisol Measurements." *Sing Med J* 33 (1992): 170.

McGregor, J., C. Hastings, T. Roberts, and J. Barrett. "Diurnal Variation in Saliva Estriol Level during Pregnancy: A Pilot Study." *Am J Obstet Gynecol* 180 (1999): S223–225.

McGregor, J., G. Jackson, G. Lachelin, T. Goodwin, R. Artal, C. Hastings, and V. Dullien. "Salivary Estriol as Risk Assessment for Preterm Labor: A Prospective Trial." *Am J Obstet Gynecol* 173 (1995): 1337–1342.

Moran, D., H. McGarrigle, and G. Lachelin. "Lack of Normal Increase in Saliva Estriol/Progesterone Ratio in Women with Labor Induced at 42 Weeks' Gestation." *Am J Obstet Gynecol* 167 (1992): 1563–1564.

Moss, H., M. Vanyukov, and C. Martin. "Salivary Cortisol Responses and the Risk for Substance Abuse in Prepubertal Boys." *Biol Psych* 38 (1995): 547–555.

Nahoul, K., L. Rao, and R. Scholler. "Saliva Testosterone Time-course Response to hCG in Adult Normal Men, Comparison with Plasma Levels." *J Steroid Biochem* 24 (1986): 1011–1015.

Navarro, M., J. Nolla, M. Machuca, A. Gonzalez, L. Mateo, R. Bonnin, and D. Roig-Escofet. "Salivary Testosterone in Postmenopausal Women with Rheumatoid Arthritis." *J Rheumatol* 25 (1998): 1059–1062.

Navarro, M., C. Villabona, A. Blanco, J. Gomez, R. Bonnin, and J. Soler. "Salivary Excretory Pattern of Testosterone in Substitutive Therapy with Testosterone Enanthate." *Fertil Steril* 61 (1994): 125–128.

O'Leary, P., P. Feddema, K. Chan, M. Taranto, M. Smith, and S. Evans. "Salivary, but Not Serum or Urinary Levels of Progesterone Are Elevated after Topical Application of Progesterone Cream to Pre- and Postmenopausal Women." *Clin Endocrinol* 53 (2000): 615–620.

O'Rourke, M. T., and P. T. Ellison. "Salivary Estradiol Levels Decrease with Age in Healthy, Regularly-cycling Women." *Endocrinol J* 1 (1993): 487–494.

Petsos, P., W. Ratcliffe, D. Heath, and D. Anderson. "Comparison of Blood Spot, Salivary and Serum Progesterone Assays in the Normal Menstrual Cycle." *Clin Endocrinol* 24 (1986): 31–38.

Raff, H., J. Raff, and J. Findling. "Late-night Salivary Cortisol as a Screening Test for Cushing's Syndrome." *J Clin Endocrinol Metab* 83 (1998): 2681–2686.

Read, G. F., J. A. Bradley, D. W. Wilson, et al. "Evaluation of Luteal-Phase Salivary Progesterone Levels in Women with Benign Breast Disease or Primary Breast Cancer." *Eur J Cancer Clin Oncol.* 21(1) (1985): 9–17.

Read, G., R. Walker, D. Wilson, and K. Griffiths. "Steroid Analysis in Saliva for the Assessment of Endocrine Function." *Ann NY Acad Sci* 27(8) (1990): 897–904.

Read, G., D. Wilson, F. Campbell, H. Holliday, R.W. Blamey, and K. Griffiths. "Salivary Cortisol and Dehydroepiandrosterone Sulphate Levels in Postmenopausal Women with Primary Breast Cancer." *Eur J Cancer Clin Oncol* 19 (1983): 477–483.

Riad-Fahmy, D., G. Read, and R. Walker. "Salivary Steroid Assays for Assessing Variation in Endocrine Activity." *J Steroid Biochem* 19 (1983): 265–272.

Rosmond, R., and P. Bjorntorp. "The Hypothalamic-Pituitary-Adrenal Axis Activity as a Predictor of Cardiovascular Disease, Type 2 Diabetes and Stroke." *J Int Med* 247 (2000): 188–197.

Ruutiainen, K., E. Sannikka, R. Santti, R. Erkkola, and H. Adlercreutz. "Salivary Testosterone in Hirsutism: Correlations with Serum Testosterone and the Degree of Hair Growth." *J Clin Endocrinol Metab* 64 (1987): 1015–1020.

Schurmeyer, T., and E. Nieschlag. "Effect of Ketoconazole and Other Imidazole Fungicides on Testosterone Biosynthesis." *Acta Endocrinol* 105 (1984): 275–280.

Schwartz, E., D. Granger, E. Susman, M. Gunnar, and B. Laird. "Assessing Salivary Cortisol in Studies of Child Development." *Child Dev* 69 (1998): 1503–1513.

Steptoe, A., M. Cropley, J. Griffith, and C. Kirschbaum. "Job Strain and Anger Expression Predict Early Morning Elevation in Salivary Cortisol." *Psychosom Med* 62 (2000): 286–292.

Stones, A., D. Groome, D. Perry, F. Hucklebridge, and P. Evans. "The Effect of Stress on Salivary Cortisol in Panic Disorder Patients." *J Affect Disorders* 52 (1999): 197–201.

Tulppala, M., U. Bjorses, U. Stenman, T. Wahlstrom, and O. Ylikorkala. "Luteal Phase Defect in Habitual Abortion: Progesterone in Saliva." *Fertil Steril* 56 (1991): 41–44.

Vedhara, K., J. Hyde, I. Gilchrist, M. Tytherleigh, and S. Plummer. "Acute Stress, Memory, Attention and Cortisol." *Psychoneuroendocrinology* 25 (2000): 535–549.

Voss, H. "Saliva as a Fluid for Measurement of Estradiol Levels." *Am J Obstet Gynecol* 180 (1999): S226–231.

Vuorento, T., A. Lahti, O. Hovatta, and I. Huhtaniemi. "Daily Measurements of Salivary Progesterone Reveal a High Rate of Anovulation in Healthy Students." *Scand J Clin Lab Invest* 49 (1989): 395–401.

Wang, D. Y., V. E. Fantl, F. Habibollahi, G. M. Clark, I. Fentiman, J. Hayward, and R. Bulbrook. "Salivary Oestradiol and Progesterone Levels in Premenopausal Women with Breast Cancer." *Eur J Cancer Clin Oncol* 22(4) (1986): 427–433.

Wellen, J., A. Smals, R. Rijken, P. Kloppenborg, and T. Benraad. "Testosterone and Androstenedione in the Saliva of Patients with Klinefelter's Syndrome." *Clin Endocrinol* 18 (1983): 51–59.

Wren, B., K. McFarland, L. Edwards, P. O'Shea, S. Sufi, et al. "Effect of Sequential Transdermal Progesterone Cream on Endometrium, Bleeding Pattern, and Plasma Progesterone and Salivary Progesterone Levels in Postmenopausal Women." *Climacteric* 3 (2000): 155–160.

Young, M., R. Walker, D. Riad-Fahmy, and I. Hughes. "Androstenedione Rhythms in Saliva in Congenital Adrenal Hyperplasia." *Arch Dis Child* 63 (1988): 624–628.

METHOD VALIDATION

Belkien, L., J. Bordt, P. Moller, R. Hano, and E. Nieschlag. "Estradiol in Saliva for Monitoring Follicular Stimulation in an in Vitro Fertilization Program." *Fertil Steril* 44 (1985): 322.

Bolajii, I., D. Tallon, E. O'Dwyer, and P. Fottrell. "Assessment of Bioavailability of Oral Micronized Progesterone Using a Salivary Progesterone Enzymeimmunoassay." *Gynecol Endocrinol* 7 (1993): 101–110.

Campbell, B., and P. Ellison. "Menstrual Variation in Salivary Testosterone among Regularly Cycling Women." *Horm Res* 37 (1992): 132–136.

Choe, J., F. Khan-Dawood, and M. Dawood. "Progesterone and Estradiol in the Saliva and Plasma during the Menstrual Cycle." *Am J Obstet Gynecol* 147 (1983): 557–562.

Clements, A., and C. Parker. "The Relationship between Salivary Cortisol Concentrations in Frozen versus Mailed Samples." *Psychoneuroendocrinology* 23 (1998): 613–616.

Dabbs, J. "Salivary Testosterone Measurements: Collecting, Storing and Mailing Saliva Samples." *Phys Behav* 49 (1991): 815–817.

Dabbs, J. "Salivary Testosterone Measurements: Reliability across Hours, Days and Weeks." *Phys Behav* 48 (1990): 83–86.

Granger, D., E. Schwartz, A. Booth, and M. Arentz. "Salivary Testosterone Determination in Studies of Child Health and Development." *Horm Behav* 35 (1999): 18–27.

Granger, D., E. Schwartz, A. Booth, M. Curran, and D. Zakaria. "Assessing Dehydroepiandrosterone in Saliva: A Simple Radioimmunosassay for Use in Studies of Children, Adolescents and Adults." *Psychoneuroendocrinology* 24 (1999): 567–579.

Khan-Dawood, F., J. Choe, and M. Dawood. "Salivary and Plasma Bound and 'Free' Testosterone in Men and Women." *Am J Obstet Gynecol* 148 (1984): 441–445.

Lac, G., N. Lac, and A. Robert. "Steroid Assays in Saliva: A Method to Detect Plasmatic Contaminations." *Arch Int Physiol Biochim Biophys* 101 (1993): 257–262.

Lac, G., P. Marquet, P. Chassain, and F. Galen. "Dexamethasone in Resting and Exercising Men. II. Effects on Adrenocortical Hormones." *J Appl Physiol* 87 (1999): 183–188.

Lachelin, G., and H. McGarrigle. "A Comparison of Saliva, Plasma Unconjugated and Plasma Total Oestriol Levels throughout Normal Pregnancy." *Brit J Obstet Gynaecol* 91 (1984): 1203–1209.

Lechner, W., C. Marth, and D. Daxenbichler. "Correlation of Oestriol Levels in Saliva, Plasma and Urine of Pregnant Women." *Acta Endocrinol* 109 (1985): 266–268.

Lipson, S. F., and P. T. Ellison. "Development of Protocols for the Application of Salivary Steroid Analyses to Field Conditions." *Am J Hum Biol* 1 (1989): 249–255.

Lipson, S. F., and P. T. Ellison. "Normative Study of Age Variation in Salivary Progesterone Profiles." *J Biosoc Sci* 24 (1992): 233–244.

Lo, M., M. Ng, B. Azmy, and B. Khalid. "Clinical Applications of Salivary Cortisol Measurements." *Sing Med J* 33 (1992): 170.

Metcalf, M., J. Evans, and J. Mackenzie. "Indices of Ovulation: Comparison of Plasma and Salivary Levels of Progesterone with Urinary Pregnanediol." *J Endocrinol* 100 (1984): 75–80.

Meulenberg, P., and J. Hofman. "Salivary Progesterone Excellently Reflects Free and Total Progesterone in Plasma during Pregnancy." *Clin Chem* 35 (1989): 168–172.

Nahoul, K., L. Rao, and R. Scholler. "Saliva Testosterone Time-course Response to hCG in Adult Normal Men, Comparison with Plasma Levels." *J Steroid Biochem* 24 (1986): 1011–1015.

Nahoul, K., and R. Scholler. "Comparison of Saliva and Plasma 17-Hydroxyprogesterone Time-course Response to hCG Administration in Normal Men." *J Steroid Biochem* 26 (1987): 251–257.

Navarro, M., J. Nolla, M. Machuca, A. Gonzalez, L. Mateo, R. Bonnin, and D. Roig-Escofet. "Salivary Testosterone in Postmenopausal Women with Rheumatoid Arthritis." *J Rheumatol* 25 (1998): 1059–1062.

O'Leary, P., P. Feddema, K. Chan, M. Taranto, M. Smith, and S. Evans. "Salivary, but Not Serum or Urinary Levels of Progesterone Are Elevated after Topical Application of Progesterone Cream to Pre- and Postmenopausal Women." *Clin Endocrinol* 53 (2000): 615–620.

O'Rourke, M. T., and P. T. Ellison. "Salivary Estradiol Levels Decrease with Age in Healthy, Regularly-cycling Women." *Endocrinol J* 1 (1993): 487–494.

Quissell, D. "Steroid Hormone Analysis in Human Saliva." *Ann NY Acad Sci* 694 (1993): 143–145.

Read, G., M. Harper, W. Peeling, and K. Griffiths. "Changes in Male Salivary Testosterone Concentrations with Age." *Int J Androl* 4 (1981): 623–627.

Read, G., R. Walker, D. Wilson, and K. Griffiths. "Steroid Analysis in Saliva for the Assessment of Endocrine Function." *Ann NY Acad Sci* (1993): 260–274.

Riad-Fahmy, D., G. Read, and R. Walker. "Salivary Steroid Assays for Assessing Variation in Endocrine Activity." *J Steroid Biochem* 19 (1983): 265–272.

Rosmond, R., and P. Bjorntorp. "The Hypothalamic-Pituitary-Adrenal Axis Activity as a Predictor of Cardiovascular Disease, Type 2 Diabetes and Stroke." *J Int Med* 247 (2000): 188–197.

Sannikka, E., P. Terho, J. Suominen, and R. Santti. "Testosterone Concentrations in Human Seminal Plasma and Saliva and Its Correlation with Non-protein-bound and Total Testosterone Levels in Serum." *Int J Androl* 6 (1983): 319–330.

Schramm, W., R. Smith, P. Craig, and H. Grates. "Testosterone Concentration Is Increased in Whole Saliva but Not in Ultrafiltrate after Toothbrushing." *Clin Chem* 39 (1993): 519–521.

Schramm, W., R. Smith, P. Craig, S. Paek, and H. Kuo. "Determination of Free Progesterone in an Ultrafiltrate of Saliva Collected in Situ." *Clin Chem* 36 (1990): 1488–1493.

Schwartz, E., D. Granger, E. Susman, M. Gunnar, and B. Laird. "Assessing Salivary Cortisol in Studies of Child Development." *Child Dev* 69 (1998): 1503–1513.

Shirtcliff, E., D. Granger, E. Schwartz, and M. Curran. "Use of Salivary Biomarkers in Biobehavioral Research: Cotton-based Sample Collection Methods Can Interfere with Salivary Immunoassay Results." *Psychoneuroendocrinology* 26 (2001): 165–173.

Shirtcliff, E., D. Granger, E. Schwartz, M. Curran, A. Booth, and W. Overman. "Assessing Estradiol in Biobehavioral Studies Using Saliva and Blood Spots: Simple Radioimmunoassay Protocols, Reliability, and Comparative Validity." *Horm Behav* 38 (2000): 137–147.

Steptoe, A., M. Cropley, J. Griffith, and C. Kirschbaum. "Job Strain and Anger Expression Predict Early Morning Elevation in Salivary Cortisol." *Psychosom Med* 62 (2000): 286–292.

Tunn, S., H. Mollmann, J. Barth, H. Derendorf, and M. Krieg. "Simultaneous Measurement of Cortisol in Serum and Saliva after Different Forms of Cortisol Administration." *Clin Chem* 38 (1992): 1491–1494.

Vining, R., and R. McGinley. "The Measurement of Hormones in Saliva: Possibilities and Pitfalls." *J Steroid Biochem* 27(1–3) (1987): 81–94.

Vining, R., R. McGinley, and R. Symons. "Hormones in Saliva: Mode of Entry and Consequent Implications for Clinical Interpretation." *Clin Chem* 29 (1983): 1752–1756.

Vittek, J., D. L'Hommedieu, G. Gordon, S. Rappaport, and L. Southren. "Direct Radioimmunoassay (RIA) of Salivary Testosterone: Correlation with Free and Total Serum Testosterone." *Life Sci* 37 (1985): 711–716.

Vuorento, T., A. Lahti, O. Hovatta, and I. Huhtaniemi. "Daily Measurements of Salivary Progesterone Reveal a High Rate of Anovulation in Healthy Students." *Scand J Clin Lab Invest* 49 (1989): 395–401.

Wang, D. Y., V. E. Fantl, F. Habibollahi, G. M. Clark, I. Fentiman, J. Hayward, and R. Bulbrook. "Salivary Oestradiol and Progesterone Levels in Premenopausal Women with Breast Cancer." *Eur J Cancer Clin Oncol* 22(4) (1986): 427–433.

Wang, D., and R. Knyba. "Salivary Progesterone: Relation to Total and Non-protein-bound Blood Levels." *J Steroid Biochem* 23 (1985): 975–979.

Wellen, J., A. Smals, J. Rijken, P. Kloppenborg, and T. Benraad. "Testosterone and Androstenedione in the Saliva of Patients with Klinefelter's Syndrome." *Clin Endocrinol* 18 (1983): 51–59.

Wren, B., K. McFarland, L. Edwards, P. O'Shea, S. Sufi, et al. "Effect of Sequential Transdermal Progesterone Cream on Endometrium, Bleeding Pattern, and Plasma Progesterone and

Salivary Progesterone Levels in Postmenopausal Women." *Climacteric* 3 (2000): 155–160.

Chapter 16

THE LIGHT AND DARK SIDES OF SOY
How to Eat Soy So That It Helps

Alexandersen, P., et al. "Ipriflavones in the Treatment of Post-menopausal Osteoporosis." *JAMA* 285 (2001): 1482–1488.

Anderson, R. L., and W. J. Wolf. "Compositional Changes in Trypsin Inhibitors, Phytic Acid, Saponins and Isoflavones Related to Soybean Processing." *J Nutr* 125 (1995): 581S–588S.

Burke, G. L. "The Potential Use of a Dietary Soy Supplement as a Post-menopausal Hormone Replacement Therapy." Second International Symposium on the Role of Soy in Preventing and Treating Chronic Disease, Brussels, Belgium, 1996. Oral abstract.

Businco, L., et al. "Allergenicity and Nutritional Adequacy of Soy Protein Formulas." *J Pediatr* 121 (1992): S21–S28.

Davies, N. T., and H. Reid. "An Evaluation of the Phytate, Zinc, Copper, Iron and Manganese Contents of, and Zinc Availability from, Soya-based Textured-vegetable-protein Meat-substitutes or Meat-extenders." *Brit J Nutr* 41(3) (1979): 579–589.

Fallon, S. W., and M. G. Enig. "Soy Products for Dairy Products? Not So Fast." *Health Freedom News* (September 1995).

Ferguson, E. L., R. S. Gibson, C. Opare-Obisaw, S. Ounpuu, L. U. Thompson, and J. Lehrfeld. "The Zinc Nutriture of Preschool Children Living in Two African Countries." *J Nutr* 123 (1993): 1487–1496.

Ferguson, E. L., R. S. Gibson, L. U. Thompson, and S. Ounpuu. "Dietary Calcium, Phytate, and Zinc Intakes and the Calcium, Phytate, and Zinc Molar Ratios of the Diets of a Selected Group of East African Children." *Am J Clin Nutr* 50(6) (1989): 1450–1456.

Fotsis, T. "Genistein, a Dietary-derived Inhibitor or in Vitro Angiogenesis." *Proc Natl Acad Sci* 90 (1993): 2690–2694.

Hargreaves, D. F., et al. "Two Week Dietary Soy Supplementation Has an Estrogenic Effect on Normal Premenopausal Breast." *J Clin Endocrinol Metab* 84(11) (1999): 4017–4024.

Hoffmann, R., W. Eicheler, E. Wenzel, and R. Happle. "Interleukin-1 Beta-induced Inhibition of Hair Growth in Vitro Is Mediated by Cyclic AMP." *J Invest Dermatol* 108(1) (1997): 40–42.

Ikeda, Y., N. Nishiyama, H. Saito, and H. Katsuki. "GABA A Receptor Stimulation Promotes Survival of Embryonic Rat Striatal Neurons in Culture." *Brain Res Dev Brain Res* 98(2) (1997): 253–258.

Kruse, F. E., A. M. Joussen, T. Fotsis, L. Schweigerer, K. Rohrschneider, and H. E. Volcker. "Inhibition of Neovascularization of the Eye by Dietary Factors Exemplified by Isoflavonoids." *Ophthalmologe* 94(2) (1997): 152–156.

Li, Y., et al. "Induction of Apoptosis in Breast Cancer Cells MDA-MB-231 by Genistein." *Oncogene* 18(20) (1999): 3166–3172.

Liener, I. E. "Implications of Antinutritional Components in Soybean Foods." *Crit Rev Food Sci Nutr* 34 (1994): 31–67.

Makela, S., M. Poutanen, J. Lehtimaki, and M. L. Kostian. "Estrogen-specific 17β-Hydroxysteroid Oxidoreductase Type I as a Possible Target for the Action of Phytoestrogens." *Proc Soc Exp Biol Med* 208 (1995): 51–59.

Petrakis, N. L., et al. "Stimulatory Influence of Soy Protein Isolate on Breast Secretion in Pre- and Postmenopausal Women." *Cancer Epidemiol Biomarkers Prev* 5 (1996): 785–794.

Sandberg, A. S. "The Effect of Food Processing on Phytate Hydrolysis and Availability of Iron and Zinc." *Adv Exp Med Biol* 289 (1991): 499–508.

Sandstrom, B., B. Kivisto, and A. Cederblad. "Absorption of Zinc from Soy Protein Meals in Humans." *J Nutr* 117 (1987): 321–327.

Santell, R. C., Y. C. Chang, M. G. Nair, and W. G. Helferich. "Dietary Genistein Exerts Estrogenic Effects upon the Uterus, Mammary Gland and the Hypothalamic/Pituitary Axis in Rats." *J Nutr* 127(2) (1997): 263–269.

Santell, R. C., N. Kieu, and W. G. Helferich. "Genistein Inhibits Growth of Estrogen-independent Human Breast Cancer Cells in Culture but Not in Athymic Mice." *J Nutr* 130(7) (2000): 1665–1669.

Vera, J. C., et al. "Genistein Is a Natural Inhibitor of Hexose and Dehydroascorbic Acid Transport through the Glucose Transporter, GLUT1." *J Biol Chem* 271 (1996): 8719–8724.

Wan, Q., H. Y. Man, J. Braunton, W. Wang, M. W. Salter, L. Becker, and Y. T. Wang. "Modulation of GABA A Receptor Function by Tyrosine Phosphorylation of Beta Subunits." *J Neurosci* (July 1997).

Wang, C., T. Makela, T. A. Hase, C. H. T. Adlercreutz, and M. S. Kurzer. "Lignans and Isoflavonoids Inhibit Aromatase Enzyme in Human Preadipocytes." *J Steroid Biochem Mol Biol* 50 (1994): 205–212.

Wilgus, H. S., Jr., et al. "Goitrogenicity of Soybeans." *J Nutr* 22 (1941): 43–52.

Zava, D. T., and G. Duwe. "Estrogenic and Antiproliferative Properties of Genistein and Other Flavonoids in Human Breast Cancer Cells in Vitro." *Nutr Cancer* 27 (1997): 31–40.

Chapter 17

HOW NUTRITION AFFECTS YOUR BREAST CANCER RISK
Making Good Choices Can Make the Difference

Badawi, A. F., and M. C. Archer. "Effect of Hormonal Status on the Expression of the Cyclooxygenase 1 and 2 Genes and Prostaglandin Synthesis in Rat Mammary Glands." *Prostaglandins Other Lipid Mediat* 56(2–3) (1998): 167–181.

Badawi, A. F., et al. "The Effect of Dietary n-3 and n-6 Polyunsaturated Fatty Acids on the Expression of Cyclooxygenase 1 and 2 Levels of p21ras in Rat Mammary Glands." *Carcinogenesis* 19(5) (1998): 905–910.

Bartsch, H., J. Nair, and R. W. Owen. "Dietary Polyunsaturated Fats and Cancers of the Breast and Colorectum: Emerging Evidence for Their Role as Risk Modifiers." *Carcinogenesis* 20(12) (1999): 2209–2218.

Capone, S. L., D. Bagga, and J. A. Glaspy. "Relationship between Omega-3 and Omega-6 Fatty Acid Ratios and Breast Cancer." *Nutrition* 13(9) (1997): 822–824.

Cave, W. T., Jr. "Dietary Omega-3 Polyunsaturated Fats and Breast Cancer." *Nutrition* 12(1 Suppl) (1996): S39–42.

Damianaki, A., et al. "Potent Inhibitory Action of Red Wine Polyphenols on Human Breast Cancer Cells." *J Cell Biochem* 78(3) (2000): 429–441.

Fowke, J. H., C. Longcope, and J. R. Hebert. "Brassica Vegetable Consumption Shifts Estrogen Metabolism in Healthy Postmenopausal Women." *Cancer Epidemiol Biomarkers Prev* 9(8) (2000): 773–779.

Gu, M., et al. "Oxidative-phosphorylation Defects in Liver of Patients with Wilson's Disease." *Lancet* 356(9228) (2000): 469–474.

Holmes, M. D., et al. "Association of Dietary Intake of Fat and Fatty Acids with Risk of Breast Cancer." *JAMA* 281(10) (1999): 914–920.

Holmes, M. D., et al. "Dietary Fat Intake and Endogenous Sex Steroid Hormone Levels in Postmenopausal Women." *J Clin Oncol* 18(21) (2000): 3668–3676.

Jasienska, G., I. Thune, and P. T. Ellison. "Energetic Factors, Ovarian Steroids and the Risk of Breast Cancer." *Eur J Cancer Prev* 9(4) (2000): 231–239.

Nagata, C., et al. "Relations of Insulin Resistance and Serum Concentrations of Estradiol and Sex Hormone Binding Globulin to Potential Breast Cancer Risk Factors." *Jpn J Cancer Res* 91(9) (2000): 948–953.

Nicholson, A., and the Physicians Committee for Responsible Medicine. "Diet and the Prevention and Treatment of Breast Cancer." *Altern Ther Health Med* 2(6) (1996): 32–38.

Owen, R. W., et al. "The Antioxidant/Anticancer Potential of Phenolic Compounds Isolated from Olive Oil." *Eur J Cancer* 36(10) (2000): 1235–1247.

Singh, A., et al. "The Regulation of Aromatase Activity in Breast Fibroblasts: The Role of Interleukin-6 and Prostaglandin E2." *Endocrinol Relat Cancer* 6(2) (1999): 139–147.

Slavin, J. L. "Mechanisms for the Impact of Whole Grain Foods on Cancer Risk." *J Am Coll Nutr* 19(3 Suppl): 300S–307S.

Trichopoulou, A., et al. "Cancer and Mediterranean Dietary Traditions." *Cancer Epidemiol Biomarkers Prev* 9(9) (2000): 869–873.

Wolk, A., et al. "A Prospective Study of Association of Monounsaturated Fat and Other Types of Fat with Risk of Breast Cancer." *Arch Intern Med* 158(1) (1998): 41–45.

Chapter 18

PROTECTING THE PRESENT AND THE FUTURE
Creating an Environment Where Cancer Can't Get Started

Baj, Z., et al. "The Effect of Chronic Exposure to Formaldehyde, Phenol and Organic Chlorohydrocarbons on Peripheral Blood Cells and the Immune System in Humans." *J Investig Allergol Clin Immunol* 4(4) (1994): 186–191.

Faustini, A., et al. "Immunological Changes among Farmers Exposed to Phenoxy Herbicides: Preliminary Observations." *Occup Environ Med* 53(9) (1996): 583–585.

Fitzgerald, E. F., et al. "Polychlorinated Biphenyl (PCB) and Dichlorodiphenyl Dichloroethylene (DDE) Exposure among Native American Men from Contaminated Great Lakes Fish and Wildlife." *Toxicol Ind Health* 12(3–4) (1996): 361–368.

Gerhard, I., B. Monga, J. Krahe, and B. Runnebaum. "Chlorinated Hydrocarbons in Infertile Women." *Environ Res* 80(4) (1999): 299–310.

Gerhard, I., and B. Runnebaum. "The Limits of Hormone Substitution in Pollutant Exposure and Fertility Disorders." *Zentralbl Gynakol* 114(12) (1992): 593–602.

Hagmar, L., et al. "High Consumption of Fatty Fish from the Baltic Sea Is Associated with Changes in Human Lymphocyte Subset Levels." *Toxicol Lett* 77(1–3) (1995): 335–342.

Nagayama, J., et al. "Postnatal Exposure to Chlorinated Dioxins and Related Chemicals on Lymphocyte Subsets in Japanese Breast-fed Infants." *Chemosphere* 37(9–12) (1998): 1781–1787.

Ross, P. S., et al. "Impaired Cellular Immune Response in Rats Exposed Perinatally to Baltic Sea Herring Oil or 2,3,7,8-TCDD." *Arch Toxicol* 71(9) (1999): 563–574.

Svensson, B. G., et al. "Parameters of Immunological Competence in Subjects with High Consumption of Fish Contaminated with Persistent Organochlorine Compounds." *Int Arch Occup Environ Health* 65(6) (1994): 351–358.

Van Loveren, H., et al. "Contaminant-induced Immunosuppression and Mass Mortalities among Harbor Seals." *Toxicol Lett* 112–113 (2000): 319–324.

Wolff, M. S., and P. G. Toniolo, et al. "Blood Levels of Organochlorine Residues and Risk of Breast Cancer." *J Natl Cancer Inst* 85(8) (1993): 468–652.

APPENDIX: THE STRUCTURE OF STEROID HORMONES

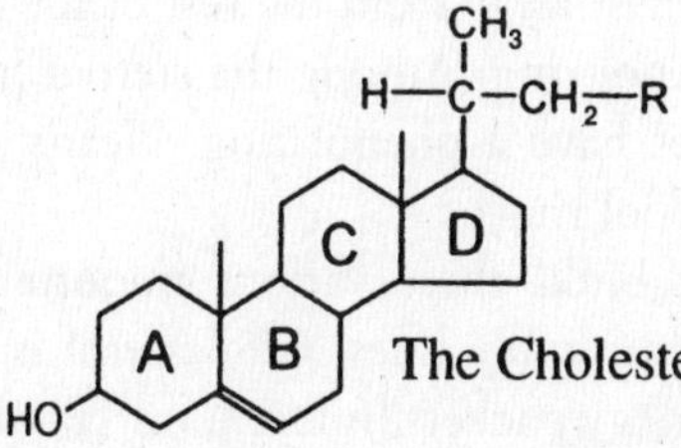

The Cholesterol Molecule

Notice the four rings, labeled A, B, C, and D, that make up the main chassis of the molecule. These are the four rings that characterize all the steroid hormones. In the following figure are three such hormones.

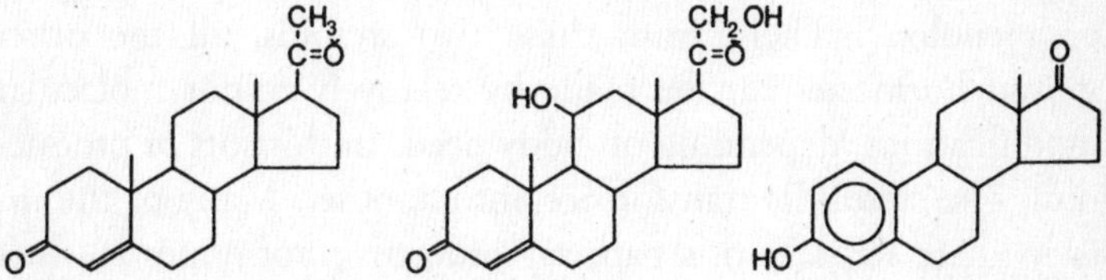

progesterone   corticosterone   estrone

Notice how the basic structure of cholesterol, the precursor to the steroid hormones, remains the same in three different steroid hormones. Slight molecular variations produce hormones that create enormous variations in humans.

Note that all of these steroid hormones retain the similar four-ring structure of the cholesterol molecule. They differ, however, in the atoms attached at various places to the basic structure. The differences appear minor, though their actions are thereby changed considerably. Others, like estrone (and all estrogens), have a different A-ring. This ring, depicted with a circle inside, indicates it has had three hydrogens removed, leaving three sets of double bonds circulating around the ring of carbon atoms making up the six-sided ring. This is what chemists call a benzene ring. However, with the presence of the -OH group at the side of the ring farthest away from the rest of the molecule, this ring is called a phenol ring. Among the steroid hormones, only estrogen molecules have a phenol ring. Nearly all of the xenoestrogens have phenol rings.

The body does not build these various important steroid hormones on different assembly lines. Cholesterol is the main building block. Tiny energy packets (mitochondria) within each and every cell of the body can substitute and rearrange some atoms at the top of cholesterol's D-ring, creating a new version called pregnenolone. As it passes through the bloodstream to the ovaries and adrenal glands, pregnenolone can then be transformed into progesterone or (almost identical) 17-OH-pregnenolone. Then, from these two steroids, all the other steroid hormones can be made by relatively minor molecular modifications, depending on body need. In this sort of production, one steroid is transformed into another. Many of the intermediate steps in this pathway are active hormones in their own right, even though they also serve by being transformed into still other hormones. At the end of the transformational paths are aldosterone, cortisol, and the estrogens, which are fated to be metabolized and excreted from the body.

Although the steroid hormones are remarkably similar in shape, each of them has markedly different effects, and these differences arise from very slight variations in their molecular structure.

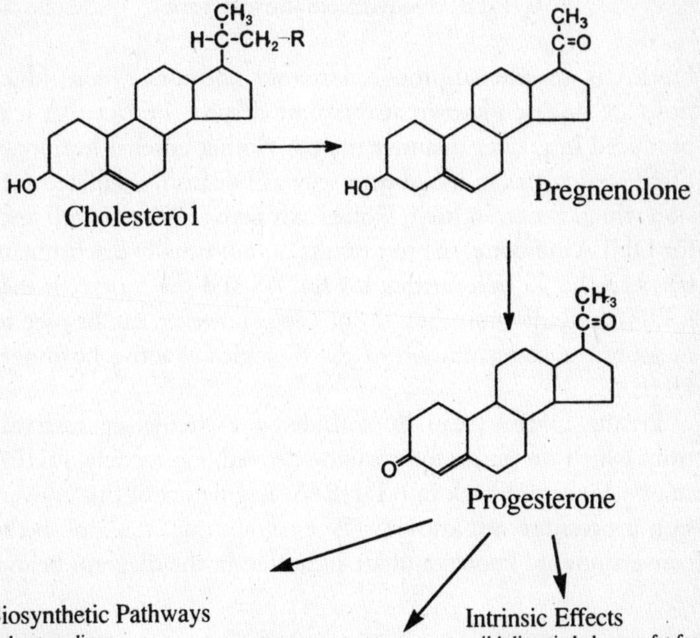

The multiple roles of progesterone.

Cholesterol → Pregnenolone → Progesterone

Biosynthetic Pathways
androstenedione
testosterone
estrone, estradiol, estriol
all cortisol and
    corticosteroids
aldosterone

Reproductive Effects
secretory endometrium
survival of embryo
development of fetus
    throughout gestation
libido

Intrinsic Effects
mild diuretic helps use fat for
    energy
natural antidepressant
helps thyroid hormone action
normalizes blood clotting
helps normalize blood sugar
    levels
normalizes zinc and copper
    levels
maintains proper cell oxygen
    levels
protects against breast cysts
protects against breast cancer
protects against endometrial
    cancer
moisturizes skin when used
    topically
counteracts estrogen side
    effects

DHEA (Dehydroepiandrosterone)

DHEA is an adrenal-produced steroid hormone whose functions are not well known at this time despite the fact that it is produced in greater quantity than any other adrenal hormone. DHEA circulates in blood primarily as DHEAS, a sulfated version which is not, in itself, biologically active. When blood tests for DHEA are done, the test results do not usually discriminate between the 95 percent that is DHEAS and the 5 percent that is DHEA. Radioimmune assay of saliva, however, can be used to measure the concentration of the biologically active hormone, DHEA.

Plasma DHEAS can be considered a circulating reservoir from which the active form can be derived. Conversely, DHEA can be converted back into DHEAS. Regulators of this conversion process are not known. The enzymes that accomplish the conversions are known and are indicated in the diagram below.

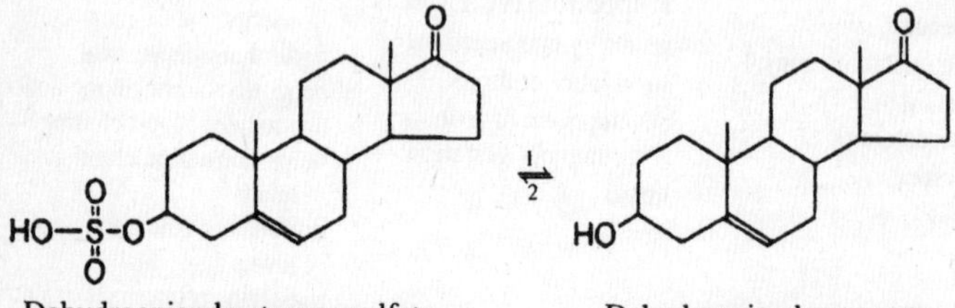

Dehydroepiandrosterone sulfate   Dehydroepiandrosterone
           DHEAS   DHEA

The enzymes that accomplish these transformations, labeled as 1 and 2 at the arrows, are the following:

1. *Sulfatases*
2. *Sulfokinases*

Steroidogenesis pathways.

INDEX

ABOUT THE AUTHORS

John R. Lee, M.D., is internationally acknowledged as a pioneer and expert in the study and use of the hormone progesterone, and on the subject of hormone replacement therapy for women. He used transdermal progesterone extensively in his clinical practice for nearly a decade, doing research that showed that it can reverse osteoporosis. Dr. Lee has had a distinguished medical career, including graduating from Harvard and the University of Minnesota Medical School. He retired from a 30-year family practice in Northern California a few years ago and ever since has been writing and traveling around the world speaking to doctors, scientists, and laypeople about progesterone. Dr. Lee taught a very popular course on Optimal Health at the College of Marin for 15 years. He is the author of *Optimal Health Guidelines, Natural Progesterone: The Multiple Roles of a Remarkable Hormone* (written for doctors) and the best-sellers, *What Your Doctor May* Not *Tell You About Menopause* and *What Your Doctor May* Not *Tell you about Premenopause* (Warner Books), and is editor in chief of the *John R. Lee, M.D., Medical Letter*.

David Zava, Ph.D., is a biochemist with extensive research experience regarding the effect of hormones on breast cancer, including published research in peer-reviewed journals, and is a pioneer in the use of saliva hormone assay to measure hormone levels. Dr. Zava has also done extensive research into the effects of food, specifically soy, on hormone balance and cancer. He is the director of ZRT Laboratory in Portland, Oregon, and is a sought-after speaker on the topics of hormone balance and salivary assays.

over . . .

Virginia Hopkins, M.A., has been a writer and editor since she graduated from Yale University in 1976. She has a master's degree in applied psychology from the University of Santa Monica. She is the coauthor, with John R. Lee, M.D., of *What Your Doctor May Not Tell You About Menopause: The Breakthrough Book on Natural Progesterone* (Warner Books, 1996), *What Your Doctor May Not Tell You About Premenopause* (Warner Books, 1999), and *Prescription Alternatives* (Keats Publishing, 1998), which she coauthored with Earl Mindell, R.Ph., Ph.D. She is the executive editor of the *John R. Lee, M.D., Medical Letter* and has written or coauthored more than 30 books on alternative health and nutrition.